Perfect weddings

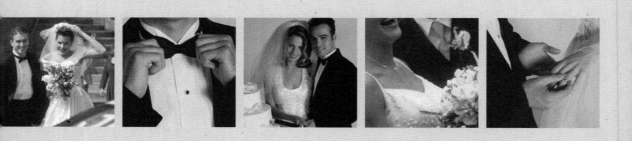

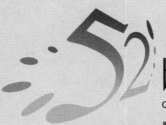

brilliantideas

one good idea can change your life...

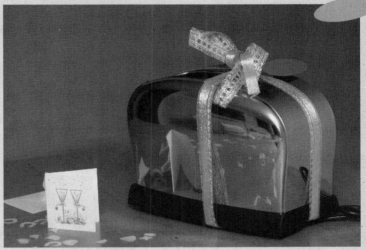

Perfect weddings

Make the most of your memorable day

Lisa Helmanis

First published in 2008 by
The Infinite Ideas Company Limited
36 St Giles
Oxford OX1 3LD
United Kingdom
T: 01865 514 888
W: www.infideas.com

A catalogue record for this book is available from the British Library.
ISBN 978-1-905940-34-9

Previously published as *Perfect weddings* (978-1-904902-25-6) and
Lose weight and stay slim (978-1-904902-22-5).

Text designed and typeset by Baseline Arts Ltd, Oxford
Cover design by Cylinder
Printed and bound in India

Brilliant ideas

   Big fluffy meringues? A dozen under-fives dressed as fairies? Or a pint and a pork pie at
   your local? Remember, there are two of you involved so deciding what kind of wedding to
   start planning is your first big hitch in getting hitched.

   Sounds simple, but there's a lot to think about. What kind of mood do you want to set?
   Where are the guests coming from? Have you elderly relatives or small children who will be
   restless if you have a long afternoon break? And will that long break find all the groomsmen
   in the pub?

   The issue of other people's expectations is possibly the most contentious factor in any
   wedding, and it will need nerves of steel and the good grace of Mother Teresa to keep all
   concerned happy.

   Everyone is so happy that they all want to say their piece. If only you could stop them. There
   is a convention, so you need to know who does the speeches and how you handle them.

Brilliant features

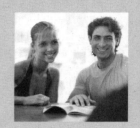

Each chapter of this book is designed to provide you with an inspirational idea that you can read quickly and put into practice straight away.

Throughout you'll find four features that will help you to get right to the heart of the idea:

- *Here's an idea for you* Take it on board and give it a go – right here, right now. Get an idea of how well you're doing so far.

- *Try another idea* If this idea looks like a life-changer then there's no time to lose. *Try another idea* will point you straight to a related tip to expand and enhance the first.

- *Defining ideas* Words of wisdom from masters and mistresses of the art, plus some interesting hangers-on.

- *How did it go?* If at first you do succeed, try to hide your amazement. If, on the other hand, you don't, then this is where you'll find a Q and A that highlights common problems and how to get over them.

Introduction

Weddings count among the all-time monumental events in a person's lifetime. In any culture, they represent hope, love and the promise of a happy and fulfilling future.

And in every culture, there are also mother-in-law jokes. That's because the same joy that goes with your desire to make a commitment to one another is usually accompanied by a set of…well, let's call them challenges, shall we? And making sure that your wedding, and the run up to it, is a time that you can cherish for all the right reasons takes some careful planning, patience and a good dollop of humour.

The current fashion for grand weddings of superstar proportions (and budgets to match) means that organising them can become a full-time job in its own right. And with other aspects to balance, such as your relationship, friends, work, family and social life, it's easy to lose perspective. (And a quick note here: a great wedding is not the same as an expensive wedding, as you will see.)

So what's the secret to getting the balance right? How do you get the fantasy wedding you want and still manage to enjoy yourself? Well, the secret is in the planning and timing, and remembering why you wanted to get married in the first place. People who get married happily (as opposed to just being happily married) share the responsibilities, share the work, share the fun. And when things get tough, they keep their eye on the prize, namely that, at the end of it all, they get to be married to the person they love.

The process of planning a wedding is often also a time when you will have to cover some big issues that you haven't had to consider before, such as joint finances, family conflict and responsibility. This book will help you get the basics right, such as communication and consideration, which will be the basis for making this wedding thing work for you. On a practical level, the book will also take a look at all of the key elements for planning a wedding, and when and how to tackle them. We will take the mystery out of it for you, dividing a mammoth task into bite-size proportions.

One of the main complaints about wedding organisation relates to the pressure of the responsibility. There are many ways to deal with this. Among the key factors (which will also stand you in good stead for the rest of your life) are learning to say no and knowing when to ask for help. Handled artfully, sharing the stress can seem like bestowing honours and building bridges, improving your relationships rather than damaging them. The book even gives you chapters which will tell your nearest and dearest what to do, so you don't have to. Try simply photocopying the relevant ideas for the key wedding party members, such as the best man or speakers, and handing them over with a smile. That way it's not you making demands or suggestions; the *book* says so. Genius.

So why do the emotions surrounding a wedding get to such a fever pitch? And when should you start to regard it as a worrying sign? Well, just about everyone closely involved in the wedding will have been dreaming about this day for many years: mums imagining their daughters in wedding dresses; fathers rehearsing their speeches; sisters expecting their infant sons to be ring bearers. Many, many hopes and dreams are brought together by a wedding, and everyone will want you to grant them their little wish (usually one of many). Families are also dealing with change, something that brings up both fear and joy in equal measure. Parents can no longer pretend that you are children (even if you still get treated like one) and you will now be shifting your focus to your new partnership. So relax – panic is normal.

And when you are not panicking, you will get to enjoy all the great stuff that makes a wedding so much fun: choosing flowers; tasting cakes; trying on pretty frocks (that's mainly the girls); catching up with old friends and long lost family; and having lots of parties.

Best of all, your wedding will give you the opportunity to bring everyone you love together to watch you make a commitment to the person you intend to share the rest of life's exhilarating and bumpy journey with. It's an amazing way to start that journey off, whether you do it on a beach in the Maldives, a tiny country church or Westminster Cathedral. Good luck and congratulations.

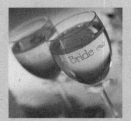 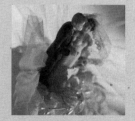 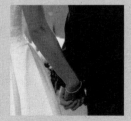

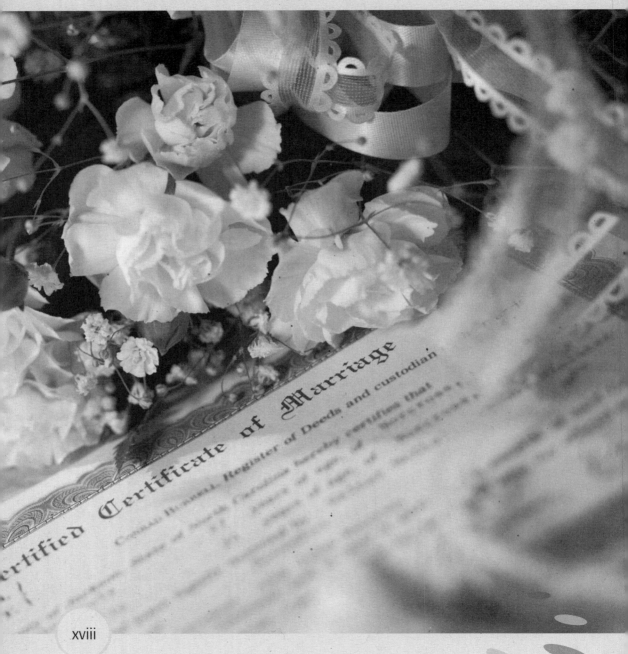

1

Who are you?

Big fluffy meringues? A dozen under-fives dressed as fairies? Or a pint and a pork pie at your local? Remember, there are two of you involved so deciding what kind of wedding to start planning is your first big hitch in getting hitched.

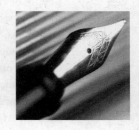

This is a time when couples often try so hard to please each other that they end up pleasing no one. The best way to prevent this is individually to write down details of your dream wedding and then swap your lists. You could be very surprised.

You may think of your partner as a metropolitan sophisticate who is actually a 'hearts and flowers, 50 pageboys' traditionalist and then find otherwise. The fact is, most people (especially the female of the species) have been fantasising about this event since they were old enough to understand the fairytales that all end in 'I do'.

Here's an idea for you...

If you or your partner are visual people or find it hard to describe what you imagine in your mind, get yourself a whole stack of wedding magazines and tear out images that appeal to you. Once you have decided on the ones you both like, keep them in a file and use them as reference material for your florist, cake designer or dressmaker. It is an ideal way to make sure that you all share the same vision. After all, words can be interpreted in many different ways.

So don't be surprised if you or your partner suddenly starts imagining glass carriages; just look at all the options before you book it – it could be your five-year-old self talking.

WHAT DO I WANT?

You will undoubtedly find that your wedding scrapbook (not a sad fanatic's obsession but an essential way to keep track of everything) seems to look like it was put together by a drunk schizophrenic. Don't be alarmed (unless you are a drunk schizophrenic) as this is often the way it goes. Instead of lamenting over the fact that you don't have one clear vision, see if there are any common denominators. Do you dither between white flowers and bright colours? Is there something connecting the pictures, like a bold use of greenery or do they all have a romantic country feel? Maybe that's the theme, rather than the specific thing you think you are looking for. Think laterally.

TOTALLY INCOMPATIBLE...

Once your list is written, if you are very lucky, you will have the same vision; more likely, you will have some similarities and some differences. Work out which are most important to you. If the bride wants several bridesmaids and the groom is a music buff, give each other an early wedding gift by handing over the decision for your favoured areas. This will also help clarify another important area, that of responsibility. Do consider consistency when sharing out responsibilities. Scrambling into a soft-top Lamborghini to head off to the reception seems more comical than romantic if the bride is sporting a vintage two-foot lace headdress.

Have a frank chat about the problems you may face ahead. Few couples make it to the big day without a few cross words, but it can be very helpful if you understand why, so take a look at IDEA 14, *How to say 'I don't' and 'you do'.*

Try another idea...

The run up to a wedding is renowned for being incredibly stressful, with one partner often feeling that they are carrying the weight of the responsibility all on their own. (No prizes for guessing which one.)

WHOSE WEDDING IS THIS?

You will almost certainly find that your wedding plans get invaded by other people's ideas. You may like the idea of running away to tie the knot on a beach but find that your family would be devastated to miss out on your big day. This is why you need to have a written 'map' of your dream wedding scenario before you announce to your nearest and dearest what your plans are. You can then refer back to it every time you feel that you are losing your way or feel bullied.

'A great marriage is not when the "perfect couple" comes together. It is when an imperfect couple learns to enjoy their differences.'
DAVE MEURER, *author*

Defining idea...

3

How did it go?

Q **My future mother-in-law is taking over our wedding and we have only just got engaged. My partner always acquiesces as she is quite a formidable woman, but I don't want to march down the aisle to her tune. How do I keep her under control?**

A *Attack is, as they say, the best defence. She has probably been looking forward to this for years, so asking her to simply 'butt out' is not going to make for a happy time. Try being proactive and giving her a list of tasks to do, none of which involve decision making. Ask her to get several quotes for harpists, locating companies that can find you a white Mercedes or gathering addresses for the invites. All of these tasks are genuinely useful so she won't feel maligned or marginalised, but will also realise the decisions aren't hers to make.*

Q **What if she keeps pushing?**

A *Keep it simple and be brave. Make sure you thank her for all her efforts and suggestions, but make it clear that you don't want to burden her with such a big job. If she still doesn't get the hint, say a polite, warm 'no' and then stay quiet. Don't explain yourself, as that would suggest she has a valid argument that you must convince her against, leaving the power balance with her. Just repeat the 'no' if she persists; if she can't respect your boundaries you will have to set them more firmly, or this problem will occur through your future relationship.*

When: date and time

Sounds simple, but there's a lot to think about. What kind of mood do you want to set? Where are the guests coming from? Have you elderly relatives or small children who will be restless if you have a long afternoon break? And will that long break find all the groomsmen in the pub?

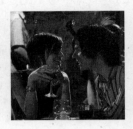

Choose your date carefully. If you want a big wedding, you need to be realistic about the amount of time you allow. And there are a few religious rites to consider too...

Ah, a summer wedding, it seems like the obvious choice. But it's worth thinking about the other options too. Autumnal weddings can be very romantic and lend the pictures the rich reddish hues of the season. Winter weddings add drama, which can be even more magical with an evening ceremony. Summer weddings also fall at the same time as many people's holidays, and can be really hot if you want the full ball gown silhouette wedding attire. If you have a summer wedding date in mind that has some special significance, be prepared to have to wait up to a year or two to get your perfect slot. Incidentally, June, the most popular month for weddings, is meant to be the luckiest for lovers, as it was named for the Roman God Juno, the god of love.

Here's an idea for you...

Is there going to be a break between the ceremony and the evening reception? You must think how your guests will spend that time. If you have grandparents, elderly or pregnant relatives or friends, then consider booking them a room in a local hotel to rest. If not, ask your reception venue if there is a restaurant or lounge area for them to relax in. Also consider that they might need some light refreshments; you mustn't leave them to fend for themselves, especially if they are in an area they don't know. If you do, you might find people retire to the nearest alehouse, and retire early from your evening a little worse for wear.

CHOOSING YOUR TIME OF DAY

Think first about the mood you want to set. Different times of day create definite moods. Outdoor evening weddings can be great in a hot summer and you can have the benefit of a pink sunset if you're lucky. A winter wedding can be given extra drama by being held at night, with great torches of fire lighting the guests' way. A spring wedding, with pretty pastel colours, can be enhanced by a morning stroll to the local church. A noon wedding can be uncomfortable if held in the midday sun, so think about the practical side as well as the romance.

RELIGIOUS TRADITIONS

Your religion may have traditions. Protestant weddings are often held in the afternoon yet Roman Catholic weddings traditionally begin at 11 a.m. or noon. If you want a Saturday wedding and you are Jewish, it will have to begin after sundown, which marks the end of the Sabbath. And you need to make sure that there are no religious holidays that will influence your choice.

AND LESS ROMANTIC...

There are slightly less interesting yet no less essential factors that need to be considered. Are you holding your ceremony in the same location as your reception? If so, you will need to ensure that the rooms will be ready immediately to move straight to the reception area. Check if there will be other weddings at the same venue on that day. Make sure there will be enough time to assemble your wedding party without confusing the guests; you don't want them ending up in the wrong room of the town hall watching another bride wander down the aisle. Also make sure that there is enough time before the service for the florists and photographer to set up. Don't be scared to ask your registry office or church how long they allow each party.

You may have to be prepared for the disappointment of finding your dream time slot unavailable, as many weddings are booked so far ahead. If that's the case, you can choose a date further in the future or accept disappointment gracefully; there is very little you can do and if you take everything to heart, you will have a rocky road ahead.

Where are the guests coming from? If many of them are coming from a long distance make sure you investigate hotels for them nearby so that they can make it to the ceremony on time.

Before you think about your time of day, consider whether or not it suits your location; see IDEA 17, *Where: choosing a location*, to make sure they work together to best effect.

Try another idea...

'We have so much time and so little to do. Strike it. Reverse it.'
ROALD DAHL, *Charlie and the Chocolate Factory*

Defining idea...

AVOID THE DREADED WEDDING LULL

There is often a natural lull when a band or DJ arrives and begins to transform the venue into a suitably festive reception area. The sight of someone humping around huge boxes and crawling around the floor looking for power points can often dampen the mood. To create a smoother flow from day to night, find out from your venue if the equipment can be set up before the reception begins. If this is not possible, perhaps there is another room that guests can retire to whilst tables are cleared and the party gets started.

How did it go?

Q   I want an evening banquet for my wedding, but my local registrar won't work past a certain time. Can I request that they work later?

A   *No, they are under no obligation, and you need to make sure you book well in advance to get the slot you like.*

Q   Are there any other options?

A   *Your best solution is to have a quiet official ceremony before the wedding, with close family as witnesses and then have a blessing ceremony when you want it.*

Q   So, can I do the ceremony again?

A   *Of course. That way you can fit it into your plans, and even have some fun writing your own vows.*

3

The world and its mother

The issue of other people's expectations is possibly the most contentious factor in any wedding, and it will need nerves of steel and the good grace of Mother Teresa to keep all concerned happy.

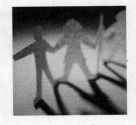

Everyone involved, from your granny to your other half's mum, will have their own list of 'must invite' cast in concrete, and don't be surprised if half of them you've never even heard of.

The best way to deal with this situation is to take control from day one. Ask all the relevant parties to write a list of their proposed guests, in order of importance. Make it clear that space and budget may mean that not everyone on their list will make it onto the final version. You and your spouse-to-be should also make separate lists, and do it as soon as you get engaged so that by the time you come to send out the invites, you've thought of everyone (rather than finding a great uncle and his brood, all the way from New Zealand, being sprung on you at the last moment, blowing both your table plan and your budget).

Draw up a map showing how to get to the ceremony and/or reception. These are becoming frequent inserts in wedding invitations, especially as wedding venues become more remote and elaborate. And it is a considerate touch that simplifies your guests' lives and saves a few marriages in the process. (Don't forget, couples trapped in cars lost on back roads don't make happy wedding guests.) Include both written and visual instructions, and account for the fact that guests may be coming from different directions. If you don't want to include it with your invitations, you could include a map reference for a web site. If you are choosing somewhere remote, you may need to design your own map, and tying balloons at relevant points will help to ensure that guests don't miss their turnings. Remember to include a reception card for ceremony guests if it is to be held at a different site than the service.

Order your invitations at least four months before the wedding, and allow an additional month for engraved invitations (instead of handwritten or printed).

The bride's parents traditionally issue invitations, but if the groom's parents are assuming some of the wedding expenses, the invitations should be in their names also.

Don't skimp when ordering; you will need at least twenty-five extra invites for last-minute invitees and the few you might smudge. It might seem wasteful, but you will spend a lot more if you have to reorder. Start addressing and planning at least two weeks before you want to put them in the post box; you will be amazed at how long it takes to collect all the addresses and mail the invitations. It'll be even longer if you're using a calligrapher or if your guest list is very large. A typical refusal rate runs at around 15–20%, so you might want to send out invites later to those people who had to be left out due to numbers. Make sure you can accommodate everyone: a standing-room-only policy might make you look popular, but you won't *be* popular. Also, take one invite to get weighed to make sure you have the right postage, and ask for pretty seasonal stamps if they have them.

MAKING THE NUMBERS ADD UP

A vital part of the invite process, and a boost for your sanity, is the response cards. These should be enclosed with the invitation and will help you determine the number of people who will be attending your wedding. The cards should be easy for your guests to understand and use, and make it really clear you want them returned. If necessary for working out the catering, it is acceptable to put a date on them by which guests must reply: a month before the wedding is acceptable. If you want to get a reply include a self-addressed and stamped return envelope to make it excuse-free for those bachelor friends who can't seem to master the art of buying a stamp. If it is being held in a different place, a separate card with the date, time and location for the reception should be enclosed with the ceremony invitation.

WHAT TO SAY?

Invitation wording can be tricky, but luckily there are lots of conventions and systems you can stick to; or break. Your preferred stationer will have examples for you to follow.

Napkins, matches and order of service may also be ordered from your stationer. See IDEA 36, *Choosing a theme for decoration*, on choosing a theme that will link them all, to create an elegant, cohesive look.

Try another idea...

'For 'tis always fair weather when good fellows get together with a stein on the table and good song ringing clear.'
RICHARD HOVEY, from *Spring*

Defining idea...

How did it go?

Q **I don't want children squawking through the wedding, but my fiancée has told her niece she can come. What can I do?**

A *The presence of children is often a big issue. Determine as early as possible if you wish to include children in the wedding party. Make it a rule and insist you both stick to it. You must be a man of steel.*

Q **So I have to look like the bad guy to her niece?**

A *It's all about the way you present it. You are being fair to all the children and parents, not trying to hurt just one. If you give in to one couple with their little precious, your walk down the aisle will met by a sea of glowers from other parents who had to leave their kids at home.*

Q **And what can I do to stop her niece being very disappointed?**

A *You may have to get around it by giving her an official role, such as a flower girl. That way you have a legitimate excuse for her inclusion.*

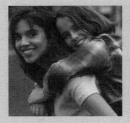
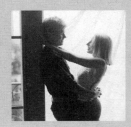
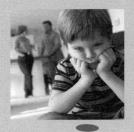

4

And so the vicar said...

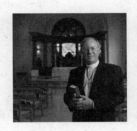

Everyone is so happy that they all want to say their piece. If only you could stop them. There is a convention, so you need to know who does the speeches and how you handle them.

Everyone looks forward to the speeches — as long as they aren't too long. Make sure everyone tries a run through and times themselves. If any of your speakers fancies himself as a bit of a performer, make your instructions very clear: this is a toast to the happy couple, not a chance to fulfil those dreams of being on the stage.

Officially, the speeches run in the following order: the bride's father's speech, the bridegroom's speech and lastly the best man's speech. Kick off the toasts with an announcement by the toastmaster or best man, who should ask for the bride's

Think about changing the rules. If the bride decides that she would like to say something, or would like her maid of honour to speak on her behalf, that's all good.

father to deliver a speech of 'health and happiness to the bride and bridegroom'. He would normally welcome the groom's parents, relatives of both families any other guests and welcome the groom to his family and say a few words about his daughter.

The bridegroom replies on behalf of himself and his bride, taking the opportunity to thank his parents and talk about his love for his bride, and thank all those present for their attendance and gifts. He will finish by toasting the bridesmaids (no, not *that* kind of toasting) and may also present them with a small gift as a token of the couple's appreciation. Next is the most awaited speech of all. It is the best man's duty to respond to the toast on behalf of the bridesmaids, and then deliver what has historically become a fun speech to warm everybody up ready for the good old knees up they should be having to give the couple a good start. And, of course, it should include a good dose of humiliation for the groom.

AND THEN I SHAVED OFF HIS EYEBROWS...

So, does the best man's feel like the most pressured speech of the day? There are tips you can give him (that might work for you, too). Firstly, relax. This is not open-mike night at your local. This audience will be rooting for you; they really want to laugh, and will even be tuned into funny bits you weren't overly impressed with yourself. Unless it's a shotgun wedding, the guests want everything to have the feel-good factor.

When faced with a blank sheet of paper, it's a good start to jot down anything that comes into your head. For the best man, writing down some facts gives an effective skeleton: how he knows the groom, when you met and how he met your partner, etc. Anecdotes about how the couple's relationship has blossomed will be well received. It is appropriate to tell stories that recall the groom's crazy, bachelor antics, but it's not the time to announce that he has slept with most of the bridesmaids. The best man will be expected to be a little risqué but not to give grandmothers heart attacks.

It may seem that every best man's speech that brought the house down was ad libbed all the way through. No such thing: always remember that no professional comedian goes on stage without any preparation so neither should any of you. Get a willing friend to listen to the speech and then consider their opinions as openly as possible. Don't get defensive if they are only trying to help.

Suggest the best man assesses his voice. If he talks in a flat, monotonous sounding way, he could practise filling it with inflection. It's surprising to discover what sounds artificial to you seems perfectly normal to others. It will also help with nerves if he feels he's playing a part rather than standing up in front of complete strangers for a rather long one-way chat. And as a general rule for all of you, slow down: most people tend to rabbit through things. If you can bear it, film yourselves with a camcorder to see which of these crimes you commit so you can rectify them as you practise.

Can you hear me at the back? Don't mumble through it only to discover that only the top table heard you. IDEA 6, *Getting readings right*, will show you how to get professional.

Try another idea...

'*Always do your best. What you plant now, you will harvest later.*'
OG MANDINO, US novelist

Defining idea...

How did
it go?

Q   **My father only has sons and is a great public speaker, and I just know he'd love the chance to do a 'father of the bride speech'. Can we cheat and do a 'father of the groom' speech too?**

A   *You can do whatever you want. Just make sure that the other speeches are short enough to accommodate an extra one. There is nothing worse than the speeches starting to resemble a Japanese endurance test.*

Q   **So how long is too long and how many speakers are too many?**

A   *As it's your big day, you probably feel as if you could listen to your loved ones wax lyrical about your good selves all day. But consider the last wedding you went to – were the speeches so long that your eyes were rolling back in your head or did they bounce along happily with lots of laughter? Based on your experience as a guest, aim for a timing that falls into the latter category. If you have concerns, get your speakers to time themselves, then add it up (you'll be surprised how quickly it mounts up). If you can see it's going to be too much of a long haul, ask them all to shave off a minute or two.*

5

The blushing bride

But are the blushes for the right reasons? Yes, you've dreamed about this day since you were a little girl, but remember you had the figure of a twelve year old back then. It's a must to be realistic when searching for the right dress.

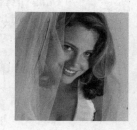

Always wanted to shimmer in silk but know going bra free is out of the question? Tried on a full skirt and looked like the Christmas fairy (tree included)? The trick is to choose a dress that you like, but a dress that suits you as well.

Firstly, you must not go into a bridal shop with any fixed ideas; that way madness lies. All kinds of married women will tell you that the dress they tried on for a laugh, the dress they would never have considered in a million years, turned out to be the one they tripped up the aisle in. So leave trawling the wedding magazines until you have had at least one major trying-on session.

Here's an idea for you...

When choosing your dress, think first about your hairstyle and headdress, or absence of one. Different necklines will work better with hair up or down, with veil or without, so consider these ideas. Tiaras are a popular choice and suit any length of hair, although you may need styling products and pins to help them stay put. If you want a headdress with a minimum of fuss, a simple silk Alice band or headband can be cute and '50s retro while also allowing for a windy day (Highland weddings take note). Coronets look wonderful with a long veil, and fresh flowers bring simple charm to any dress; a single exotic bloom can add real glamour. Hats need a more formal outfit, but can look dynamite with a chic trouser or skirt suit. Just bear in mind you might want to take it off later, and you'll need a hairdo that can handle it.

Your wedding dress is unlike any dress you will ever have worn. For starters, it is likely to be white or cream, and much longer, and a much more unusual shape, than anything currently hanging in your wardrobe. So throw away your preconceptions of what will suit you: you'll be wrong. Try on every shape you can get your hands on, even if you don't like the style. You are guaranteed to be surprised by what flatters you. And that goes for your complexion, too: pure white doesn't work for everyone so make sure you see the dress against your skin in daylight as well as in the shop, because your guests will.

When you have found a style that suits, compare the cost of materials. (A plain silk shift is likely to differ from a boned, beaded bodice with full skirt.) This will give you an idea of what you need to consider when setting your budget. Now you can look at the wedding magazines, to help you find variations on your theme. Bear in mind, you will need to order at least three to four months before your big day and, if you are indecisive, work back from this date to make sure you don't end up panic buying.

ANYONE COVERING YOUR BACK?

You need a dress buddy to talk you out of any childish Cinderella fantasy and give her free rein to say, 'Yes, your bum does look big in that'. (When you say your vows, most guests won't be looking at your face.) And make sure one of you remembers to bring some heels, unless you will be wearing flat (or no) shoes. Having your dress cut a few inches too short could be devastating, sartorially speaking.

SOME NOT-SO-EXCITING PRACTICAL CONSIDERATIONS

A lace shift in December? Nice idea; miserable wedding. Think about the season of your wedding. In high summer, cool silk, chiffon, pure cotton or lace; cooler winter months call for heavier fabrics such as brocade, velvet and duchess satin. And be practical: hiking a huge skirt through fields to a marquee might seem funny at first but will soon lose its humorous appeal.

Be positive. Write a list of all your best assets and those which you would like to show off to full advantage on the day. (Not all of them will be suitable for showing off.) A lovely off-the-shoulder number is ideal for a high neck, and a pear shape can be hidden with a slinky waist, flaunting a full skirt and nipped-in bodice. You will never have a chance to hide your disliked bits so skilfully again! And don't forget that budgets often get stretched by essentials such as underwear, stockings, shoes, jewellery, bags, scarves, etc. All will add finishing touches and complete your look, but will they bust your budget?

Think about whether you want a theme to your wedding (colour, period, style), as this will make your choice of dress easier. See IDEA 36, *Choosing a theme for decoration.*

Try another idea...

'I...chose my wife, as she did her wedding gown, not for a fine glossy surface but such qualities as would wear well.'
OLIVER GOLDSMITH, *The Vicar of Wakefield.*

Defining idea...

19

How did it go?

Q **The wedding is off. I've found my dream dress and *he* says no, it's too expensive for a one-off. What can I do?**

A *Ah, men and frocks. There are ways of reining in the costs whilst letting your dreams run free; consider man-made fabrics instead of silk. If you want to feel the real McCoy of silk on your skin, consider hiring your dress. Before you shriek in horror, you can pay about the same to hire a designer dress as you would to buy a mass-produced one. If you must have it, you could recoup some of the cost of a designer dress by selling it after the wedding. Lots of agencies and web sites offer this service (unless you've covered it in red wine). And how often will you wear it anyway?*

Q **No, I can't bear to part with my dress. What should I do now?**

A *Then something might have to give. Offer to compromise on another area of the wedding and tell him the dress will be a family heirloom. Preserve your dress by having it expertly cleaned and boxed, ready for your offspring's big day. Or cut it short and dye it red, and take him dancing...*

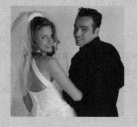 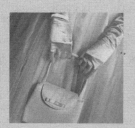 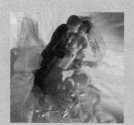

6

Getting readings right

Readings can be a wonderful way to express what's in your heart without having to emotionally put yourself on the line (especially if you are a blubberer). And the best thing is, someone has already done the work for you.

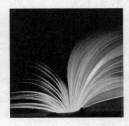

Choosing the right readings is essential because they set the tone for the whole ceremony. So, don't be too hasty in making your decision — it could help you say a great deal in a very short time.

Timing is a key factor. Make sure your readings are concise, but long enough to express your personal sentiments fully. They must not be so long that guests zone out and start reading the prayer book for relief. At the same time, anything too short will sound like a limerick, and those should be saved for the best man's speech. Get a friend to time them as you read them out – you might be surprised how quickly three stanzas can seem like a stroll through eternity.

Here's an idea for you...

Think about where and when the reading will take place. If you want to do it during the ceremony, rather than have the reader step into the place vacated by the clergyman, try having her stood slightly to the side. If the reading is long, you can break it up into sections relevant to the running of the ceremony. There are no rules here; you can even move the reading to the reception to keep the ceremony shorter, and you can drop the reading altogether if you don't feel that it works for you. And consider putting a copy of it in with guests' favours as a sweet keepsake.

WHERE TO LOOK

There are plenty of books out there dedicated to wedding readings, but spread your search wider. Is there a favourite poem or book from your childhood that has special memories? You don't have to stick with Kahlil Gibran's *The Prophet* or Shakespeare to have a meaningful reading. And think hard about what you are trying to communicate: are you trying to express your feelings for each other through the reading? If so, why not consider choosing a reading each, to be read as responses. Lots of couples choose readings that express their feelings about their relationship or what they think marriage should be about.

Readings are a lovely way of communicating your intentions towards each other and how you hope to relate to one another in the future. This is not to say you should go as far as including the lines such as 'And I will take control of the laundry basket as long as the dishwasher gets stacked straight after dinner'.

However, a light touch can be just as poignant as a seventeenth-century romantic poet. Make sure that you understand each other's tastes. Get your partner to choose three poems they like, and you do the same, and see which are the most similar in tone. You could even consider writing a reading yourself – try a witty list of intentions, or a love letter you have kept (just make sure it's one from the person you're about to walk down the aisle with).

Looking to include everyone? Check out IDEA 26, *The supporting cast*, when you are considering your reader.

Try another idea...

CHOOSING YOUR READER

Just because Aunt Maude was in amateur dramatics, it's not a good reason to let her step up to the mike. Similarly, as much as you love your gran, if she can't read your chosen passage without 2 ft cue cards, you may have to think again. You need to consider how comfortable your reader will be. Don't strong-arm a reluctant friend into participating or you will get the reading you deserve – mumbled and raced through. Choose someone who will relish the task and put some thought into its delivery; many an exquisite Shakespeare sonnet has been murdered by a lack of intonation and inflection.

'I wish thee as much pleasure in the reading as I had in the writing.'
FRANCES QUARLES, English religious poet

Defining idea...

How did
it go?

**Q   I love a poem that my partner hates. How can I get him to agree
to what I want?**

A   *It's the 'c' word that keeps coming up again and again: compromise. You
need to ask yourself why you would want a reading he will be tutting
through, rather than something that represents how you both feel. You will
have to resume your search. Watching him smile at you lovingly during the
reading, rather than seething, will be worth it. Ask him to get involved in
the search so that you get a better idea of what he likes more quickly.
(He might even let you have your way if that seems like too much effort.)*

**Q   And he really wants his sister to do the reading. I think she has a
speaking voice like a distant hover mower. She has no intonation
and will send everyone to sleep. What can I do about that?**

A   *This is where being benign bears fruit: after all, if you are willing to give in
on your reading, it's his turn to be reasonable. If it is truly important to
him, gently remind him of his sister's flat, dull tone and suggest, for
everyone's comfort, she has a couple of classes in public speaking. It's
something most people could benefit from (few of us get up in front of a
room to deliver speeches on a daily basis). If that's too controversial,
suggest all of the wedding speakers get together to practise and let the
others help her (and point out her weak points).*

Q   So I might not get my way?

A   *It's not my way anymore, it's our way.*

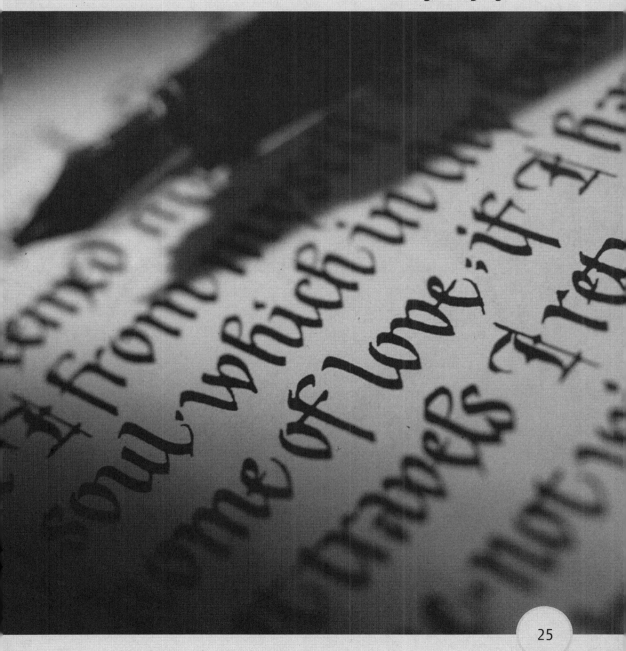

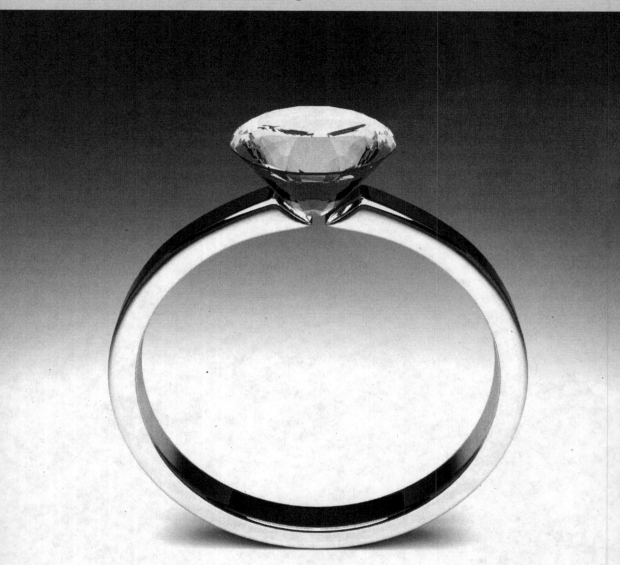

7

Ring the changes

Tradition has it that you are supposed to hand over two months' salary for an engagement ring, and spend whatever you want on the wedding rings, which are usually cheaper because they are usually more simple. It's a big outlay so be sure you make the right choices.

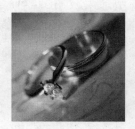

You need to get to grips with some jewellery facts to make sure that you get the best sparkler for the light of your life. So how do you know what to look for?

The cut is the most essential element of the 'sparkle' and there are many of them. There are also fashionable cuts (such as a baguette cut), so you need to get yourself acquainted with them by spending a few afternoons flicking through bridal magazines and visiting a decent jeweller's. You don't want to present her with something a dowager would have loved, but she is already planning to lose.

The cut refers to the number, placement, and shape of the 'facets' (flat, polished planes) that create a finished diamond. The shape into which the stone is cut determines its brilliance (white light reflection or sparkle), and fire (reflection of

Here's an idea for you...

Think of messages you could have engraved on the inside of your rings – perhaps a pet name, the date you met, the date of your marriage or both of your initials.

rainbow colours). A good cut can release a stone's beauty, just as a bad one makes a stone dull. The next aspect to consider is the clarity, which is how clear the diamond is. The imperfections on the outside are called blemishes and the ones inside are called inclusions. This may seem like a horrifying prospect, buying a less than flawless diamond for your beloved, but most diamonds have imperfections. Another thing that may surprise you is that they are not always white, even if you might think they are. The majority are white or yellow, though they come in most colours of the rainbow. Yellow diamonds tend to be cheaper, although they don't reflect light as well. The weight of your diamond is measured in carats, which is equivalent to 200 milligrams.

So, now you know what you need to spend money on, you need to think about the style of setting. Once again, now is not the time to think about what your mum has worn. Do a bit of James Bond style spying on her. What colours does she like? Rifle through her jewellery box; does she have mainly gold or silver? If it's a mix, were some presents that she doesn't ever seem to wear? Is she an ostentatious character or does she loathe fuss? You may want to buy her a rock that has her arm dragging along the floor as a sign of your adoration, but she might feel much more appreciated and understood if you get her a simple vintage setting that reflects her style.

There are many settings to choose from, and all of them can bring something different to the stone. If you want it to really sparkle, choose something that allows as much light through the stone as possible. Traditionally, you would choose to set the stone/stones in one of the three most popular precious metals. These are gold (which comes in various shades; the silver appearance of some rings often being white gold), platinum and titanium. There are the same choices for wedding rings. When it comes to paying for these, it is traditional for the bride to pay for her husband's wedding band, and for him to purchase hers.

Do you know what your bride has in mind? If you are at a loss, get talking: look to IDEA 1, *Who are you?*, for ways to work it out.

Try another idea...

MAKING IT SPECIAL

Commissioning your own design can bring an extra special slant to your union, and will be a gesture greatly appreciated by your beloved. Although it might seem like an expensive and time-consuming approach, it could end up giving you the best value. Unmounted diamonds are by far the best deal, and you could get a setting copied if you really like it. Plus, buying a diamond already mounted means that you cannot check its quality. However, it can take weeks to get your ring made up, or to settle on a design if you are commissioning a designer, so build that into your proposal or wedding day schedules.

HOW MUCH?!!

Determine your budget and then play with the different components to get the best combination for you. Is size king or a band of smaller, well cut super sparkly gleamers that you can see from three streets away? Decide what shape, carat weight, and colour you want. And be prepared to haggle; there is often a margin for play built into the price. Then get it home, and please insure any rings before you give them to the best man.

'With this ring, I thee wed, with my body I thee worship and with all my worldly goods I thee endow.'
Wedding vow, *Book of Common Prayer*

Defining idea...

29

How did it go?

Q **In her will, my grandmother left me her engagement ring to present to my future wife. We were close, and I would love to do that, but it's a rather old-fashioned cluster in a gold setting; my bride is a modern blonde who only wears silver. What should I do?**

A *Lucky you. This is easy to fix. You can have the stones removed and reset. Depending on your taste, you could take the larger central stone and have it set in a silver band, and then take smaller jewels and have them turned into earrings for your wedding to her.*

Q **Isn't it disrespectful to break up the old ring?**

A *I'm sure your grandmother would rather the jewels were worn in some form than not at all. Why not take a photograph of it and write the lineage of it on the back as a keepsake, and your wife might choose to bequeath it to one of your kids – a family tradition could be born, but one that keeps up with the times.*

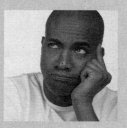
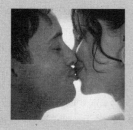
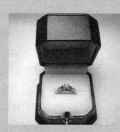

8

How to be the best best man

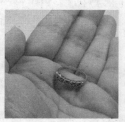

So, what's this best man lark all about? There is more to it than ensuring the groom is never left with an empty glass at his stag do. Traditionally, it was the best man's duty to protect the groom from bad luck, and ensure that once he had begun his journey to the church he actually got there (no matter how substantial the bribe).

Sorry, but if anything goes wrong, it kind of is the best man's fault. So here is a simple guide to what you should be doing to prove your mettle.

You should start by getting the contact details of the maid of honour or chief bridesmaid. This way you'll be able to liaise on arrangements and queries (such as "Where is the bride?!"). And although the jokes about the best man having first crack at the bridesmaids might be funny, they are just that: jokes. Those posh dresses they are wearing are not wrapping paper, and you will have to talk to them a lot in the run up to the wedding, so leave any indiscretions until the reception (where you can make a hasty retreat).

Here's an idea for you...

Offer to look after the distribution of corsages, which are part of the groom's responsibility. You should also be willing to help him choose his suit, shirt and tie. If he is the superstitious type, or if you are, arrange for the groom to carry a small mascot or charm in his pocket on the wedding day for good luck. And remove any ladders from the nearby area.

You also need to sit and work a few things out with the groom. He may ask you to help to choose the ushers and explain their duties to them, and even oversee them on the day. Compile a list of close family members who should have special seating arrangements at the ceremony and pass it on to the ushers. Transport is part of your domain too, so visit the ceremony and the reception venues to check on timings and parking arrangements; you don't want to discover the bride's limo can only stop to let her out two blocks away. (For extra points, check the traffic conditions on the big day.) You will also be expected to attend the wedding rehearsal and arrange the going-away car for the bride and groom from the reception if required. (Stick an emergency list of taxi companies on your schedule list so you can save the day should needs must.)

The day before, you are your groom's wing man, but you really need to be available to him for the whole week before and do things such as collect any hired clothing and accessories. You'll have to badger the groom to make sure he has all the necessary documents for the ceremony and the honeymoon. You also need to organise decorations for the going-away car, which can be as simple as a single ribbon, tastefully tied, or something more along the jovial theme of tin cans and shaving foam. Just make sure that the driver can still see where he's going.

Some best men also organise decoration for the honeymoon suite, especially if it is in the same location as the reception. Remember, the adult, sensitive approach to this tends to involve a bottle of chilled champagne and some soft lighting, not putting water-filled condoms in the bed. (Anything has to be an improvement on the best man who filled the couple's Jacuzzi full of washing up liquid, and then filled it full of ushers (still in hired morning suits), and filled *them* with the contents of the mini bar. The not so happy couple came in to find them all fast asleep buried in foam.)

The stag do used to be the groom's problem, but it has begun to be the best man's headache instead. This means more work, but also more opportunities for devilment. (Bear in mind, though, that no one will love or thank you for a wedding picture missing a groom. Or his eyebrows.) Try IDEA 47, *Tied to a lamp-post in Germany*, for some guidance.

Try another idea...

During the ceremony you carry and present the rings to the groom, and follow the wedding procession down the aisle after the last bridesmaid, and keep following them until you hit the reception. There you will be part of the receiving line and greet the guests. You might also be expected to carry cash to pay the band or DJ, and it is traditional for you to pay the church minister's fee, adding an odd sum to bring luck to the couple.

The next day, collect and return any hired clothing and accessories. And the chief bridesmaid.

"Friendship is mutual blackmail elevated to the level of love."
ROBIN MORGAN, US writer

Defining idea...

How did it go?

Q   **I really want my brother to be my best man but he is notoriously lazy. I know he would be offended if I asked someone else but I don't want to end up having to organise everything for him. What can I do?**

A   *Hand him this book. If he is too lazy to read it, you may need to print out a laminate for him showing a list of required responsibilities. If he won't even engage with that, maybe you need to rethink. Try telling him that you want him to have the role, but if he won't take it all on, the responsibility as well as the privilege, then you may have to ask someone else.*

Q   **If I've asked my brother to be best man, and he's accepted, but I can see that he's shirking, what should I do then?**

A   *If you must have him in the role, name someone as head usher and ask him for help in explaining your situation and getting the best out of your brother. Remember to make sure the third party gets suitable appreciation – a yacht might do – for his thankless behind-the-scenes toil.*

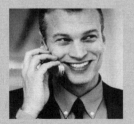 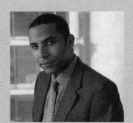 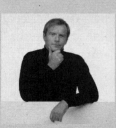

9

Ladies in waiting

Once you've charted the shark-infested waters of choosing your bridesmaids, the real work begins. You need to get them looking great, feeling great, and even being great to each other.

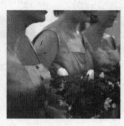

The bridesmaids play a pivotal role. As well as looking great (but not too great), they should be offering help, support and planning, and giving the single you a decently decadent send off. But, of course, there is one essential area that will influence how happy all of you are: the bridesmaids' dresses. Friendships have floundered over pink shantung silk and puff sleeves.

There are several variations to consider. Firstly, unless you are a member of the jet set with only models for attendants, all of yours will be different sizes, and ages. Start by asking everyone what they feel comfortable with: adult bridesmaids often feel a bit self-conscious in a full-length outfit and might prefer knee length. Empire

Here's an idea for you... **Get swatches from your dressmaker or shop, one for each bridesmaid (and a couple over in case they lose them) so each can have one to use when looking for shoes and make up.**

line is great for tummy hiding, and those endowed with larger breasts might not be comfortable with spaghetti straps that rule out the support of a bra. Rather than drive yourself insane, why not choose a colour and fabric and ask them to choose variations on that theme? That way you can ensure the fighting is kept to a minimum. (And remember when choosing your fabric that flowing, clingy satin shows no mercy.) If colour matching is a problem, choose a dress style and let them pick colours from a complementary range, or different tones of one shade. Try two in one shade and two in another. But when planning your colour theme, do consider that not everyone can pull off canary yellow.

IT'S YOUR DAY, SO IT'S YOUR WAY

Don't let yourself be bullied by your bridesmaids when it comes to outfits. All women know how it feels to dislike the way you look, so it's easy to give in to their demands. But do not let them pull you in several directions. The best way to do this is to allow them their individuality by letting them choose their own shoes, bags and jewellery. You can even make their posies a little different from each other, or if one would rather not carry a posy, have a corsage in the same flowers. This way they will still feel like themselves on the day. And don't be forced away from your original idea. You don't want people looking at the wedding photographs and wondering if the bride in the Edwardian lace dress had borrowed the funky, super-modern bridesmaids from someone else's wedding just for the pictures.

HITTING STICKY ISSUES

Appointing a maid of honour might seem like unnecessary favouritism, but it is a good way of making sure that someone is keeping tabs on your lovely handmaidens other than just you. Ask her to collect the bridesmaids' measurements and to ensure that everyone has suitable underwear – your dizzy college friend wearing a black bra under her pale pink dress because she hadn't thought things through may be endearing, but will ruin the photographs. The maid of honour can also intercede if there are any disputes.

Make sure the bridesmaids are involved from the beginning so that they can raise concerns early on. Also ask them to be realistic: you need exact measurements, and do not let them claim they will lose that extra half stone only to find yourself surrounded by acres of straining seams. Bear in mind bridesmaids' dresses can take up to six months to arrive if they are being ordered from abroad.

A problem can often arise over who pays for the dresses. It is not uncommon for the bridesmaids to buy their own dresses, but think that through. Don't ask them to splash out on outfits they couldn't wear again, except to fancy dress, and don't choose something ridiculously pricey. If they can choose something they can wear again they may be happier to cough up. You need to weigh up everyone's present financial situation before settling on a style, and you may have to help out your cousin struggling through college with a donation.

Try another idea...

Got a bridesmaid who has bird's nest hair and puts eye make up on like a five year old? Get her to read through IDEA 18, *Crowning glory*, **with you to help her sharpen up her act.**

Defining idea...

'Love is blind, friendship closes its eyes.'
FRIEDRICH NIETZSCHE

HAIRSTYLE

You may consider using artificial flowers for the hairpieces as long as they are in keeping with the flowers carried by members of the bridal party. Since it is not always easy to find good artificial blooms, other types of hairpieces may be more satisfactory, durable, and attractive.

How did it go?

Q **My future husband's sister is a very pretty, very thin 21-year-old who's insisting on wearing a strapless, short dress that my friends, who are slightly older and more self-conscious, hate. I want everyone to be comfortable but how do I get her to relent?**

A *She sounds pretty self-absorbed so appeal to her ego. Tell her that your friends are anxious about the comparison and you need to find a compromise for all. Agree that she can have strapless but nix the clingy shift; a structured dress or separates with boning is more accommodating for a range of figures.*

Q **What can I do for my friend who is uncomfortable with her upper arms?**

A *A pretty wrap draped over the shoulders will provide a little extra coverage.*

10

The outlaws

The old adage that you can choose your friends but not your family will never ring so true as in the run up to your wedding – especially when it's other people's family. With the right balance of honesty and firmness, you can cope.

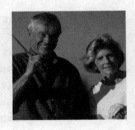

Weddings bring up a lot of intense emotional feelings for all involved, and you may find yourself on the receiving end of some pretty unreasonable demands. Add to this the fact that your own emotions will be running pretty high, and you have a rather volatile situation just waiting to explode.

Often parents may be divorced and sometimes with new partners. All of them will be pressing you to be sensitive to their feelings. They will all feel that they have a special claim on you in some way.

Here's an idea for you... **Invite all of the parents or immediate family out, or round to your house, for dinner. This way they will have some kind of rapport before you get to the big day, and maybe learn to appreciate that there are other close family members who have vested interests.**

BE HONEST

The more you smile and nod whilst secretly plotting to lock your relative in the potting shed, the more complications you make for yourself. A slight smile and shrug will mean that they take for granted your agreement; we all see what we want to when we are looking for it. Try to be friendly but firm from the start. It will be much harder to tell the prospective father-in-law that you don't want his brass band to play marching tunes at the reception if he's already booked it and bought new uniforms to match your bouquet than telling him as soon as the idea is mooted that you'd rather have him charming your guests than stuck behind a euphonium.

MAKE SURE YOU INVOLVE THE SPECIAL PEOPLE

Although you have a guest list to try to manage, be considerate about the others' feelings. You may not know the best friends of your in-laws, but they will have watched your partner grow from being a child and probably been babysitters many times. They will have shared the experience of parenthood with your in-laws and no doubt talked about this moment repeatedly. They are also probably the people listening to the concerns and excitement of your future family regarding the wedding, so if you can possibly include them in some way, it will be no doubt appreciated.

When it comes to family, be clear about their involvement. Ask them what they feel; they may not want to feel like they are adding to your hassles. If you are the bride, ask your fiancé's mum if she would like to come and see

Make sure that whatever problems arise you keep chipper – see IDEA 42, *Arguing*, on making it a happy time.

Try another idea...

the dress or if she wants to help you buy the shoes or accessories. This will be appreciated, even if declined, especially if she doesn't have any daughters of her own. Don't be frightened to bring in the reserves. Ask your mum if she wants to coordinate wedding outfits and you could all shop together for them. You must also ask your partner for help. Make an agreement that you are responsible for difficult discussions with your own families. You don't want to be asking your future father-in-law for deposit cheques.

If they are of a different religion, be sensitive to their requirements. You can ask a celebrant, a respected family figure or a friend of the family to introduce elements of their religious beliefs, such as a blessing, as part of the ceremony. It may mean very little to you if you are of a different religion or an atheist, but a great deal to them. Ask them which part of the ceremony they would feel it is most important to include, and this way they may be more understanding about having to relinquish other elements. If your partner is of a different religion, you may have to consider two ceremonies rather than one. This consideration should stand you in good stead further down the line (like when you are looking for babysitters).

'*One would be in less danger
From the wiles of the stranger
If one's kin and kith
Were more fun to be with.*'
OGDEN NASH, from *Family Court*

Defining idea...

WHO ARE THEY?

Are the outlaws confident, bold types or are they timid people eager to please? Make sure that you really do consider precisely who they are, and don't assume if they're keeping quiet that they are uninterested – they may be trying to avoid adding to your stress. The flip side of this are the very overbearing type of in-laws, who want to force their own vision onto your wedding. You can always tackle this by giving them a part of the wedding to manage that plays to their strengths. Are they great at time keeping, for instance? If so, ask them to organise the cars and transport arrangements.

How did it go?

Q   I really like my future mother-in-law but I feel quite remote from her. How do I move our relationship forward before the big day?

A   *Consider carefully what kind of person she is. Is she uncomfortable with big displays of affection? Look at the way she treats her son; you may notice that she is not a very tactile person, so don't bombard her. You are marrying her pride and joy, and so you should accept that she will be sizing you up. So use a softly, softly approach. Ask her to go shopping with you and have lunch and go from there.*

Q   But I want to feel like she is excited for me at the ceremony. How can I try to enthuse her?

A   *She might well already be excited: don't judge her displays of affection by your own standards. At the end of the day, it's better that her affection is hard won and genuine than gushing and two faced.*

11

Coming up roses

Your florist could be your saviour! They may be able to help with more than you think, so learn to ask for what you want and get the best from your blooms.

If the florist keeps pushing you towards arrangements you can't afford, move on. Make sure that you interview them properly, and ask to see their portfolio. If you want to compare prices, choose a simple flower, like a single white rose corsage and a white rose bouquet, and use that as your guide.

A popular, or just good, local florist will know the main venues in the area and should be able to make suitable recommendations. They should also be able to rent table mirrors, vases and candleholders. And it's worth asking if they can provide silk flowers for hair arrangements (or an allergic wedding party member). Some florists charge a fee to deliver flowers to the ceremony and reception sites and to arrange them on site, so check if that is included in your costing.

Here's an idea for you...

As well as looking great, you need to consider the fragrance of flowers. Scented flowers on the pews can enhance a spring wedding but can fight the smell of your wedding feast on the buffet tables. And certain flowers look stunning but might not really work in a bouquet or table centre (the lilac globes of alliums are visually arresting, but they are part of the onion family, and smell like it too). Get down to the florist's and familiarise yourself with the scents before you start making decisions about your floral displays.

SO JUST HOW MANY FLOWERS DO YOU NEED?

The bride and her maids aren't the only ones sporting flowers. The groom wears his boutonniére on the left lapel, nearest to his heart. The groom often chooses a flower for his buttonhole that also occurs in the bride's bouquet. To make sure no one mistakes him for the best man (including the bride if she's had a little Dutch courage to steady her nerves), make sure that the groom's arrangement is more elaborate or larger than the other males' buttonholes. The groom gives each man in the wedding party a boutonniére to wear on his left lapel, often including the officiant (if male; a corsage if female).

The groom is also responsible for providing flowers for his mother, the bride's mother, and the grandmothers. Make sure they match the outfit each is wearing. (Ask the chief bridesmaid to find out the colour of each outfit.) He can also win a few points for being exceptionally considerate by planning corsages for the bride's going-away outfit.

As well as people, you have to bring some floral flair to your special occasion. Whether you are in a church or civil ceremony, you will have a main altar where you will be married. As this is one of the most prominent locations for flowers, it's a nice idea to use blooms reflecting the theme or colour of the bride's bouquet. Make sure they are tall or elaborate enough to be seen by guests seated at the back. Check if the church is happy for you to choose your own display, as sometimes you may be expected to have their existing creations, which might clash. Ask if you (or your florist) can talk to the regular flower arranger who can tell you which flowers suit the space and which get lost – some sweet country blooms can seem ineffectual if you are marrying in Westminster Cathedral. You could be better off using two main displays at the altar, rather than the ends of the pews. These are often decorated with flowers, candles, ribbons or pew cards. If your ceremony is outdoors, you could marry under a favourite blossom tree, or hang blooms sewn onto twine from its branches. If it's a winter or autumn wedding, or candlelight ceremony, use candelabra decorated with flowers or greens for a dramatic mood. Obviously, you can add or subtract depending on location and budget.

A strict, limited colour palette can enhance the effect of your flowers, as will choosing a suitable variety of blooms. See IDEA 36, *Choosing a theme for decoration.*

Try another idea...

GETTING A GOOD RECEPTION

The head table is where the wedding party will sit during the reception, and is the most important in terms of decoration. It should be decorated with a dramatic centrepiece to mark it out from the others. As it is often a rectangular shape, it looks wonderful with garlands draped around the edges, which also allows guests to see the wedding party. The bridesmaids often place their bouquets in front of their places, so also make this a feature when

'Flowers always make people better, happier and more helpful; they are the sunshine, food and medicine to the soul.'
LUTHER BURBANK, naturalist

Defining idea...

45

planning. The guest tables often have flower arrangements. These need to be low enough for the guests to chat over, or high enough for them to see through (like large fluted vases).

If you are having buffet tables use floral tables to keep them in theme with the rest of the room. Use the food to its best advantage, too, such as piling fruit like a cornucopia, adding to the feeling of celebration. Think laterally: pumpkins might sound like a strange choice but can be striking as part of an autumnal display, as can herbs.

How did it go?

Q   I love flowers and don't want to skimp on them, but my quote from the florist had me reaching for the smelling salts. I've decided not to decorate the church but can't find anywhere else I'm willing to miss out. Any ideas?

A   *There are lots of ways round this. Ask your florist to come up with a similar arrangement but supplementing some of the flowers with more readily available, less expensive blooms. As long as you are willing to budge on the flowers you choose, any florist worth their salt should be able to do this.*

Q   What if I don't want to change to more affordable flowers?

A   *Consider doing the table centres for the reception yourself, or enlist a talented friend or relative. An elegant, tightly packed head of roses in a plain vase can be very effective; just remember this will take a bit of time. And don't skimp on your bouquet or anything vital and elaborate.*

12

The bouquets

The bouquet needs considering almost as soon as your dress, and choosing the right one will be essential to the success of the overall effect of your wedding day look.

Hopefully, by now, you have an idea of what kind of wedding you want. Is it a romantic vintage inspired do, or a very Modern Millie affair? Your bouquet should be a perfectly distilled version of this theme, whilst complementing your look (and, if you are very clever, your figure too).

First you need a suitable partner in crime. It's time to bring in your florist: you need to ensure that you are, ahem, singing from the same hymn book. If you do not feel a rapport with your florist, or they are trying to force their vision onto you rather than letting you call the shots, move on. They may want a chance to recreate the Eiffel Tower in carnations but unless that's your dream too, you can say 'no'. That said, a good florist should be able to guide a confused bride towards their dream

Here's an idea for you...

The orange blossom is the original bridal bloom, symbolising beauty, personality and fertility for hundreds of years. But there are many other ways to florally express your feelings for your loved one. Learn how to use the language of flowers:

Almond blossom, hope; **Apple blossom,** good fortune; **Camellia,** gratitude; **Carnation,** fascination; **Chrysanthemum (red),** I love you; **Chrysanthemum (white**), truth; **Cyclamen,** modesty; **Daffodil,** regard; **Daisy,** innocence; **Gardenia,** joy; **Heather,** good luck; **Heliotrope,** devotion; **Honeysuckle,** generosity; **Hyacinth,** loveliness; **Iris,** burning love; **Ivy,** fidelity; **Japonica,** loveliness; **Jasmine,** amiability; **Lemon blossom,** fidelity in love; **Lilac,** youthful innocence; **Lily,** majesty; **Magnolia,** perseverance; **Mimosa,** sensitivity; **Orange blossom,** purity; **Orchid,** beauty; **Peach blossom,** captive; **Rose,** love and happiness; **Snowdrop,** hope; **Sweet pea,** pleasure; **Violet,** faithfulness.

blooms by asking a few pertinent questions. Always take along reference material (don't worry if it's inconsistent, you can talk that through too) and be open to their ideas. That is, after all, what you are paying them for. If you have any doubts, however, always ask if you can call back the next day; a bit of space will let you see if those ideas were exactly what you want, or exactly what you think you should have. It is also easy to get carried away in the moment, so be wary. And don't forget to ask if they can preserve your bouquet should you choose to.

LET'S BEGIN

There is no set way to do this, but you need to start somewhere, so make it colour, shape, flower or theme. Traditionally a bridal bouquet is made of white flowers, but few brides stick to that rule. If you do want to do that, a nice way to bring colour in is to have your bridesmaid's bouquet made up in a smaller version, using the same flower but in a colour. (With grown-up bridesmaids, you may want to opt for wrist corsages instead, or vary the colours.) If you want to choose your bouquet by colour, or a mix of complementary colours, your florist should be able to present you with a selection of blooms available in those shades. The main shapes are a loose and hand tied arrangement, a flowing cascade (which is full at

See IDEA 18, *Crowning glory*, for how flowers can be used to great effect in your hair.

Try another idea...

the top and trails to a point), a tight cluster, a pomander (a ball of flower heads carried by a ribbon) or a nosegay or basket filled with flowers, or arm bouquet that rests naturally in the crook of the arm. You may have a love of a certain flower that you want to build your bouquet around, or be holding a 1920s themed wedding, in which case flowers popular in that era, like Calla lilies, are a good choice.

HELPING YOU BLOOM

The bride usually holds flowers at waist height, and this needs to figure in your plan. If you are petite, an overwhelming cascade bouquet will overpower you (and possibly tip you over), so choose something in proportion to your size. Similarly, if you have a fuller figure, a small pomander might look a bit inconsequential whereas a cascade will lengthen your silhouette. As with your dress, keep an open mind about the shape you want until you have explored the options. The colour you choose must also flatter your skin tone, especially if you intend to also have them in your hair. Whatever you choose needs to work with the flow of your dress and not obscure you – this is decoration, not camouflage.

'There are always flowers for those who want to see them.'
HENRI MATISSE

Defining idea...

FORGET ME NOT

Smell is the most evocative of the senses, and the most likely to trigger memories, so include a scented bloom. A lovely way to make your flowers special to you for more than just the day is to choose seasonal blooms, so that the daffodils will always remind you of your spring wedding (and hopefully remind your groom that your anniversary is nigh). Another advantage of choosing seasonal blooms is that they will be able to withstand the weather conditions. If your bouquet includes delicate flowers that can wilt, make sure your arrangement can incorporate a bouquet holder to keep them fresh – your hand-tied posy won't look quite so great if it's turning brown at the edges. If you want exotic or off-season flowers, make sure this is discussed well in advance. And make sure you are clear about whether the flowers are to be collected or delivered, and at what time.

How did it go?

Q **I'm a bit of a tomboy and feel uncomfortable with flowers. Do I have to have them?**

A *You may find yourself unsure what to do with your hands, so do carry something. Consider a single stem or a little handbag with a bloom through the clasp.*

Q **How can I get over feeling all girlie and self-conscious?**

A *Look for something with a bit of attitude and wit. Try using a thick, soft velvet ribbon, a collar of net or lace or a frill of grass to add some structure.*

13

Something old...

No, not your gran, but a guide to wedding traditions and their origination. Just why do you need to wear something blue, and why shouldn't the bride walk over the threshold?

There are many customs and superstitions associated with weddings. In the past a wedding was seen as a time when people were particularly susceptible to bad luck and evil spirits and the rituals were supposed to help. They can be fun, too.

You may be the most practical and level-headed of people, but remember that most people enjoy indulging in the rituals and customs of weddings. Even weddings incorporating religious or cultural differences can join in the fun. Make your own rules and put together a combination that means something to you as a couple.

It seems to be that although we still practise these customs few people know what they symbolise, beyond 'good luck'. Here are some pointers.

Here's an idea for you...

If you have different faiths marrying, think how to incorporate traditions from both. As well as good fun, they will get guests talking to each other about what the traditions mean. They are also a great way to make families feel recognised if you are having a non-denominational ceremony.

WHO'S NEXT?

Every woman knows the meaning of tossing the bridal bouquet: whoever catches the bouquet is the next to be married. If you want to keep the bouquet as a memento, have a smaller, less expensive bouquet specifically made for aiming at your best friend. Let's just hope she isn't pushed to the ground in the scramble. If she is, she gets another chance with the throwing of the garter. This is not just a cheeky chance to show the assembled wedding party that you are wearing stockings, it was originally meant to keep back the guests who were overly anxious to disrobe the newlyweds as they made it to their bed. A parallel custom is for the groom to remove the garter worn by the bride and throw it back over his shoulder toward the unmarried guests. Again the one who catches it will be the next to marry.

'SOMETHING OLD, SOMETHING NEW, SOMETHING BORROWED, SOMETHING BLUE...'

...And the final line many forget from this Victorian rhyme: 'And a silver sixpence in your shoe'. The 'something old' refers to the past, the couple's family and friends. The 'new' is their new life as a couple. The 'something borrowed' is often lent by the bride's family and is an item much valued by the family (hopefully not a grand piano) and must be returned for her good luck to be collected. 'Something blue' is an ancient Israelite custom: the bride wore a blue ribbon in her hair to represent fidelity. The sixpence in the bride's shoe was to ensure wealth in the couple's married life. Although you can use modern currency if you are clean out of sixpences, it's probably best to stay away from some of today's plate-size coins. The garter is often given to represent one of these items too.

Like the symbolism of traditions? See IDEA 12, *The bouquets*, and learn how to say it with flowers, symbolically.

Try another idea...

DRESSING THE PART

This has always been very important. However, white wedding dresses are a new invention; many brides wore coloured dresses in times gone by. The rich started the tradition of white, which symbolises maidenhood, in the sixteenth century. Despite its pretty, irreverent use these days, the veil, which became popular in the UK in the eighteenth century, was originally worn by Roman brides as a camouflage to disguise the bride from evil spirits. This is also why bridesmaids were dressed in a similar way to the bride – they were decoys. It's not very often that you get to ask your mates to act as your protectors against the powers of evil sprits, so enjoy it. However, the etiquette of how to handle them getting the bad luck that was aimed at you is unclear. Maybe you could buy them a bottle of wine.

Strangely, shoes have also played a big part in weddings. The bride's father used to give the groom a pair of the bride's shoes to symbolise the passing of responsibility for the daughter to the husband; a modern version of this could be the handing over of her unpaid Visa bill which she ran up buying shoes. Even the throwing of

'Tradition is a guide and not a jailer.'
W. SOMERSET MAUGHAM

Defining idea...

53

the bouquet over the shoulder was originally performed by her throwing one of her shoes over her shoulder; if they are expensive, however, be prepared not to get them back. And, of course, shoes are still tied to the back of the wedding car for good luck.

We can thank the Italians for confetti, which translates into sweets, which are thrown over the couple after the ceremony and symbolise prosperity and fertility.

The final tradition, which has been seen in thousands of Hollywood weepies, is the carrying of the bride over the threshold. The fact that she usually has been paying her share of the mortgage on that threshold for some time is neither here nor there. After the wedding, the groom is supposed to carry the bride over the threshold when they enter the marital home for the first time. One explanation is that the bride will suffer bad luck if she falls when passing over the threshold or enters with her left foot first. She can thus avoid both dangers by being carried. The modern explanation is that she may just be a bit too merry to make it home on her own.

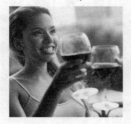
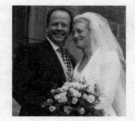

Q **Since I was a child, my mother, who's a strict Catholic, has always told me that she'd like me to wear her family heirloom, a garter, at my own wedding. I'm having a pagan ceremony, though, and feel like a fraud. How can I say no?**

How did it go?

A *Why do you have to? Although the rhyme is Victorian, the traditions that surround weddings are from much earlier; so much so that we are unsure of the origins of most of them.*

Q **So can I adopt other traditions too? I've always loved the Jewish breaking of the glass.**

A *Well, you will need to put your own spin on it, or acknowledge its origins so you don't offend any Jewish guests, but why not? It's your day, so have it your way.*

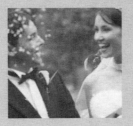 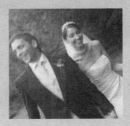

55

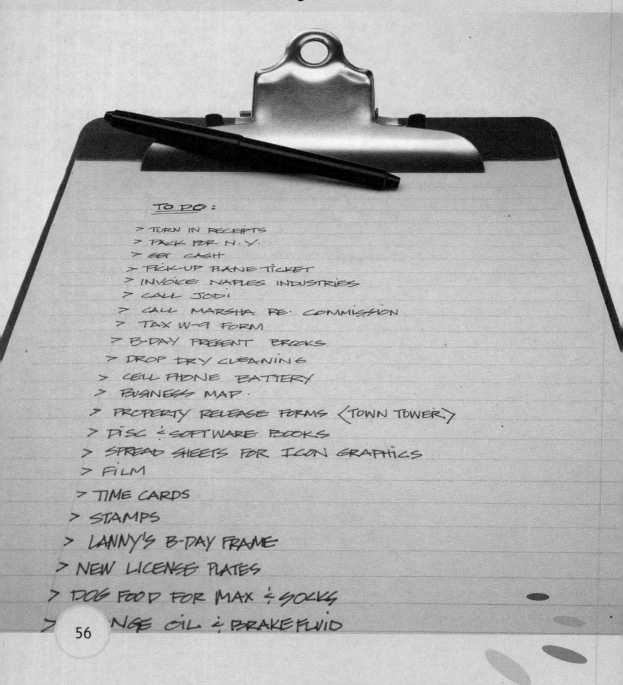

TO DO:

> TURN IN RECEIPTS
> PACK FOR N.Y.
> GET CASH
> PICK-UP PLANE TICKET
> INVOICE NAPLES INDUSTRIES
> CALL JODI
> CALL MARSHA RE. COMMISSION
> TAX W-9 FORM
> B-DAY PRESENT BROOKS
> DROP DRY CLEANING
> CELL PHONE BATTERY
> BUSINESS MAP.
> PROPERTY RELEASE FORMS <TOWN TOWER>
> DISC & SOFTWARE BOOKS
> SPREAD SHEETS FOR ICON GRAPHICS
> FILM
> TIME CARDS
> STAMPS
> LANNY'S B-DAY FRAME
> NEW LICENSE PLATES
> DOG FOOD FOR MAX & SOCKS
> NGE OIL & BRAKE FLUID

14

How to say 'I don't' and 'you do'

The key to a happy wedding, a sane bride and a wedding that won't be annulled is to master two ancient and rare arts: saying 'no' and delegation.

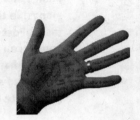

If you can share responsibility and refuse to take on too much, it will stop you from cracking under the pressure, and it may also allow you a little time to sit back and enjoy the ride.

Finding suppliers, venues, a reliable and tasteful caterer: the things-to-do list can seem endless. However, you have a much bigger resource at your hands than you think. How many of your friends are already married? Ask them about their disasters as well as their triumphs, and collect their recommendations. Get all the names and numbers you can from them.

If you have friends who are especially good at certain tasks, tell them that you admire their talents, and then enlist their help. Got a shopaholic sister? Tell her you need her help to find silver ballet shoes for the flower girls in miniature sizes and

Here's an idea for you...

Design a spreadsheet with names and contact details alongside the delegated list of tasks. Post it on the web so people can access it, or print it out and hand copies to all concerned so they can coordinate if necessary.

watch her go. This isn't really manipulation, just an efficient way of getting the best out of everyone whilst making them feel good about it. And if someone has a task they enjoy, they are much more likely to excel at it.

By the same token, a night in with some fountain pens, a bottle of wine and your mum will give her a warm glow of being involved, and a chance to get all those invitations addressed. Then there will be all the RSVPs to deal with; so you need to ask people to chip in there, as there will be a lot of chasing. Perhaps one of the bridesmaids can be given this as a single responsibility; it is a big job and one that can become more complex if you try to split it.

Rather than being a huge burden, asking for help can be a great way of including slightly marginalized people, such as a favourite aunt, who has no official position but would like to be involved. Make sure that you show appreciation to whomever you ask, and don't dump a dull task on somebody while you skip off with the bridesmaids shopping for underwear and a long boozy lunch. Most people will be happy to help if they feel appreciated.

Now you have to start saying no. You must set out clear boundaries with all involved so when you hear the words 'Oh, I'm busy, can you do it?' you are very clear that, no, you can't. Do not explain why not; just be firm. It may seem tough to start with, but the more you do it the easier it gets, and it will save you a lot of problems, and resentment, further down the line.

Find it hard to say no? Get yourself a wedding coordinator who can take over the tough bit of putting up boundaries. Your mother-in-law may find it acceptable to bully you into matching thrones at the reception but the professional distance a wedding coordinator can bring will make it impossible for her to win.

Want to make sure that your partner understands how much there is to do? Make them read IDEA 50, *Time lines*, so they get with the programme.

Try another idea...

Don't micromanage everything: The key to successful delegation is trust, so do not peer over people's shoulders, metaphorically or physically. The classic way to de-motivate someone is to check up on him or her all the time. It is reasonable to ask for a progress report but appreciate that other people have lives and that your wedding isn't the centre of theirs like it is yours. Try not to delegate anything time sensitive, like booking the church or reception.

Many hotel venues have wedding organisers who are on hand during the day, so find out how much you can rely on them and what they are responsible for. Will they be on hand to let in the florists? Do they oversee the setting up of the bar and putting favours on tables? Clear this up as soon as you start discussions, or you could end up duplicating work. You may also need to ask your bridesmaids to have a spot check on the day. If you are planning on doing some of the catering or table displays yourself, make sure that someone else is overseeing the final implementation when the big day arrives. If you give yourself too much to think about, it will end up feeling like you've thrown a great party but you didn't get to enjoy it.

'The art of leadership is saying no, not yes. It is very easy to say yes.'
TONY BLAIR

Defining idea...

If someone else in your party is overseeing aspects such as the flowers, make sure that they come to the meetings with you so that they know exactly what they are meant to be doing, and what things are meant to look like. Many a disaster has occurred when two people interpreted the same set of words in different ways.

How did it go?

Q **I think about all the details of the planning constantly. No one seems to be helping and time is running out. How can I fire them up?**

A *Sounds like you are running on Bride Time. To other people, six months away sounds like a lifetime, but you want to tick things off the list now. You need to be patient with them but explain your concerns firmly to turn up their sense of urgency.*

Q **But I feel like no one cares and I am the only one taking this seriously. What if they just tell me that I'm being overly worried?**

A *It is a simple case of getting your communication right. Explain to your helpers how stressed you feel rather than pointing the finger of blame (or you'll find them even less willing to help). Let them know that the sooner these things are taken care of, the sooner will come the time that you can relax and enjoy the run up to your big day.*

15

Smile!

One thing is for sure, your big day will pass in a complete blur and seem to last four minutes rather than twenty-four hours. So, you will be relying heavily on your photographs and video to remind you that you didn't just dream the whole thing.

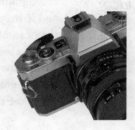

When you start looking for your photographer, you should cast your net wide and see as many portfolios as you have time for. Remember, there is only one chance to capture the magic of this day, so you need the right eye behind the lens.

There is a huge range of styles and options to consider, and making the right choice means that you will be able to reflect the very personal feel of your own day. With that in mind, you will by now be aware that there are a lot of other people to consider – you may want more reportage-style shots whereas older family members want more posed, traditional shots as mementos of the day. It is a good idea to set

Here's an idea for you...

It's common to have a videographer at weddings too, and if they are filming digitally they can often produce great stills as well as videos. Look at their show reel (their version of a photographer's portfolio) to see what they can do.

aside some time before your reception to make sure that everyone has the combination they would like. (Make sure you order extra sets of these prints for sending out; putting them in a frame as special gifts for grandparents would be a nice touch.) Brides sometimes like to have a posed portrait before the wedding, so do ask if that is available too.

KEEPING IT STRICTLY BUSINESS

Be wary of allowing eager amateurs to help out. Specialised wedding photographers will understand wedding procedures, ceremonies and receptions, so they can anticipate your next move and be in the proper place at the right time to capture all the special moments. Make sure that your photographer is someone you feel comfortable with; if they remind you of a sergeant major and your dream wedding is more along the lines of Glastonbury, but with more mud, you will clash terribly. Make sure they are happy to cajole merry family members along for the group shots and can keep things moving along. Imagine how devastated you would be if your cousin's kind-hearted attempt to help went wrong and you had no decent pictures of the day.

Look at his or her work. See if the photographer captured the excitement and emotion of the bridal couple. Don't be frightened to take along pages torn from magazines or photographs you have that capture a feel that you like. It is also reasonable to ask them about their attire: they may think that trainers are acceptable or come in full morning suit, so check. Also check if they bring an assistant with them, and enquire after their attire too.

EXTRAS! EXTRAS!

Once you like someone's style, you need to clear up a few grey areas. This is where some less reputable photographers make their money. How much do extra prints cost? Is processing included in the cost? Who gets the negatives, you or them? Many photographers keep the rights to the negatives, so you can only get extra prints through them. If so, see if you can negotiate a fee to release them to you after a certain time. Ask the photographer how soon after the wedding you will get the prints. You should also ask if they could do retouching. A good photographer should have liability insurance, offer a money-back guarantee and make references available if you require them.

In terms of style, it's often nice to get reportage shots of the bride in preparation before the ceremony, so consider whether or not you would be comfortable with a male photographer catching you or your fiancé in your smalls. Be clear about the amount of time you expect them to spend at the wedding, and if you want them at the reception. In case things run over, check what the cost per additional hour of shooting would be. A good photographer will be prepared for this eventuality, and not skip out before you are happy. Be wary of booking someone who has booked a second wedding later that day. It's just an added pressure for you and will prevent them from being entirely focused on your day.

Try another idea…

Photographs can make a great 'thank you' for nearest and dearest. IDEA 27, *Thank yous and gifts*, shows you how.

Defining idea…

'We do not remember days, we remember moments.'
CESARE PAVESE, Italian novelist

FEELING GOOD

You will be expected to select the finish for the printed pictures, which are usually gloss or matt. There is a huge range of effects that can alter the way your photographs look and feel, such as adding a white border or making a small print on a large sheet of paper. The photographer should also be able to offer your colour prints in sepia or black and white, but remember that they will not have the same level of contrast as photographs taken in black and white film. Ask your photographer to shoot using both types of film if possible. Don't forget to check if you need to order extras for family and friends.

How did it go?

Q   The vicar says we can't have any photographs! What can I do about it?

A   *Make sure you understand exactly what he is saying; many vicars are simply referring to the obtrusive flash photography by some over-eager amateur photographers.*

Q   Can the vicar stop us?

A   *Well, you could do it anyway but annoying the vicar wouldn't set a very nice tone. It is vital that your photographer understands the rules and regulations of your church before planning the ceremony shots. Some churches do not allow photographs to be taken during the ceremony, but most allow shots before and after.*

16

Make an entrance

How do you imagine your big entrance? Helicopter or horse and carriage? Or are you so in love you are just going to sprint to the church? Get there in style, and on time.

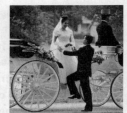

As sexist as this is going to sound, the fact is, if you want the groom to pull his weight in the preparations, the best thing to do is give him something he might enjoy sorting out, like the transport. Of course, it might be the bride that's the petro-head, but there does tend to be a grain of truth in any stereotype.

If you want to keep the wedding vehicles a surprise, start by talking themes. Vintage or modern? Four legged or two wheeled? Also, there are a few practicalities to consider before you commit. An open-top, low-slung Jaguar could look incredibly chic and fitting if the bride is wearing a sharp cream trouser suit. However, the same bride, in a huge skirt and petticoats, would look like an upside down

Here's an idea for you...

A white car can make cream or ivory dresses look dirty in photographs, so compare scraps of sample fabric against the car to check for a clash. If you are not sure what you are looking for, it works like this: a 'warm' white or cream has a yellow undertone; a cold white has a 'blue' undertone. The two together clash. Different shades can go together as long as they are both 'warm' or both 'cold'.

lampshade after she'd squeezed through the door. Same bride, white '60s style mini dress and huge veil – she'll need the veil to cover her mortified blushes after displaying more than she'd like to the assembled wedding party as she climbs in. It won't be a great wedding night if the bride has been humiliated, purposefully or not.

This is the first step on your life's biggest journey, so get it right. Do you want something to remind you of the era you were married in? A white Bentley may be a classic choice, but what about a sky blue Mini for that something blue? You might also want the close family in matching transport that could make for a grand exit. A little thought makes the difference between adding another special part to the day and something perfunctory that drearily gets you from A to B.

CHECK IT OUT

Make sure you go and see the cars, as a brochure or web site can be deceptive. Are they well maintained, will it be used by other weddings that day and, if so, will they valet it in between so the bride doesn't turn up with other people's confetti on her dress? Do they include the ribbons and flowers; can you be involved in choosing them or selecting something different? You may want to carry the theme of the wedding flowers through.

There are other options that don't involve petrol, such as ones that involve aviation fuel. A small plane or helicopter would be a memorable way to leave your guests, and get hats fluttering. This could be less expensive than you might think.

Make sure your transport suits the theme. Look at IDEA 36, Choosing a theme for decoration.

Try another idea...

Some prefer the four-legged way of getting around on their big day. However, if you are shy you might want to reconsider, as it's not exactly speedy. And a horse and carriage is not suitable for getting you long distances across town in the rush hour. If you don't have far to go to reach your reception, consider having the bride riding side-saddle as you lead her on a horse – a pretty romantic gesture. You might give up on transport altogether, if your reception is nearby, and stroll with your wedding party in a grand procession. A nice touch here would be to provide some pretty parasols against summer sun for your beloved and your attendants (and grannies and mums), or some umbrellas to be carried by the ushers just in case.

Whatever you decide to do, you need to book well in advance, perhaps even a year before, especially if you are looking at a Saturday in the summer. If you can't get the car you want through a hire agency, try approaching a classic car or collectors club. Don't forget to reconfirm and check your route by driving it in advance. It would be a disaster if you give everybody a route taken from a street map which turns out to be all one

'Take most people, they're crazy about cars. I'd rather have a goddamn horse. A horse is at least human, for God's sake.'
J. D. SALINGER

Defining idea...

way; the wrong way. And make sure that everyone knows where the reception is – don't rely on convoys as they only ever work if no one else is on the road. You can always have extra reception cards on hand with one of the ushers in case of emergency (someone is bound to have forgotten them). Also make sure someone has a cab number in case of rain emergencies.

How did it go?

Q   I've booked our wedding car, and now she tells me I have to do all the others. What others?

A   *It is the groom's responsibility, although often the best man will help, to book cars for both sets of parents, your attendants, and of course, one to take you to the airport or your first-night hotel. You may also want to include other close family members such as grandparents in that equation. And don't forget, cars are needed to collect everyone and take them to the ceremony, and then take them to the reception.*

Q   Blimey. Sounds expensive. Is there anything I can do to rein in the costs?

A   *It's not necessarily a fortune. You often can book by the hour, and if you don't want a whole row of priceless white vintage Fords you can have a set of sleek black London-style cabs that look elegant (but make sure that they are not emblazoned with ads when booking). What about a London bus for the second stage of the journey? Use your imagination, not just your chequebook.*

17

Where: choosing a location

A location must be more than a pretty backdrop for the photos. It will have a direct influence on how many guests you can invite, the kind of entertainment you can have, and whether or not you can do a full waltz for your first dance.

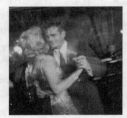

For most, a key consideration in deciding on the 'where' will be your budget limitations. But that doesn't mean you can't have some fun; there is still lots of scope within that for some imagination.

Think bigger than the local church: what about a cathedral with spires and stained glass, a glamorous hotel ballroom, a public park, a rooftop, marrying on holiday or even your own back garden strewn with a hundred balloons? There are endless possibilities, so don't just opt for the obvious without a little research.

WHERE TO START

What will suit the kind of ceremony and reception you want? Your location should be a reflection of your overall theme. If it's formal, your local grand hotel may be a

Here's an idea for you...

Outdoor ceremony or reception? Make a plan to enclose 'If rain stops play...' cards with your invites, informing guests of an alternative location in case of bad weather. It might simply mean moving to a room inside the hotel or, if you are marrying at home with a garden reception, a local pub. Just make sure the wording is clear – you don't want to lose half your guests to the King's Arms when they should be at the King's Head.

suitable location (and should be licensed for civil weddings), with plenty of space for ceremony and guests. But make sure you have free rein to make your own choices – they sometimes insist on using their own favoured caterer. And check there's enough parking space.

If you plan to hold a church wedding, you may need to book up to two years in advance for the date that you want. If you want something a little more unusual, such as a ceremony with your own vows in a ruined castle, try a quiet registry office and a second ceremony; that way you are free to make all your own style choices.

Make sure you have a dry run well in advance of the big day. You must make sure that you know which door the band will use, and that they also know which one it is, unless you want everyone moving tables to allow equipment to be lugged through your reception meal. Will the fire regulations allow for the hundreds of tea lights you have planned to dot all around your tables? Is there room for you to greet your guests? Can they make sure that there is a safe place for the wedding gifts to be left, or can they be locked away and collected the following day by your parents if you are going on honeymoon straight from the reception?

ALL THE HELP YOU CAN GET

The first question that you ask of the person who manages your venue (even if it's your mum and her back garden) is 'What exactly can you do for me?' If you are opting for a more traditional venue, there should be several resources on hand: the church might take care of the altar flowers, a hotel might have a valet who can handle the parking, a banqueting hall might have a toastmaster that they can recommend. The added bonus of following recommendations is that these people will have worked together before and already be familiar with the way things run. One less thing to tick off your list.

Hotels will sometimes offer the use of extra rooms, or even discounts on group bookings for the wedding party, so it's worth asking. Make sure you keep asking. Even if you are marrying a sports buff and holding your reception in the cricket club, they may be more than happy to string the place with bunting or put your names on the scoreboard. You will also find that quite quickly your organisational list becomes very long, so clear up the areas of responsibility early; if the venue has a great relationship with a reliable cab firm why worry about tracking one down yourself? Local knowledge is a wonderful thing.

Try another idea…

As you are choosing the venue, consider the time of day that you are hoping to marry and hold your reception. A medieval banqueting room might look a bit bleak and lost in the middle of the day, but at night will come alive with warming points of flickering candlelight. See **IDEA 2**, *When: date and time*, for more ideas.

Defining idea…

'*Luck is being in the right place at the right time, but location and timing are to some extent under our control.*'
NATASHA JOSEFOWITZ, US script writer

How did
it go?

Q **I went to my local church as a child and it would be very special for me to get married there, but there is nowhere nearby to hold the reception – it's all very rural. Is it unreasonable for guests to travel 40 minutes to a decent venue?**

A *It depends on how you expect them to get there. You could take the stress out of it by hiring a couple of old fashioned buses and ushering the guests onto them. Keep the festive feel by adorning them with ribbons and balloons.*

Q **But what about the guests collecting their cars later?**

A *Well, those not drinking would probably prefer to drive themselves to the reception anyway. Have a good think about alternatives. Is there a nice meadow nearby, owned by a friendly farmer who might be willing to let you set up a marquee? If it is very close by, you could even make a nice show of a good old-fashioned wedding procession. Just remember you will need generators for power, unless you are going to go very rural and just stick to candlelight (not advised in a marquee). And check the field for bulls.*

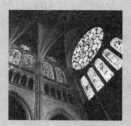
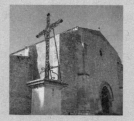

18

Crowning glory

Some things are a matter of life and death; some are more important – like gorgeous hair. And that isn't achieved overnight. Take responsibility for looking fabulous.

You can spend all the money in the world on good cuts, but if you don't give your hair the appropriate TLC in between you won't get the results you hope for.

From the minute the engagement ring is slipped on your finger, you need to start getting serious about your mane. Take the time to work out your hair type (ask your hairdresser if you aren't sure) and start using the appropriate shampoo and conditioner and a weekly treatment pack.

Bear in mind that getting your hair into its premium condition isn't just about splashing out on the products (and splashing them on). Have your hair trimmed regularly to guard against split ends (ideally every six weeks; if you find yourself fiddling with them while you are on the phone, you've left it too long) and avoid overusing heated appliances and styling aids. Consider giving your hair a 'day off' every week. Consider hiding it under a cute headscarf on a Sunday: after all, do you

Here's an idea for you...

Little bridesmaids or flower girls often wear a wreath of flowers as a hairpiece, and can look adorable in them – if you can get them to keep them on. If they are very young and have silky and fine hair, have the flowers made into a crown to rest on the hair with slides or grips. This is where your maid of honour comes in: make her responsible for carrying a damage limitation kit, including hairspray and spare grips for all, to protect against mishaps and the elements.

really need to straighten it to within an inch of its life whilst you wash the car or do a supermarket run?

ATTACK OF THE WEDDING RINGLETS

You probably should head straight for the salon anyway, but if you've had a skinhead on a playful whim and you want an up-do for your big day, you need a plan, and fast. Hairdressers can always tell that your fantasy style will make you look like an extra from Dallas, and how long it will take (at least a year to six months if you need to grow out a fringe or a perm). If you are thinking of any radical changes, consider doing it now so that there's still plenty of time to limit the damage if you then decide it's really not you. And try to avoid the strange phenomenon that is wedding ringlets – you might be unpleasantly surprised how they can sneak up on you. Although no grown woman sports them in normal life, a flick through any wedding photographer's portfolio will show a rash of them.

When you have ordered your dress, show a picture to the hairdresser and see if they agree that your chosen style will work with your neckline. About six weeks before the wedding, book a practice session with your hairdresser, taking any tiara, headdress, hat or veil you might have. If you're going to wear a veil and you plan to take it off during the day, let them know, as your style needs to be able to stay intact and still look elegant.

Wash your hair the night before your wedding – freshly washed hair is hard to work with especially if you intend to put it up. Get friendly with styling products, and don't leave it until the last minute to try them out; there are many different ones to choose from and your hair type will suit certain brands better than others. You can also easily overload hair by using too much or not get the result you want by being too timid. Practice here is key.

Your bridesmaids' styles need to reflect the general theme of your wedding. Try a night of pampering together, to talk through ideas that everyone can be comfortable with. Take a look at IDEA 9, *Ladies in waiting*.

Try another idea...

And remember, have colour treatments or perms done a few weeks in advance to allow them to settle down (no one wants the stench of perming fluid wafting down the aisle as you do).

HONEYMOON HAIR

Depending on your honeymoon location, it's unlikely that your honeymoon hair is going to resemble your wedding 'display'. More often than not, you will be tackling a whole new set of challenges, such as sun damage, chlorine and humidity. And there is little reason to spend months getting your hair in shape before the big day only to let it flop as soon as you've said 'I (up) do'. Surely you should wait until at least the first anniversary to let yourself go. Make sure you pack the appropriate products to combat the stresses to tresses.

'And forget not that the earth delights to feel your bare feet and the winds long to play with your hair.'
KAHLIL GIBRAN

Defining idea...

How did it go?

Q **I'm utterly distressed – my hair is falling out and it's gone dull and miserable. And I've been nurturing it better than any time before in my whole life but it's never looked worse! What's going on?**

A *It's probably stress. Give yourself a day off, do something entirely unrelated to weddings and treat yourself to a reconditioning and strengthening treatment. You also probably need a good boost of vitamin B to help beat the stress too.*

Q **But what about the shedding? My hair feels so thin.**

A *Don't panic, we can rebuild her. When you condition, keep conditioner to a minimum so you don't weigh it down. Wash the night before, and on the big day use volumising spray. If it really is very thin, consider wearing your hair up; and don't be frightened of a little backcombing to add body and staying power. Just remember to smooth it over, or you might look a little frightened.*

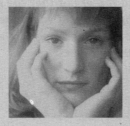 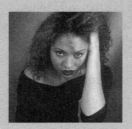

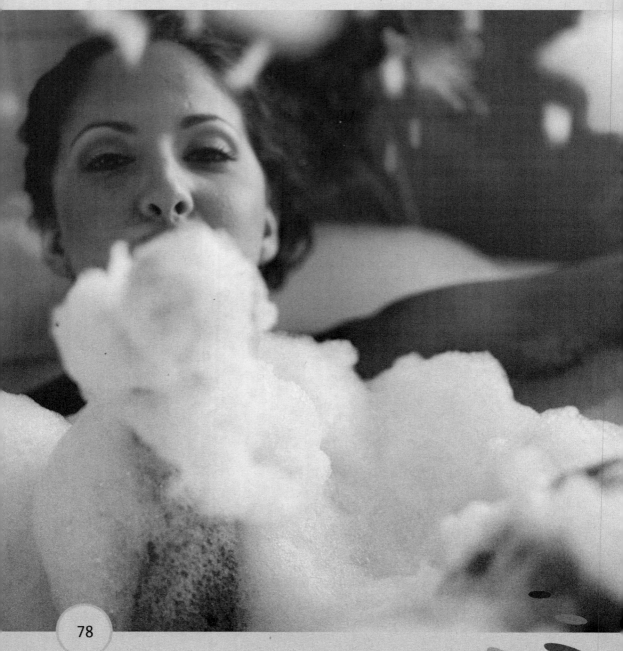

19

Get glowing

Even if you think of yourself as a natural kind of girl, to get away with the bare minimum on the day will still probably take a lot of planning beforehand. The good news is that you'll have a legitimate reason for pampering yourself.

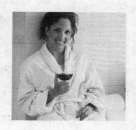

It's always a good idea to get on first name terms with your beauty therapist. She can help you get some understanding of your body and cycles. Do you have any particular triggers that give you problems?

The first tip for great skin couldn't be simpler. Everyone needs to drink more water – it's not hard to get hold of and it will help clear your complexion. Good basic skin care is also a must, so make sure you cleanse, tone and moisturise morning and night. Use products designed for your skin type (most beauty counters offer a free type analysis, so seek them out if you are unsure). Facial exfoliators will help to make skin more radiant so use one at least once a week. For serious problems, or

Here's an idea for you...

Get your hands in shape. Not only will your hands be shaken and kissed, but also your new sparklers will be admired. The last thing that you need is to try to show off your ring with the claws of a crone. Make sure you keep a hand and nail treatment cream by your bed to keep them in tip top condition. And don't forget that pedicure.

ones that don't respond to these routines, visit your doctor and ask them to refer you to a dermatologist. Now is also the time to tackle any dental issues you want to address, as a treatment plan could take some time.

IT'S YOUR DUTY TO TREAT YOURSELF

Treat yourself to a monthly facial, and plan the timing so any eruptions caused as the skin begins to renew itself don't happen near the big day. It will also help calm your nerves and create a bit of vital personal time that will help keep you balanced. It is also important to splash out on some new pampering products, such as new make-up, fragrances and lush body cream. It will help to make you feel special and suitably princess-like.

PUT ON A HAPPY FACE

This is a perfect opportunity to give your look a real overhaul. Many women stick to the habits they formed as a teenager, which may have worked well for some time, but our skin texture, face shape and pallor change throughout our lives and, therefore, so will the colours and styles that suit us.

You should think about this at least several weeks, preferably months, before your wedding. You need to get used to the new you, and other people need time to do so too. After all, you don't want to look like a stranger walking down the aisle. Get the professionals in if you are unsure. You can always have a make-up lesson, or head once again to your department store's beauty counter. Make sure they know you want a bridal look and are not planning to do a rain dance. If you will be doing your make-up on the big day, it's best to keep your colours fairly neutral and make sure it's something you feel you can replicate. If your bridesmaids will be making you up, take them to the store with you.

Even if you don't normally wear make-up, you might want to consider it for your nuptials. Flash photography can be very unflattering and bleach the colour from anyone; even a touch of foundation can even out your complexion to great effect.

Have a complete run through of your make-up from start to finish so that you can gauge exactly how much time you will need to allow on the day, and make sure you do any eyebrow plucking the day before, so you don't have an unpleasant, red Vulcan v between your eyes.

If you have a facial in the week before your wedding, don't try anything new as you could have a reaction. On the day, stick to your practised routine and don't deviate from it; you could create a monster you don't know how to repair. Make sure someone close to you, physically and emotionally, carries some touch-up products and is on hand to help you when you might be expected to look particularly fabulous.

Why not use your treatment times as a way to involve your in-laws, or relatives who don't have any special role, by asking them to come along with you. Or see IDEA 27, *Thank yous and gifts*, for ideas about how to make them feel special.

Try another idea...

'Beauty is in the heart of the beholder.'
AL BERNSTEIN

Defining idea...

Q **I'm someone whose emotions are always written all over her face. And I know I'll be crying like a baby off and on. What can I do?**

A *You need a waterproof mascara and some make-up pads impregnated with remover tucked in your bridesmaid's handbag, just in case when the flood gates open even the waterproofing can't cope.*

Q **It gets worse: my neck gets blotchy and bright red. What can I do about that?**

A *You could get away with a green tinged concealer from a regular make-up brand, but you may have to go for some serious coverage. Try stage make-up, or make-up designed for scar coverage that has special green pigmentation to neutralise redness. Make sure you brush with loose powder to fix it afterwards.*

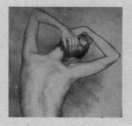
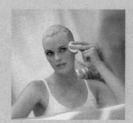
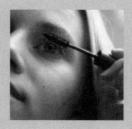

20

The body beautiful

There are some women who love their bodies with steadfast conviction. Then there are those of us who are awake. This is the time when most women finally get serious about getting in shape.

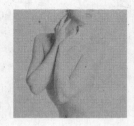

Be realistic. How much time have you got? What is achievable? With a combination of diet and exercise, quite a lot, actually.

Don't pin all your hopes on a silk slip designed for a willowy sylph if you're a classic English pear. Instead, choose a gown that plays to your strengths and then work towards that. There have been many disastrous tales of brides who order their dress a size too small only to have to face heading down the aisle like a trussed-up turkey shoved in a carrier bag. So keep it real.

FULL BODIED

A fuller figure that is firm and well looked after is far preferable to a crash diet bag of bones (which can also make your skin's appearance grey and cause energy levels to hit an all-time low). To lose weight you need an exercise regime and a good diet, so plan them properly. Don't set unrealistic Olympian goals with exercise regimes if

When selecting your wedding fragrance, make sure you can get matching body cream and bath oil; you don't want five fragrances fighting as you lean in to kiss your new husband.

you work long hours, or your failure to stick to them will demoralise and de-motivate you. And get to know your diet weak spots: empty the house of all bad stuff rather than spend all evening trying to resist the siren song of that chocolate in the cupboard, and don't try a diet that insists on fresh seaweed for lunch if you work in the middle of a land locked city centre. The key to success is always suitability.

Don't just try to shed the pounds through diet. If you do, you will miss out on the other main benefits of exercise; namely that it helps to relieve stress and ensures a good night's sleep when you need it most.

DRESSING SLIM

What is your dress like? Ask your gym to create a program that bears that in mind. Maybe you will be wearing a strapless gown, and would like slender, toned arms and shoulders to show off. An A-line dress looks best on trim hips, so make this your target area.

If motivation is a problem, stick a photograph of your dress on the fridge and get yourself a diet buddy; maybe one of the bridesmaids who also wants to shape up for the big event. You can talk each other down from the chocolate biscuit ledge and force each other to the gym – maybe at gunpoint.

If money isn't an issue, then consider paying for a grown-up gym babysitter. A personal trainer will make sure you hit the exercise machines whatever the weather, or favourite TV show repeat. They often charge by the hour so if you can get a couple of others to join in the sessions, you can make it that bit more affordable.

Make your body regime work with your new beauty discipline. Have a look at IDEA 19, *Get glowing*, for suggestions.

Try another idea...

FEELING GOOD

You also want your body to feel sleek and soft to the touch. Keep a bottle of body scrub in the shower so it will quickly become part of your daily routine. Start at your feet and work up the body in small circular motions, always moving towards your heart, and then slather on the body cream. Massage is also good for improving the circulation and expelling toxins from the body, and as a result will improve the look and feel of your skin. Make it an aromatherapy massage for the added benefit of calming and relaxing your slightly frayed soul.

A few days before the wedding, book yourself and your chief bridesmaid or mum into a beauty salon to take care of any waxing and tanning. Fake tans all work differently on different skin types, so try a few before deciding which looks the most natural on you. You need to find out the specifics too: some work best applied on moisturised skin; some 'slip' and cause streaks if applied on top of a body cream. It is advisable to do this a few days before the big day, as they last a few days and it allows a margin for error.

'I always wanted to be somebody, but I should have been more specific.'
JANE WAGNER, playwright

Defining idea...

85

How did it go?

Q **I'm doing a quickie wedding in Las Vegas and have no time shed the half stone I want to lose. Any quick fixes? I go in a month.**

A *A low carbohydrate, high protein diet will help, but you need to couple it with exercise. Walk for half an hour before work (maybe to a further away bus stop), always use stairs (even for ten floors), and use your lunch hour to speed walk around the local park.*

Q **I've heard giving up drinking will help weight loss. Is that right?**

A *There are a horrifying number of calories in alcohol so definitely shelve it for now. However, you should also get yourself to the gym for a tailored programme and if all else fails get a light fake tan (everyone looks better with a bit of a glow). To be honest, a beaming grin will do far more to make you look like a blooming bride than a diet. That's what everyone will be looking for as you head down the aisle.*

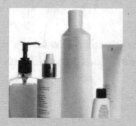
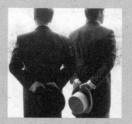
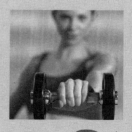

21

Grooms grooming

Weddings: they can make a man do the funniest things, like dress up in top hat and tails, and wear moisturiser. This is the chance for more life-style improvements.

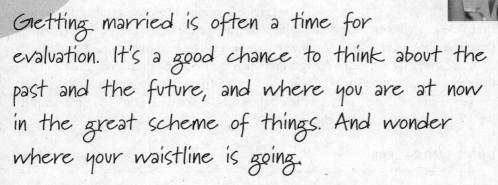

Getting married is often a time for evaluation. It's a good chance to think about the past and the future, and where you are at now in the great scheme of things. And wonder where your waistline is going.

Most of us work better with a deadline, so if you have always thought that you would like to regain your slender youth's figure, or try a different hairstyle, why not use this time as an opportunity? It also gives you a chance to muscle in on some of the girls' good stuff. Massages, manicures, and any general chances to be pampered are nothing to be ashamed of if you are simply doing it to look the best for your beloved on the big day. And it feels great.

Here's an idea for you...

Feel unsure about your foray into the world of grooming? Enlist one of your ushers or your best man as a wing man to try these ideas out with. It also means that they won't be able to use it against you at the stag night.

FIT FOR A KING

You may need to spend a little more time lifting weights, instead of lifting pints. You will know what your body responds to most, but a general rule is cutting back on drinking alcohol, processed food, and upping the exercise quotient. Most men store fat around their waists, so if you want guests whispering about the dash you are cutting, rather than speculating on who the father of your beer pregnancy might be, then there is no other option. Essentially, doing a little exercise does not mean that you can therefore eat what you like – or you won't lose a thing (except the will to live). Visit your gym and ask for a session with a trainer who can create a tailored programme for you, including a sensible diet plan.

DON'T SMILE PLEASE

Do small children run screaming from you in the street when you give them a friendly grin? It may be time to take a trip to the dentist and have a look at your gnashers. For more serious work, you may need to start a dental plan that may take up to at least a year. Whitening can take years off your appearance, as teeth discolour as you age. Don't overdo it though, as you may end up looking like an overgrown Ken doll. And people may be able to see you in the dark.

CLOSE SHAVES AND FINAL CHECKS

If you have ever fancied trying out a good old-fashioned barber's, now is the time. A close shave by a professional, with warm towels to open the pores and a super sharp blade brandished by someone who understands which way the grain goes, is a great way to relax and feel special. See if you can book into a good barber on the morning of the wedding. Some of the grander hotels have them on site, so do check.

You will also need to make some basic checks on the big day. Make sure that you have a brush to remove any specks of lint from your suit. Your shoes need to shine like never before. (Dad in the army? Re-enlist him.) Make sure new underwear and socks are laid out with your new suit, shirt and neck tie the night before. Even your cufflinks should be put out ready so that you don't find yourself on all fours in your new bib and tucker emptying drawers looking for them. Your hands need to be clean, as well as your nails which should also be short as they will be playing a key part in the day. Consider a manicure before the big day so you have less to worry about. If you will be having a haircut, don't do it the day before as it will still have that just scalped look, and don't try anything too radical in case you hate it (twenty-four hours isn't exactly long enough to grow it back).

Make sure that you choose a suit that plays to your strengths. Take a look at IDEA 39, *Choosing a morning suit*, for advice on how to select one.

Try another idea...

'I'm tired of all this nonsense about beauty being only skin-deep. That's deep enough. What do you want, an adorable pancreas?'
JEAN KERR, novelist

Defining idea...

How did
it go?

Q   **I always look rubbish in photos, like I've been dug up. I know it
bothers my girlfriend but she pretends it doesn't, although I've
noticed all the pictures she has of me around her flat are black
and white, even if they were taken with colour film. Is there
anything I can do?**

A   *You may be being over-sensitive; she could just be the arty type. Remember
that your professional photographer will have the equipment and skill to
produce top-quality pictures. It would be a good idea to talk to him or her
to raise the problem and learn some tricks of the trade.*

Q   **What could I do to improve the chances of the guests' photos
turning out better? They might look back and think they were at a
zombie wedding.**

A   *OK, you have the unfortunate pallor of a corpse, then. In that case you
need to consider a fake tan, either from a sun bed or out of a bottle. And,
no, it doesn't have to be humiliating. You can now get fake tanning
preparations that don't need a beauty therapist to apply them, as they are
in a spray form and very accurate. If that idea is still a bridge too far, try
buying one you can apply at home from the chemist. If you are
exceptionally pale, try mixing it with a bit of moisturiser first to get a more
subtle result. And do have a test run before the wedding day so you don't
accidentally turn up looking as if you are appearing in panto.*

22

I married a-broad!

People used to run away to Gretna Green to tie the knot; now it tends to be Mauritius or anywhere else with an azure blue sea and some swaying palm trees. If the exotic appeals to you, make sure you understand what it'll mean for your big day.

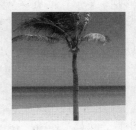

Who do you want with you on the beach as you say 'I do' under a radiant sun? Will you be husband and wife legally when you get home? What will you wear?

Consider who you would like present, and for how long. For a long-haul destination it is only fair to expect guests to be around for a week, as they will probably have to eat into their annual holiday. You need to allow for this if you are staying in the same destination for your honeymoon (perhaps marry half way through the week so you don't have your new in-laws as chaperones the entire time). Consider the cost of your destination, too; you must be prepared to accept that some guests will be unable to make it due to the expense.

Here's an idea for you... **If you are keen to have guests at your wedding, suggest that they give you their attendance as a wedding gift; flights, hotel rooms and food soon add up, so this could be your way of showing your appreciation.**

'WE'RE NOT RUNNING *FROM*, WE'RE RUNNING *TO*...'

You'll have to handle the announcement of your plans carefully. Some friends and family will be very disappointed, so be prepared to deal with their feelings sensitively. You could take them for a meal or hold a party on your return to give everyone the chance to share your good fortune. Importantly, let them know that you are going away to fulfil a dream, *not* choosing to leave them all behind.

MAKING IT LEGAL

To ensure that your marriage is legal in the UK, you have to be sure that you fit the UK criteria: you must not be underage, awaiting a divorce or married to someone else. To make it legal in your country of choice, then you must ensure that you fit their criteria. It is important to find out the legal requirements. These can include a minimum period of stay in the country (and often a certain number of days before the ceremony can take place). For example, in America you need a blood test, and some countries have religious restrictions. You also need to be aware of the country's public holidays and festivals; you don't want to arrive and discover everyone is out at the carnival. Each country will also demand documents – birth certificates, passports and evidence of single status (e.g. divorce documents or death certificate of a former spouse) – and the embassy or consulate can help you determine which.

HANDING OVER THE STRESS

There are now many reputable tour organisations that offer wedding packages. They can take care of everything from ceremonies to honeymoons. This is a good option if you are planning to marry somewhere very exotic or with a language you don't understand because they can provide someone with specialist local knowledge who can help out with any problems that might occur.

The tour company can often organise the ceremony and find the celebrant, and even offer wedding cakes, photographer, flowers and champagne. Make sure you check what you're getting, though – the local Chateau de Gastric '89 might not be to your taste. As you often have to be in your chosen location for a few days before the ceremony, you might prefer to make your own arrangements for flowers and decoration – a collection of seashells from the beach and some local blooms, for instance.

Most tour operators ask for photocopies of the required legal documents (e.g. birth certificates) to be sent to them around two months before travelling. The original documents should be carried on the journey.

You need to take care of your skin too when hitting the sun, so check out IDEA 19, *Get glowing*.

Try another idea...

'Remember that happiness is a way of travel – not a destination.'
ROY M. GOODMAN

Defining idea...

93

JUST A G-STRING EACH

When choosing what you want to wear, remember that your outfits need to be comfortable and not too hot, so if you're off to Jamaica for a beach wedding, leave the wool morning suit at home, along with the fifteen metres of French Chantilly lace veil. You may favour a slinky, tiny white bikini and cowboy hat, but if you want something more elaborate you need to make sure it travels well. This may have a strong influence on your choice – remember that stuffing fifteen layers of petticoat in a suitcase will cause the kind of damage to the dress that might never bounce back. You should check with your airline if there is somewhere your outfits can be hung; if not, you need to choose something that can sustain a little stress, such as synthetic fabrics, which crush less. You can also get small hand-steamers to take out creases, or book ahead with your hotel for the laundry service to primp and preen your outfits.

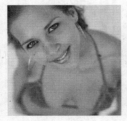
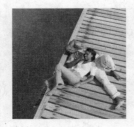

Q **My boyfriend and I are going to get married in St Tropez and sent out our invitations ages ago, but so far we've had very few RSVPs. I feel very frustrated that people are taking so long to get back to us. What should I do to stimulate the responses?**

How did it go?

A *It's not a cheap destination, so maybe they are waiting to see if they can afford it before committing. You need to ask yourself what you would do in their shoes and how you can help them make their minds up.*

Q **But we would make the effort for them. So what help should we give?**

A *Even if you would put yourselves out if the roles were reversed, remember that they may have several other family commitments – perhaps other overseas weddings – during the year, all of which chip away at meagre savings. Have you included a list of alternative accommodation for them in the invite and booking details? To give your invitees the best idea of what to expect, give one in each price bracket: sweet B&B, middle range and super luxury hotels. You have to allow for every pocket. And be graceful if they say no.*

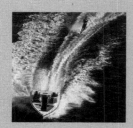

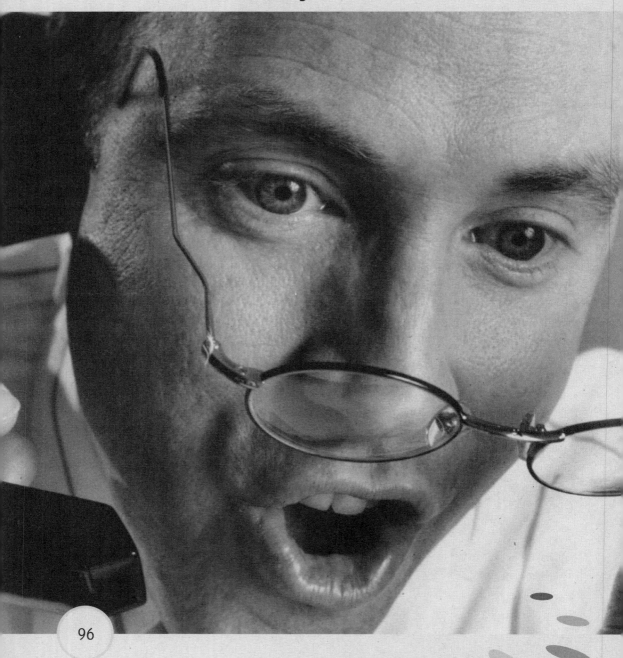

23

Getting your bank manager to say 'I do'

Given that the average UK wedding now costs £15,000, you need to get a handle on your budget, finances and wedding insurance before they get you in a headlock, and find some sneaky ways to save your pennies.

Sensible budgeting will take the stress factor out of the planning, and help you enjoy your big day to the max.

So where does it all go? The honeymoon, reception, and bride's dress amount to approximately half of the total cost. The single biggest expense is usually the honeymoon, with the most popular destinations being the Caribbean and USA. If you are planning something more local, you may have a little more to play with. Just remember that getting yourself into debt will take the edge off your magical day and leave you with a long-term headache that will overshadow your happy memories.

Here's an idea for you...

Early on in your planning, talk to your partner about your priorities. They may see the honeymoon as the big spend, whilst you want top and tails for all the male family members. It's best to consider at the outset what you are happy to compromise on, as budgets can quickly spiral out of control.

SHOW ME THE MONEY

Although it was traditionally the bride's parents' responsibility, many couples now pay for their own wedding. However, it is also common for the bride and groom's parents and the couple to split the overall bill into thirds. Regardless of how you choose to cover the costs, it is advisable to discuss this with all the parties from the outset; and that includes the deposits that will be required to book everyone from the harpist to the vicar. Losing your dream venue because you are too overdrawn to cover the deposit your future in-laws were meant to pay will not bode well for happy relations.

WHEN DO YOU PAY?

Most of your suppliers will expect a deposit to ensure that the date that you want is secured. You will be expected to pay some of them, such as the band or DJ, the remainder of the balance on the day of the wedding. Make sure the best man has the necessary cash to pay the appropriate people.

MAKING THE MONEY WORK HARDER FOR YOU

Need to make some budget savings? See IDEA 35, *Ways to save*, for a few hints.

Try another idea...

If you have some money saved, make sure you place it in a high interest account so that you are getting a little extra. However, you need to ensure that you can get access to it easily. Do check, because some accounts won't allow immediate withdrawals and these could only work for you if you are super-organised and are planning way ahead and won't need access within the next year or two – but withdraw early and you might have to pay a penalty.

If you need to rely on credit, don't just hand over the old card that has been collecting dust in your wallet since time immemorial. There are lots of great new credit card services that offer interest free deals, so don't be financially lazy, as you could keep your debt interest free if you move your money from card to card every time the interest free offer is up. Just try not to ramp up your borrowing too early on, as you may still have bills rolling in after the big day.

If you are a homeowner, you can also release equity from your mortgage, as it can be a good way of getting a low interest loan to keep your debts in one manageable lump. Your mortgage lender can help you understand the options.

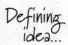

Defining idea...

GETTING SET FOR THE FUTURE

A joint account set up specifically for the arrangements can be a great way of managing the finances relating to your wedding. That way there is no doubt that the spending is fair and controlled, and you can keep up to date with all the expenses. If one of you is a good saver whilst the other is an impetuous spender, make sure that you are both joint signatories. There are different types of account available so shop around for the one that best suits you. Check out overdraft facilities; you will probably need them for a while.

Let your families know that you have set up an account for the wedding, and suggest that they make their contributions to the wedding directly into the account. This will ensure that you don't have to keep harassing them for deposit cheques. If they cannot place a lump sum in the account, perhaps a direct debit that helps cover expenses as they come up is the best way to go.

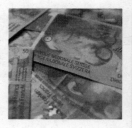

Q **I want a nice wedding, but my fiancée is obsessed with staging something grand enough for the royal family. I have tried to explain to her that we can't afford it but she doesn't seem to listen. How can I open her eyes to the reality?**

A *You need to get out some pen and paper, and your bank statement. Show how the spending and borrowing will affect your future life. She might not be keen to go from princess to eating beans for breakfast, dinner and tea.*

Q **Done that; didn't work. She still insists on the spending. What else can I do?**

A *It sounds like she is suffering from a reality blind spot. In this case, insist that she gets involved in finding a suitable loan or best deal re-mortgage. Once people start to understand money, and its implications on their everyday life, they often get more realistic about it.* '

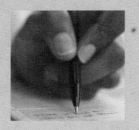
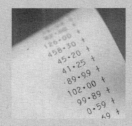

Try
another
idea...

101

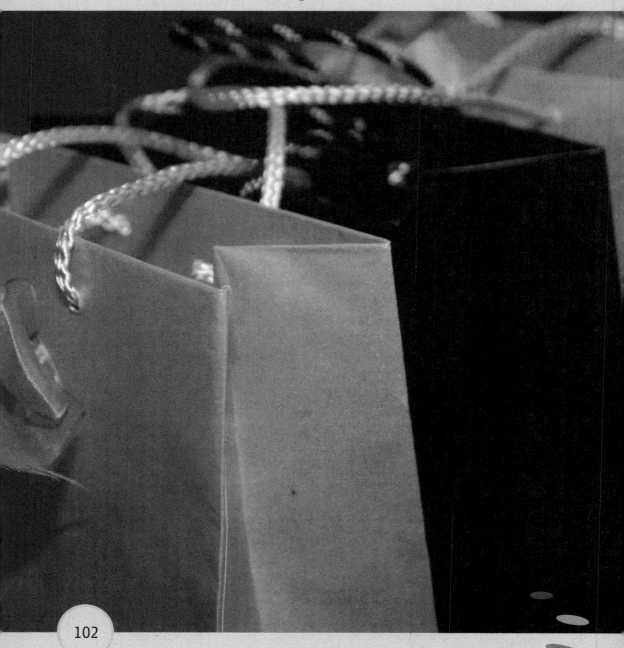

24

Gimme, gimme, gimme

Getting married has some great perks (apart from a lifelong commitment from your soul mate, of course). One of them is the gift list.

Already got two of everything? Or do you want to upgrade to more expensive stuff but can't bring yourself to ask for that Italian glassware? Make your gift list work for you.

Traditionally, guests gave the couple gifts to help them set up home. However, depending on your age, whether you already have your own home or if it's your second wedding, your needs will probably be different.

If you are living together for the first time, then you need to cover all the basics from wooden spoons to linen. Rather than mercenary, gift lists are a good way of making sure that you don't end up with seven toasters and no cutlery. The way to make sure that your list is inclusive is to make sure you include everything from an egg timer right through to a DVD player. Make sure that you know exactly who gave you what, so that you can thank them. It is important that you should be able to tell your Aunt Phyllis when she pops over that you use her teapot every morning (unless she got you a garden swing).

Here's an idea for you...

Commission a special piece of furniture by a local craftsperson. Why not a bedstead, so that your guests can present you with your marital bed?

You can get things for the house and still be a little adventurous. As it is a given that many couples often have the things that they need, most people are prepared to buy something a little different. You may ask people to make a contribution to a piece of art or a piece of furniture. You can even consider a trip: hot air ballooning or holiday, or even the honeymoon.

But, before you start visualising yourself climbing into your scuba suit, ask yourself if you *really* have everything. After all, couldn't some super-soft, huge waffle bath sheets replace those towels? And what about a full set of china that actually matches? This is an opportunity to select items you would never normally think to splash out on (like a proper dinner service, which can cost hundreds of pounds) that you will be able to enjoy for years to come. And your own kids will probably be more excited to be presented with a cherished family heirloom than a photo album of your diving trip in the Maldives.

Make sure that you do the list together, and go to the relevant department stores to choose things together. This should be one of the fun, relatively stress-free tasks in planning your wedding. And try to give each other a couple of free passes to choose something totally self-indulgent. Take a visit to some of the other departments in the stores; if you really have all the pots and pans you will ever need, what about a leather backgammon set or tennis racquets? (Then you can tell your guests that they bought you your six-pack.) A great investment, and a slightly more elegant approach than asking for cold cash, is to ask for donations towards a cellar of good wine. Guests can ring up and buy wines in multiples of bottles. If you are uncomfortable with asking for specifics, then you could consider using one of the wedding lists that allow you to redeem your gift values in vouchers. (However, you may have to deal with some disappointment from those who would prefer to see their gifts being part of your marital home.)

If you want your guests to travel abroad for your wedding, ask them to make this your wedding gift: see IDEA 22, I married a-broad!

Try another idea...

When choosing a list, you also need to check other details, such as how and when the store can deliver the gifts and if they can exchange unwanted items (or doubles). Make sure that the delivery is after your honeymoon so that your house is not full of unattended gifts. Some lists like to deliver before the wedding but make sure that it all works within your time frame.

SAY PLEASE WITH EASE

The easiest way to let your guests know that you have a wedding list is to include it in your invitations, on a separate card. You must make it clear that people know they can make their own choices of gifts. It might seem a little mercenary, but it is a lot less uncomfortable than making friends call and request the list – and it is now standard practice.

SAYING THANKS

It may seem old fashioned to write thank you cards, but it is essential if you want to make people feel special and appreciated. You may want a design printed that reflects the theme and style of the other wedding stationery.

'Man's best possession is a sympathetic wife.'
EURIPIDES

Defining idea...

105

How did
it go?

Q My aunt wants to buy us an antique for our wedding, as she believes it will hold its value. But our style is very minimal and it just won't go in our flat. Is there a tactful way we can put her off?

A I believe that it is wrong to turn down a gift, as the giver should derive just as much pleasure as the receiver. For some, ticking things off a list isn't an expression of their style. Try getting involved with the purchase: ask for a painting or a jewellery box – something that's a manageable size and you can get out when she comes over.

Q How rigid should we be with the items specified on our list?

A It depends on how much respect you have for your friends' and families' taste. If there are definite items and brands you want, spell it out on the list. There will be some people who will relish the shopping challenge, so it would be nice if you include other present ideas that give them the option of buying something they think you will like.

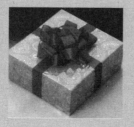
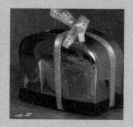

25

Drink and be merry

It's an ancient tradition that guests raise a glass of the hard stuff to congratulate the happy couple – these days, it tends to be several. Get your wine right and the party will flow.

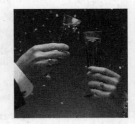

If you are having a sit-down meal, you need to provide wine, water and soft drinks. It is also standard to provide champagne for the toast, and often as the guests arrive and are milling around.

When planning your wine order, for a start you need to know that there are six standard 12.5 cl glasses to a bottle. Some people will drink more than a bottle, some less (children under five, perhaps), so when making your calculations base it on one bottle per person. Soft drinks and mineral water should be available for people who have to drive, teetotallers and children. If you want to be especially nice, consider having a special alcohol-free cocktail for the non-drinkers. And if you make it a tasty option, it will also encourage other guests to pace their drinking – no one wants to see your gran start the dancing on her own after a sherry or two too many, especially if there is no music.

Here's an idea for you...

Look into having a cocktail made in your honour to serve to the guests on arrival. If you have a colour theme, why not ask a great mixologist at a good local cocktail bar or hotel to create one for you? The same staff might be available for hire themselves, which would give you a bar with real flair.

TO PAY BAR OR NOT TO PAY BAR?

You may begin your planning by intending to pay for all the alcohol at the wedding. However, you could be unpleasantly surprised at how quickly that tots up. Don't worry, though, whatever configuration of free/pay bar you choose, it is pretty standard these days for guests to buy their own drinks after a certain point.

A good way of splitting the responsibilities is to put a set amount behind the bar, which then becomes a pay bar after it runs out. You should, however, make provisions for a welcome drink for all the guests as they arrive at the reception. A nice way to do this is to have waiters with trays of champagne and soft drinks at the room's entrance. This makes it clear that it is a welcome drink, rather than a moveable bar to revisit.

CRUISING FOR A BOOZING

A fun part of the wedding preparations can often be a quick nip across the Channel to top up on the wedding wines. It can save you a great deal of money, although you need to ensure, before you do your sums and spend the savings on shoes, that you check the corkage costs if you are holding your reception at a venue.

This can vary from as little as 50p to a few pounds. Don't be frightened to ask for a special deal – and if you're holding your do at your parents', refuse to pay, point blank! If you have a caterer, check if they have a corkage fee, too. And remember that a licence is needed to sell alcohol in most hired halls and even at home. So you would need to provide all the drinks or apply for a special drinks licence. Get in touch with your local council if you are unsure.

If you're using a local vineyard or wine shop, ask if they can offer discounts on bulk orders and if they will take returns of unopened bottles. Let them know you are getting married and ask what they can do; they may offer to lend glasses, supply free ice or recommend a good toastmaster.

GLASS HIRE

Presentation is vital, so you might also want to try glass hire from your local wine shop or supermarket; that way everything will look sharp. Check if there is a supplement for returning dirty glasses; often there isn't, which will make life a lot simpler. Organise a rota of people to serve at the bar if this is not one of the caterer's duties. Most people will be glad to help for a short period.

You need to consider the menu as soon as you start thinking about wine. Look at IDEA 28, *Food of love*, so you can plan in tandem.

Try another idea...

'From wine what sudden friendship springs.'
JOHN GAY, from *The Squire and His Cur*

Defining idea...

109

How did
it go?

Q   I'm a bit confused about which wine to choose. I don't like red wine but we are having fillet of beef for the main meal. Can we ignore the norms?

A   Firstly, unless you are drinking all of the wine yourself, it's perfectly acceptable to have both, especially as there will be other white wine lovers and red wine haters in the party. And it's not the colour of the wine that should be the defining element when choosing wine; it's the body and flavour.

Q   If I can have white wine with red meat, what should I look for?

A   When choosing wedding wines, go for crowd pleasers: something dependable and drinkable, something that won't give everybody a nasty hangover and is a well-known name that guests are comfortable with. Don't spend too much money as it won't be appreciated. People are looking for something pleasant to quaff, like a quality southern hemisphere (Chilean or Australian) brand. Go for reliable all-rounders, like a good Cabernet Sauvignon and a Chardonnay.

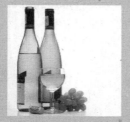

26

The supporting cast

The wedding party is more than just the two of you, unless you are running away to Gretna Green. You need to work out who you want to do what, and how to get them to do it.

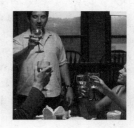

If you are remotely popular, there will be people jostling for the top roles like a rugby scrum in stilettos. Your talents for organisation and diplomacy will have to shine.

Luckily, some of the roles in the wedding day bandwagon are naturally taken care of – like the role of father of the bride (unless your mother was rather too popular herself). If you don't have someone to fill this role, consider another close family member or a special friend, man or woman; their key qualification is that you love each other.

Bridesmaids are usually either a sister of the bride or groom, a close friend of the bride or a niece or nephew. Choose who you want, but remember you can always fall back on this tradition if you need to dissuade an eager friend who keeps hinting heavily. When choosing someone to play these roles, consider that the maid of honour should be someone responsible and willing to help, as you will need

If you want everyone to pass by the receiving line, you may end up with a glut of people waiting to enter the reception. To make sure that the natives don't get restless, plan to have waiters circulating with welcome drinks and nibbles.

support and some hen night organising. She can then ask the other bridesmaids awkward questions, like what their hip measurements are, and pressgang them into doing errands – so you can play the good cop, bad cop game. Little ones and ring bearers will not be expected to take an active part in the planning stage but their mothers may get involved instead.

A way for the groom to soothe the egos of those not voted into the best man slot is to appoint them as ushers. (If it seems too hard to pick between choices for the top slot, choose a brother or other male relative.) These positions were normally given to the bride's brothers, but these days anything goes; for a church wedding you will need at least three and make sure one is delegated the job of pampering the close family members. They should hand out orders of ceremony and herd people into the correct pews. They should also be made to oversee any transport arrangements and help band members, speakers and any other 'turns' for the ceremony know their place – physically and in the running order.

Attendants are often flower girls and boys, or ring bearers (although strictly speaking this term also applies to bridesmaids too). They can be nieces, nephews or just children of close family friends. Just make sure that you don't overwork them or expect them to be all that well behaved. They probably don't realise that you are meant to be the star of the show, so if they decide to wander off half way down the aisle in the wrong direction, don't be surprised or annoyed.

Mums have been pivotal in your entire existence, yet the old-fashioned rituals of the wedding feast mean they tend to have little to do. You can always change the rules and let them give a speech, and at the very least you should present them with flowers at the reception in front of your assembled guests, probably just after the speeches.

You'll want to show your appreciation to your special helpers by giving them gifts – IDEA 27, *Thank yous and gifts*, will tell you who should get what.

Try another idea...

HELLO!

Another way of making the family and attendants feel special is with the receiving line. It's a great way of making guests feel important and welcomed too; some will have travelled a long way to celebrate with you, and it ensures that they get their chance to chat to you all.

A traditional receiving line includes the bride's mother and father, the groom's mother and father, the bride, and the groom, and it is also quite common for the bride's maid of honour and best man to be there. These days, it is quite common to create a more varied line: many families don't follow the traditional format, so many receiving lines won't either. Approach this with tact: you need to bear in mind that some divorced parents may be remarried while others are still single, so mix them up amongst other celebrants so

'The ritual of marriage is not simply a social event; it is a crossing of threads in the fabric of fate. Many strands bring the couple and their families together and spin their lives into a fabric that is woven on their children.'
Portuguese-Jewish wedding ceremony.

Defining idea...

people don't end up doing a married 'who's who'. You may also want to include brothers, sisters and grandparents – just don't make your list so long that the guests finish the line looking a bit stunned from all the small talk.

How did it go?

Q **What do I do if I know I'm going to upset some friends by not giving them a key role?**

A *There are so many different aspects to arranging your wedding that it's likely you will be able to involve all of your nearest and dearest if you can let them share some parts of your decision-making processes, and perhaps enlist their help. Use a reasoned argument, if needs be – if your aspiring best man lives 200 miles away, point out that you really need a local best friend to get the job done. It's never personal between true friends.*

Q **I have a huge extended family of half brothers and sisters, and really don't want a reception line that is bigger than the rest of the accumulated guests added together. But how do I choose? They would all be seriously offended to be left out.**

A *Forget honesty; sometimes it is far from the best policy. Why not create your own moving reception line? Tell them you are worried about people not knowing each other and mixing, and ask them to circulate amongst the crowd and start to warm things up.*

27

Thank yous and gifts

Much as you feel it should be just your special day, it can't all be one-way traffic. There are a few little nods of gratitude and appreciation you need to make to your nearest and dearest for all their hard work.

You will probably feel that you have said thank you a thousand times during the day, but an elegant couple will write a thank you note for every gift and message received.

PUTTING IT ON PAPER

It makes sense to order your thank you notes along with your other stationery. It's fine to have 'thank you' printed across your cards, and any motifs you included in the other wedding stationery, but you must hand write a personal message yourself. You will need to make them all slightly different: there will be guests who can't make it, who need to be told they were missed; thanks have to go to those who gave you money or vouchers, who need to be told what their contributions will be used for; and there are people who will have given you specific gifts, which need to be acknowledged by name.

Here's an idea for you...

Consider thanking both sets of parents with their own albums of the wedding. These albums could contain a special configuration of prints that focus on them and other family members more than just a replica of yours. Include on the opening page a special thank you note, with the dates and all of your names, plus a special message to show your appreciation.

As a standard guide, thank you notes are sent within two weeks to acknowledge gifts that arrive before the wedding. Although you may feel that you have a lot of other things to consider, it will save you time and spread good will in the long run. Gifts received after or during the ceremony have a longer period of grace to allow for the honeymoon and the couple settling in, but you still need to send them within two months of your wedding day.

When wording the card, mention the giver by name and the gift that you received. Tell them why you like it and how useful it will be. Don't be too stiff, even if you had a really formal wedding. Be chatty and warm, and, if you can, include a personal memory of them on the day or a picture of them at the wedding. Try splitting the task: get a bottle of wine on a Friday night and try to work through them together. Also, don't automatically say 'we' as it adds to the formal theme – you could always write half the note each. Another approach would be to try writing a few letters each evening for as long as you can keep your enthusiasm fresh and perky. Make sure you don't feel resentful as you write them; it will show in the tone and feel you give the notes.

SPECIAL THANK YOUS FOR SPECIAL PEOPLE

The groom has on his list of responsibilities gifts for the bridesmaids, attendants, ushers and the best man. These don't have to be extravagant but do need to be serious rather than flippant to show your appreciation. Consider necklaces or bracelets for the bridesmaids. You may want to give such gifts out on the morning of the ceremony so that they can wear them on the day and forever associate them with your marriage. You should consider getting the chief bridesmaid a slightly more elaborate gift, or a larger version, for all her extra efforts.

For flower girls and ring bearing boys, you should expect disappointment, but it probably means you have chosen something with appropriate *gravitas*. Your four-year-old niece might not seem very excited about a silver locket that isn't (a) pink or (b) plastic, but her parents will appreciate it, and so will she in later years.

As for the ushers, consider something matching to keep, like cufflinks or silk ties that they can use again. For the best man, as for the chief bridesmaid, give something with a little edge over the others, such as a leather wallet or gold tie pin. You could even have your gifts engraved to remind them of your special day. If they aren't the type to appreciate a sartorial gesture, picture frames with a snap of you all in your finery might be a nice idea; after all, you may never see it again.

Choosing your stationery? Take a look at IDEA 34, *Start spreading the news*, on what you'll need.

Try another idea...

'If the only prayer you ever say in your whole life is "thank you", that would suffice.'
MEISTER ECKHART

Defining idea...

How did
it go?

Q **Complete horror! I've just found a new stack of cards from wedding gifts that I haven't replied to, from my wedding six months ago! Can I ever make amends?**

A *Of course you can. Get out your address book and start writing. It is not uncommon for couples to send out thank you cards in waves, as there are so many to send out. Something pleasant, that isn't in a bill format, hitting the doormat usually erodes any bad feeling immediately on contact.*

Q **But isn't six months a rather excessive delay?**

A *Just don't try to hide from the truth – give a reason for the delay and explain how mortified you feel. Emphasise that the gift was appreciated just as much as all the others that you received.*

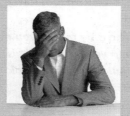
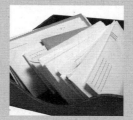

28

Food of love

**You might be too happy to eat, but your guests will
certainly expect a little nourishment. But will a sit-down
meal for 200 or a ham sandwich in your local fit the bill?**

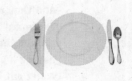

The format of the meal will greatly
influence your menu. Your choice is almost
limitless if you choose a formal meal, but bear in
mind that large numbers will require dishes that
can also be made comfortably en masse — so,
no soufflé for 300. Three courses are usually
standard.

To begin with, you need to decide what part food will be playing in your festivities,
and then make a decision about how that will be achieved. If you would like a
proper feast, your options are formal sit-down meal or buffet. The first will require
waiter service; a formal buffet will, too, since it will be eaten with knives and forks,
sitting at proper tables, and therefore need to be cleared afterwards. Another idea is

'I only eat reindeer.' Of course, some of your guests will have special dietary requirements, and they need to be catered for. There are a variety of food foibles these days, so just having a vegetarian option won't cut it. Find out if any of your guests are gluten intolerant, have seafood allergies or must avoid certain dishes on religious grounds. Always make sure you have a few extra portions of the vegetarian options; someone is almost guaranteed to have forgotten to make their needs known on their RSVP.

the more casual finger buffet, which is eaten whilst standing and will not need to be cleared away immediately. Obviously, for weddings held at home, the last is the most suitable option, unless you are planning a marquee.

A sit-down buffet will allow you to plan the seating arrangements, but is a slightly more affordable (and often less stressful) option than the banquet. It used to be a collection of cold foods, but now they often include hot dishes too. A finger buffet allows people to eat and mingle, and is often a great choice when you are pressed for time or squeezed by your budget. Remember, though, that you still need to provide some chairs for children, pregnant ladies and the elderly. (You should make provisions for these people throughout the day whatever format you decide on.)

Canapés are an elegant way to look after your guests as they await the formal sit-down dinner, and also as a means of ensuring that evening guests are catered for. Your caterer should be able to offer you a selection of options, so plan a tasting session and see what you like. Ask to see photographs of previous events, as presentation is essential.

HIRING CATERERS

If you plan to use the catering services of the venue you have hired – hotel or restaurant – try them out before confirming. That way you can see their approach. (Extra staff may be hired in on the day for your wedding, but at least it gives you a feel for things.) If the food is dreadful under normal service conditions, you are unlikely to get a good standard when the kitchen has to cope with a hundred covers at once.

Thinking of doing it yourself? Ease the burden by considering the easiest way to handle the liquid part of the refreshments: see IDEA 25, *Drink and be merry*, for some options that will help you out.

Try another idea...

For outside catering companies, seek recommendations from everyone you know. Eaten fabulously at a friend's wedding? Ask for the number. Great canapés at the work Christmas party? Find out who organised it and raid their address book. A reputable caterer should also be able to give you references.

Caterers (and hotels) will also have sample menus that cover different price ranges. They are a great place to get inspiration: ask if you can mix and match from their sample menus, and don't be afraid to make special requests. Do remember, though, that the dishes will need to be made in hefty quantities within a strict time frame, so be reasonable.

Look at the venue's recommended caterers; they will know the layout of the kitchens and therefore should be able to make things run smoothly. If the venue is new to the caterers, they should carry out a site visit to ensure that they have all they need to prepare the menu you have planned.

Defining
idea...

'A good cook is like a sorceress who dispenses happiness.'
ELSA SCHIAPIRELLI, French fashion designer

For a marquee, they will need to bring all of their own equipment, such as ovens, and be able to handle all of the disposal and clearing of waste and bottles. Make sure that you know what you are both responsible for. Make sure that they have a head waiter who can act as intermediary between your best man and the kitchen so that the cutting of the cake, champagne toast and clearing are all done efficiently. You may even want to give them a copy of the schedule. Many of us have been to a wedding that is so delayed that everyone is too tipsy to take any interest in the starter that arrives two hours late.

Ask your caterers what extras they can provide: can they organise extra staff to do the coat check and run the bar after the meal is over? They also will have contacts for chairs and tables, cutlery and linen, so ask, but you needn't stick with their suppliers.

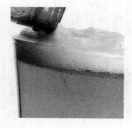

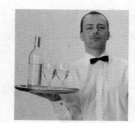

Q **We're having a budget crisis, and need to cut back drastically somewhere. The obvious choice is the buffet at the evening reception, but I feel it's mean to have guests travel – some from a long way – and not cater fully for them. Will they think us terribly unwelcoming if we do?**

How did it go?

A *If you've not stated that you'll be serving food at the reception on your invitations, then anything you provide will be an added bonus. Why don't you consider a compromise by providing substantial canapés and roping in some keen younger cousins as your waiting staff?*

Q **In the early planning stages, how can we keep some flexibility in the catering costs of our evening bash?**

A *Your caterers should be able to provide you with something special on a budget so ask them for ideas. If you are doing the food yourself, make sure you choose something that can be made well in advance and stored easily. Consider employing someone to do the heating and final preparation on the night – after all, you can't expect your mum or friends to spend hours in the kitchen when they should be enjoying themselves.*

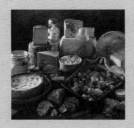
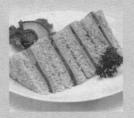

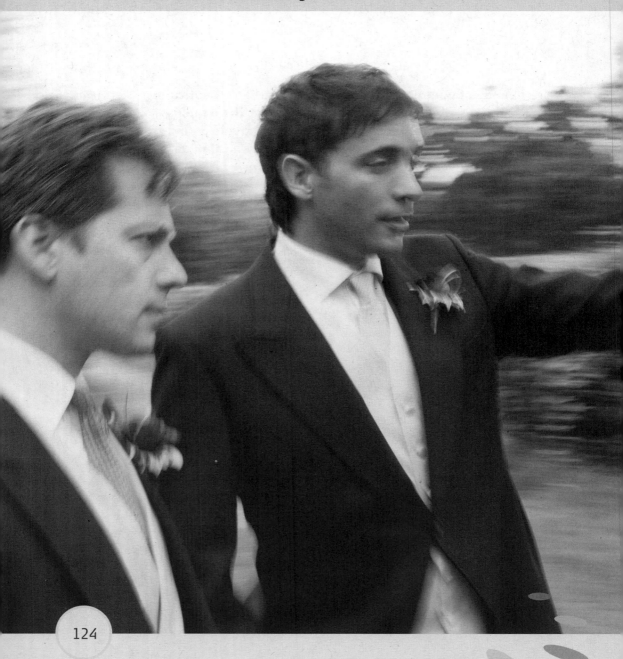

124

29

Be the best guest going

There are many stories of guests from hell, falling from grace as they collapse over the top table onto the bride's mother. Oh, how we laughed. The bride and groom didn't, though.

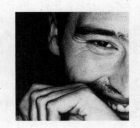

The wedding day belongs to the bride and groom and all of the guests should remember that. The warmth of their support and love will make sure the couple's enjoyment of their big day is complete.

The best way to start accruing good guest points, is to RSVP promptly. The couple will have a lot to think about already, and as a lot of decisions they need to finalise will be based on numbers, it is very impolite to leave them hanging.

WISHING THEM WELL WITH A BIG BOW ON IT

When choosing a gift, make sure you choose them something from the list. You may feel it is a bit impersonal, but at least you know you will be getting something

Here's an idea for you...

When it comes to alcohol, be mindful of your limits. It is entirely inappropriate to get drunk during the meal and heckle during the toasts. A lot of hard work, thought and consideration has gone into these speeches, so resist your witty asides. You must pace your intake. Drinking during the meal, the toasts, all often before six o'clock? Make sure that every other drink is a soft drink, as it will help you stay perky and also make the next day easier by keeping your hangover to a minimum.

they really need and like. It is very easy to give them something you like, that you *think* they should like. However, it's very possible that they will hate it and be too polite to say. So stick with the plan unless you know them very well and could stake your life on the premise that they will love your surprise.

Weddings are becoming increasingly expensive, so you can factor that in when choosing your gift; don't feel pressured to choose something you can't afford just because the list they have put together is very expensive. If the gifts in your price range have gone from the list, why not try and partner up with some friends to buy a bigger gift? Don't get it monogrammed unless you know that they are certain to keep it, as they won't be able to exchange it. When buying from the list ask for gift wrapping and delivery so that you don't have to take it to the wedding.

Any questions that you have, if possible, should be addressed to the bridesmaids or best man, so that you don't inundate the probably not-so-happy, stressed-out couple. As a rule, don't assume that you can take children unless they are specifically listed on the invitation. If you do take them, make sure provision is made for children during the evening – unruly, overtired nippers are almost never welcome.

Stick to the dress code that has been stated. If you are unsure, dress up. It's better that you make too much effort than not enough.

Not sure what to get them? Check out IDEA 24, *Gimme, gimme, gimme*, for some unusual suggestions.

Try another idea...

If you are invited to the ceremony, make sure you are there with at least fifteen minutes to spare; the only big entrance should be made by the bride. If you are unsure of the proper place to sit, see the ushers. If there is a receiving line at the reception, make sure that you don't hog the wedding party – you may be bursting with joy and a monologue of only a thousand words that you prepared earlier, but they have a lot of people to say hello to. By the same token, don't be offended if you only manage to see the back of their heads most of the time, as they will be very busy.

Wait for the bride and groom to hit the dance floor before you do. Do *not* do a dramatic slide across the floor and try and knock them down like dominoes – no one besides you will think it's funny. This is meant to be a treasured moment, so try and act with some decorum.

Bear in mind that this is also meant to be a celebration with a purpose; a celebration of two people and their families coming together. The best guests show consideration to the other people around them. Make sure that you mix, and talk to your neighbours at sit-down meals. Include any single guests in your party and make sure you seek out key family members, like parents and grandparents; it's a special day for them too.

'True friends are those who really know you but love you anyway.'
EDNA BUCHANAN, novelist

Defining idea...

How did it go?

Q **I'm a single woman and I've been invited to a friend's wedding. But I'm told I can't bring anybody with me. I feel so annoyed because my friends in couples are allowed to take their partners, so why should I be penalised?**

A *I can appreciate your feelings, but the main problem with weddings tends to be money, and extra guests equal extra money. You'll have to try not to take this personally and focus on the happiness of the bride and groom.*

Q **I appreciate that but I don't want to go alone. Can I ask them about this?**

A *You could quietly request that they give you the opportunity to bring a guest, if they have room, once they've received all their RSVPs. If they still say no, you need to consider whether or not you would be able to go and enjoy it, or if you should bow out gracefully and just send them a gift. There's no point in going if you will feel uncomfortable all day.*

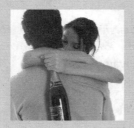
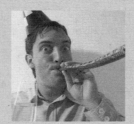

30

Honeymoon

The stuff of Blackpool postcards, but that doesn't make it your dream destination. You need to plan carefully if you are hoping to find your ideal blissful bolthole, with guaranteed sun (or snow).

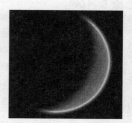

Just so you know, it is traditionally the responsibility of the groom to plan the honeymoon. However, times change and the bride often wants equal involvement.

So what exactly does 'honeymoon' mean? It originates from the times when a man captured his bride and they would hide from the bride's parents before marrying. They would remain in hiding for a further cycle of the *moon* after the wedding. During this period they drank *honey* wine.

You will probably need a break after the wedding to recover from all the stress and chaos of the run up to the big day. In which case, plan the honeymoon carefully and make sure you splash out on a few extras like cars to meet and transport you, and nice comfy airline seats. Tell everyone that you are honeymooners because you will often get free upgrades with rooms and flights if they are available, and nice touches from the hotels, such as complimentary champagne in the room.

Here's an idea for you...

Ask your friends and relatives about their honeymoons. As well as some great ideas for your holiday, you might get an idea of some places to avoid (not to mention a few great stories for the speeches).

You can always choose one of the specialist packages on offer. Most companies have a specific brochure that relates to honeymoons, but different companies may offer the same hotels with different rates and packages so make sure you shop around before settling. If you are using a travel agent, make sure that they present you with some options and earn their commission; don't just always settle for the first option that they come up with. Some hotels often insist that you produce your marriage certificate to qualify for special treatment, so don't forget to take it.

If you are booking directly, make sure you are very clear about what is included. The images you will be shown do not necessarily reflect your room, so ask if you will get a room of a comparable standard. Don't take anything for granted, such as a sea view, as you need to get written confirmation from the hotel about what you will be offered.

WHERE TO?

Make sure you have a serious think about all the honeymoon options. You don't have to go with the traditional destinations in the brochures. It may be sold as the fantasy of every new honeymooner, but if you are usually rock climbing or clubbing at the weekend, is being marooned on a sleepy island really right for you? It can be huge pressure for you to go from busy working lives to suddenly staring at each other every day across cocktails in coconuts. If you do choose a resort holiday, make sure you take time off from each other with the odd spa treatment or round of golf, so you can look forward to seeing each other again.

If you have ever wanted to take a longer break, many companies offer the option of a lengthier getaway than your usual two-week allowance. You could always use this as a chance to visit the rainforest in Brazil or go whale watching in the North Pole.

When planning to leave your reception, make sure you do it in style. See IDEA 16, _Make an entrance_, to make sure you get yourself a suitable carriage.

Try another idea...

MAKING IT STRESS FREE

When planning your honeymoon, consider the location of your wedding and the reception. You might like the idea of jetting off straight away, but a four-hour car journey to the airport can take the edge off your exciting day. Consider booking a special hotel nearby so that you can still leave the reception, but don't have to turn up in a flustered state. Have your suitcases delivered to your wedding suite in the morning so you don't have to think about it as the honeymoon begins. Make sure it's a special suite, and a pretty location. You might not see much of the grounds or spa on this visit, but you might want to return there for your anniversary.

Practically speaking, you need to make sure that you have all you need before heading off. Some more exotic locations may require special jabs and documentation, so ensure that you have this covered before you hit the airport. As soon as you have chosen a destination, get a list of required vaccinations and make sure you have time to get them done; you might need to take a course, or have them spaced out, so allow enough time.

'Only passions, great passions, can elevate the soul to great things.'
DENIS DIDEROT, French philosopher

Defining idea...

How did
it go?

Q **I'm already stressed out and the wedding's months off. I really want some time off to look forward to on the honeymoon, but my spouse to be – who, I have to say, has managed to duck all of the hassles – wants to do something adventurous. What can I do?**

A *Be clear and tell your partner how you feel. Then there are three ways of getting round this. First, you could choose a location that offers activities as well as a great pool or beach to lounge around. That way you can slob out until you have recovered and then join him in the more active pursuits. Second, you can try a twin-centre holiday, where you visit a beach location like the Seychelles, and then try taking a short hop over to Kenya for a safari.*

Q **And the third option?**

A *Separate honeymoons.*

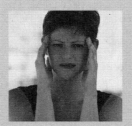 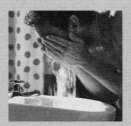

31

Let them eat cake

Most women regard themselves as experts when it comes to cake, but there is a bit more to this one than meets the eye. It is as important to foodies as the dress, and usually takes centre stage at the reception. So you need to get it right.

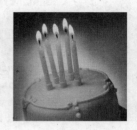

The ritual of cutting the cake is also a key part of the marriage: the couple's joint first slice into it symbolises their shared future. Announced by the toastmaster, this usually happens after the speeches.

Wedding cakes have had all kinds of formats and recipes over the years, but the modern shape, with three tiers of iced cake, was believed to have been inspired by Saint Bride's Church in London. Tradition has it that bridesmaids who sleep with a piece under their pillow will dream of their future husbands (and wake up with cake in their hair, and possibly having their faces licked by the family pet). The top tier of the cake is often kept by couples for the christening of their first child.

Here's an idea for you... **Half and half? If your gran is adamant that her family cake will grace your reception table, but she is a little out of touch with contemporary decoration, get it finished by a professional. Alternatively, if you don't want the stress of making it taste good but want the chance to make it look pretty, get it baked elsewhere and do the fun stuff yourself (as long as you do so well in advance).**

Traditionally, it is a fruitcake with royal icing decoration, but many couples don't adhere to this nowadays – it is perfectly common to have a sponge cake, or a tower of profiteroles, and even a cheesecake. (Honestly!) It really is a matter of preference, but if you want to carry on with some of the classic cake traditions, such as the saving of the top layer for new arrivals and sending some to absent guests, it needs to keep and travel; bear this in mind when you order the cake. You need to add this factor to the calculations of the appropriate size of cake for the number of guests.

CHOOSING THE STYLE AND DECORATION

Symbols that often graced wedding cakes traditionally include horseshoes and tiny models of brides and grooms. These days though, your only limitation is your imagination. Consider incorporating fresh flowers, exotic colours or graphic shapes. Why not have your names spelled out in letters or a stack of fairy cakes replicating a traditional wedding cake silhouette? Stock up on heaps of wedding magazines and gorge yourself on the styles and variety available. Make sure you rip them out and keep them in a file, but try not to include every single one that you see. If you choose your own pastry chef, they will have a portfolio that will show their previous commissions and styles. These should only be guidelines, though, which they should be happy to tailor in terms of size and style to fit your wishes, number of guests and budget.

FINDING A PASTRY CHEF

Wedding fairs are a great place to find a
suitable pastry chef, and they also give you the
chance to munch cake legitimately while you
wander around looking at wedding portfolios.
(It's all in the name of research, you understand.) If you are having the catering
provided by a professional outside company or hotel, they may also be able to
supply the wedding cake or have a contact who can.

When you have found a pastry chef that you like, you should be able to enjoy a
tasting with them. Once again, this is in the interest of the greater good. Tell them
what your concerns are, your requirements and budget. The wedding cake should
be ordered at least three months in advance. The cake is usually delivered to the
venue on the morning of the reception, where they should add any final touches in
situ. When it comes to the cutting of the cake, make sure that you have organised
with your caterers if you want them to cut the cake for guests. You need to let them
know how many pieces you need (including
the absent guests) and if you want to keep the
top layer uncut. Your pastry chef should also be
able to tell you about the proper way to store
this cake for future use.

**Make sure that your cake suits
your theme or picks up the
motifs of your flowers: see
IDEA 12, *The bouquets*, on
selecting blooms to decorate.**

Try another idea…

*'Qu'ils mangent de la
brioche.' [Let them eat cake.]*
MARIE ANTOINETTE

Defining idea…

MAKING YOUR OWN

In spite of it being considered as bringing bad luck, it is not a completely crazy notion that you could make your own cake. However, if you are well known as a disaster area in the kitchen, it probably would be crazy. If you do decide to bake the cake yourself, then you need to plan to make it at least a month before the wedding. This gives you plenty of time to tick it off your list before the day draws near. You can hire any necessary equipment, like outsize cake tins, from events companies and specialist cookery shops.

How did it go?

Q I love the idea of having a traditional cake, but my partner's family are strict vegetarians and they've given me a huge list of things that can't be included in the recipe! Can I keep all of us happy?

A *Don't panic, there are lots of substitutes for traditional ingredients these days. Try having a look through a couple of veggie cookery books to get some ideas.*

Q How about accommodating people with intolerance to specific foods?

A *It can be done. However, if you really feel like it will spoil your plans, then why not make a separate cake for them? You can always make a point of asking the other guests with food intolerances to state any specific needs and then you can handle them and the vegetarians all in one go.*

32

Keeping hangovers at bay

Even the most abstemious of us may get a little tipsy in the face of a happy union and end up being distinctly foggy the next day. However, you can easily help yourself and your guests avoid the worst.

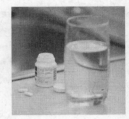

Prevention is without doubt the best cure for hangovers. With commonsense regulation of what you all eat and drink you'll minimise those 'morning after the night before' feelings.

The first major weapon on the front line in the battle against hangovers is good old H_2O. Dehydration is a major factor so make sure that there is a free and plentiful supply of water for all your guests. Another key strategy in avoiding a hangover (mainly that horrible uncomfortable acidic stomach) is eating. Starchy food is best, such as bread and pasta, which will absorb the alcohol. You can't ensure that everyone arriving at your reception is going to have followed this rule, but you can help them by arranging for canapés to be circulated.

You can also make sure that your cocktails are not super alcoholic – make them long drinks, with plenty of mixers and lots of lovely clinking ice (freeze lemon rind inside for extra effect). Make sure that they actually taste like grown-up alcoholic

Are you from the kill-or-cure school? Some people believe in taking their medicine and getting back under the duvet to watch some no-brainer kids' TV. Others think that exercise will restore well-being – pushing the toxins out of your pores will help, as will taking in extra oxygen, to eliminate the rubbish swilling around in your blood. Whatever your preference, allow your body some down-time while your remedies kick in.

drinks, if that's what they are – if you don't want to see your mum face down in the flowers on the top table by half six, don't try to disguise the flavour of killer drinks with fruit juice.

Elderflower cordial is the classic soft drink for English weddings, and when mixed with sparkling water is so delicious it's a great alternative to champagne, so have lots on hand. You can also rein in the pain by making sure that you serve a truly decent wine. If you want to pay for all the drinks yourselves but are worried about the budget, remember that no one will appreciate the gesture if any spilled wine strips the varnish off tabletops. They would probably prefer to have a pay bar and miss out on the pain that follows every free glass.

Inform your bar staff to have glasses of water on trays so people can grab them – they might not consider ordering one but are likely to pick it up if it's there. Your guests will thank you in the morning.

You might feel that you are treating your guests like children, but weddings can be like starting a heavy-duty Saturday evening out at nine in the morning. This is not something most people are used to dealing with, so things are bound to be a little harder to control.

THE DAMAGE IS DONE

Oh-oh. It came, it saw you to the floor, it conquered your head. So, what now? Most of the symptoms you'll be experiencing are down to dehydration; not impossible to believe when you consider that we are made up mainly of water. Then there are the toxins in booze – they'll be where your headache's coming from. These leach essentials from your system. The hangover treatments you can pick up from chemist's are full of vitamins to help your depleted reserves.

Considering a main effect of dehydration is losing the ability to think, you should try to follow these simple steps. Drink plenty of water before bed, with some orange juice if possible (waking up in the middle of the night in a panic is due to a sugar crash and dehydration; the orange juice will stop that happening). As soon as you awake, force some water down, and then some more.

The following day, do you need to keep going, catch a flight, or are you just worried about guests travelling home? Make sure you have coffee on hand and, better still, encourage even more water intake. Although coffee and tea may make you feel more perky, they add to the dehydration (which is why coffee shouldn't be used to sober people up).

You might not fancy fruit; you may be yearning for a full-blown fry up instead. However, all those good vitamins are badly needed, and they will be easy for an upset stomach to process.

Thinking about the best way to cause that hangover in the first place? Take a look at IDEA 25, *Drink and be merry*, on how to get the mix right.

Try another idea…

'Let us have wine and women, mirth and laughter, sermons and soda water the day after.'
LORD BYRON, from *Don Juan*

Defining idea…

139

How did it go?

Q **I want everyone to enjoy a drink at my wedding, but I don't want people getting drunk. How can I control the situation?**

A   *By controlling the flow of alcohol, although I can't imagine why you want to rein them all in. If you try and limit their consumption too much, they may think you're being stingy or a control-freak. The best way to handle it is probably control the flow in the day and then resign yourself to the fact that your guests are adults for the evening.*

Q **I think drunkenness is undignified and I don't want a wedding video of people with ties on their head doing air guitar. What's the best way to manage the flow of alcohol?**

A   *Well, weddings tend to be a time for people to let go, so you may have to be prepared to loosen up a little. On a practical level, you can have waiters circulating in the evening with soft drinks and gentle cocktails. Instruct them to take their time between topping up people's glasses (the same rules applying for a sit-down meal) and fill up the water glasses more frequently. If you have a pay bar, there is little you can do realistically – and bear in mind that people will have their own ideas about how much they can, or want to, imbibe. It's a good idea to have the wedding video shot early if you're that worried.*

33

And to your left...

Who sits on the top table; should couples sit together; should you engage in a little subtle matchmaking with the singles table? Seating plans are surprisingly tricky and important.

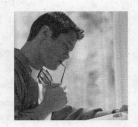

Mix the right people together and you have a recipe for an unbeatable atmosphere at your reception. Putting ample effort into working out that mix is a must.

When it comes to planning your seating, you should allow at least five years, maybe six. Only joking – the point is, though, seating plans will definitely take up more of your time than you ever thought possible. You will need to employ a lot of subtlety and grace to get it right. A great seating plan will have strangers laughing along together and boosting the general feeling of joy and good cheer. A bad seating plan will lower the temperature in the marquee by about fifty degrees and see tumbleweed rattling between the tables.

Want your wedding feast to run as smoothly as a five-star restaurant's VIP room? Then ensure that you brief your caterer properly, with a full copy of the seating plan. Clearly mark all the vegetarian/special requirements on it, so that waiting staff don't have to constantly ask. It will make those guests feel extra appreciated.

With a finger buffet, you can definitely avoid this stress, but any kind of formal meal should have a proper plan. When deciding where to place guests, remember that, rather than a college reunion, this is meant to be the joining of two sets of families and friends, so mix people up. There will be plenty of time for old friends to hook up later in the evening. If something terrible happens, and guests don't arrive for whatever reason, you will still be liable for the cost of the food but, more importantly, you should quickly re-arrange the tables to stop any gaps from becoming apparent.

Special consideration needs to be given to guests who are single or unaccompanied. Don't corral them all on one table – you may as well cover it in snow and flag it 'social Siberia'. The same goes for guests of different ages. It is common to seat children together but you shouldn't put all of your elderly relatives on one table. Be considerate. Although you shouldn't start pimping your single guests, it is a well-known fact that many couples meet at weddings so don't be scared of indulging in some gentle matchmaking.

Little people also need some special thought. A table for small children is a great way of keeping the mess and chaos to a minimum, but really little ones will need to be sat with their parents so make sure provision is made for them. Take into account that children are not known for their patience, so placid, thoughtful consideration during the speeches is probably out. Put them somewhere they can cause a little bit of trouble (like doing headstands on the dance floor) without disrupting the proceedings too much.

ROUND OR SQUARE?

Or even one big u-shape, to avoid favouritism. Whatever you go for, just make sure that your tables have a good mix of guests on them; people who, ideally, are comfortable talking to more than just their immediate neighbours. You may find, however, that your table shapes and sizes are dictated by the space and shape of your location. Remember that waiting staff and guests will need to be able to move freely, and the bride will also need to be able to circulate and mingle. Traditionally, most top tables (where the wedding party sits) are rectangular and face the guests, but you can have a round table if you would like to be less formal (or conspicuous, you shy brides).

The basic running order of the top table goes like this: maid of honour, groom's father, bride's mother, bridegroom, bride, bride's father, groom's mother, best man. Of course, you may have step-parents, siblings, ushers and bridesmaids you want to include too. If so, just make sure that the members of the different families are mixed up and have the opportunity to get to know each other better.

Of course, there is a limit to how many can head up the top table. It is usual for the partners of those on the top table, such as the

> While they are waiting to be seated, keep your guests happy with a special tipple. See IDEA 25, *Drink and be merry*, for ideas.

Try another idea...

> '*Food is our common ground, a universal experience.*'
> JAMES BEARD, US chef

Defining idea...

bridesmaids and best man, to sit together on a table nearby. However, if there are tensions about top table honours, why not break with tradition and have special party members host the tables? They can also take on the important task of getting everyone chatting and at ease.

SIT DOWN!

As guests enter the venue, it is a good idea to have a table plan displayed; even better, two: one on either side of the entrance. This will allow guests to find their places easily and without causing a glut of bumping bodies in the doorway and around the tables. You can use all kinds of methods to differentiate the tables: numbers, vases of different flowers, coloured balloons or ribbons, even naming them after different family pets.

How did it go?

Q   **When we're designing our seating plan should we have couples sitting together or apart?**

A   *If you want your guests to integrate, you should sit them on the same table but apart; maybe opposite each other.*

Q   **What if there are guests who are shy? My sister couldn't be less gregarious and won't talk to anyone if I sit her away from my brother-in-law.**

A   *Then it's probably best not to torture her; sit them together. It's a celebration, not an endurance test.*

34

Start spreading the news...

You've met the person you want to be with for ever, proposed and, hooray, they feel the same way too. All you need to do now is tell the world. There are quite a few details worth thinking about to get the ball rolling.

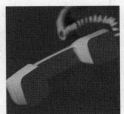

Start as you mean to go on — the way you announce your engagement is a great way to set the tone for your whole wedding. And why not have a big party while you're at it?

It is not unusual for brides to choose their own wedding and engagement rings these days, especially as they will be wearing them together. If you want to present your partner with something when you propose (bearing in mind that lots of thoroughly modern women do the asking nowadays), you could present them with a keepsake to mark the occasion, and then pick the rings together. A piece of jewellery such as a necklace or watch might be appropriate and something they could still show off. If you want to present a ring, a nice piece of costume jewellery could be a pretty and memorable stand in. Alternatively, the way you pop the question could be that special something to tide them over until they get their sparkler. Consider taking them to a favourite spot, filling a room with flowers, or

Here's an idea for you...

Get the key elements in place before you get onto the fluffy, enjoyable stuff. Start with date and location for your wedding (which will be the hardest to secure), then your reception venue or marquee hire.

having your proposal grace the notice board at a football stadium. Whatever you do, make it good – this is the story you'll be telling your kids in years to come. A drunken 'Shall we get it over and done with, then?' takes the edge off the romance somewhat.

HOLD THE FRONT PAGE

Are you retiring types who would happily let the news spread by word of mouth, or are you planning a banner trailing behind a plane? An announcement in a national or local newspaper is a popular way of spreading the news. Bear in mind, though, that you pay by the word so this is not the time to write lengthy and profound statements of love (unless money is no object). If you are unsure of the wording, take a look at their announcements page or ask if they have a formal style that you can use.

A whole glut of information is out there waiting for you to find it. There are lots of great web sites to use for ideas. You should also get yourself a big pile of wedding magazines. Try a range of different ones at first to give you a flavour of which ones suit you best. Even if you already know exactly what you want, the web and magazines are a great resource to show you where to find it. And your ideas might need a little overhaul – lots of women last seriously planned their own weddings when they were 12. That replica Princess Diana puff sleeve number that you dreamed of might not look so very 'now' anymore. The same can be said of cakes, dresses and shoes.

Wedding fairs are also hugely useful. These are usually held at a local hotel or popular wedding venue, and are a great way of getting to see local talent in action. Harpists, string quartets, pastry chefs, photographers and florists are among the service providers present at these events. Although you should always look around, a company's regular presence is often a good sign – it shows they are obviously organised and motivated, qualities you will come to appreciate as you undertake a project as time-consuming and stressful (and fun!) as planning a wedding.

Can't decide on where to have your wedding and the reception? IDEA 17, *Where: choosing a location*, will give you lots of ideas on how to select the perfect places.

Try another idea...

'SAVE THE DATE' CARDS

A great way to ensure that you have all your special people with you on your big day is by sending out 'save the date' cards. You don't need to have planned anything further than who you're marrying, and when, to issue these: people's summer weekends can quickly become booked up, so you will certainly want to make sure your wedding goes into their diaries first. These cards can be bought from most stationer's, or you can order them from a printer in the same style that you want for your invitations. If the wedding is to be intimate, you can always rely on a less formal phone call or email.

'Happiness isn't something you experience; it's something you remember.'
OSCAR LEVANT

Defining idea...

How did
it go?

Q **We want to have a huge engagement party and really raise the roof, but does that mean we will have to invite everyone who will be coming to the wedding?**

A *Of course not. Many older relatives certainly wouldn't mind missing a boozy night shaking their booties to thumping hip-hop. On the other side of the coin, it's often a great way to include all your pals in the celebrations if you are thinking of having a small wedding or going away.*

Q **And can we ask for specific engagement presents?**

A *Certainly not; it's not appropriate at all. In fact you should accept anything and nothing with the same grace. Just be glad they turn up to wish you well.*

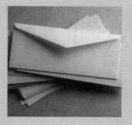
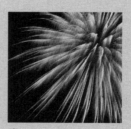

35

Ways to save

One thing that often stays with a couple long after their first anniversary is the overdraft. However, there is no reason for getting yourself hitched to a massive debt when you get hitched. You don't need to compromise on style just because you need to compromise on cost.

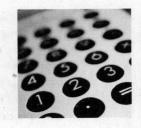

No matter how hard you try, things can often seem to spiral out of control. But there are things that you can do to get yourselves back on track. You need to get money savvy.

If you have to borrow money to finance your wedding, get reading the financial pages in the Sunday newspapers and make sure you get the best deals. (It might seem daunting at first but you will soon get the gist of it all.) You can use interest free credit card deals, release equity from your mortgage or get a low interest loan. Make sure your decisions are informed, and don't just go to your bank – they won't always be offering the best rates. By making good choices from the start, you can save yourself a lot of stress and money later.

Here's an idea for you...

Look into taking out wedding insurance to help ease the fear that goes with splashing out so much money in advance. But remember, too, that any suppliers you book should also have their own liability insurance. If a photographer with a technical hitch ruins all your photographs, you want to know that there will be some way to claw the costs back. And although no one likes to think about the worst, you should always ask about the supplier's cancellation policy.

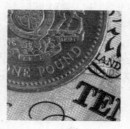

Check the business hours of your suppliers: sometimes the cost of out-of-hours delivery can really push up your bill. You may even be able to save a small fortune by taking over the collections and deliveries yourself – or, rather, getting a willing helper to take them on. Bear in mind that some things might also have to be returned.

THE GREEN STUFF

Flowers are a prime area for saving. Start by thinking about your venue: does it seem huge and yawning? Do you imagine that it would take Kew Gardens to fill it? If so, try some clever tricks with the lighting. Spots of candlelight can create an intimate glow on tables, and push cavernous high ceilings out of focus.

If another couple will be marrying on the same day as you, save money and time by sharing the cost of ceremony flowers and aisle pew displays. (Some churches include these anyway as part of the service.) Aisle pews don't always need to be decorated, or perhaps you can tackle every second one, alternating with ribbon. When choosing the flowers, make sure they are in season, as they will be much cheaper. If you really want some more exotic blooms, limit them to your bouquet and altar flowers, and give the displays more body and presence with less expensive blooms in the same shade. Vivid, large displays of greenery or hired trees can be used with – or instead of – flowers to great effect.

Take a look at IDEA 2, *When: date and time*, for choosing a time of day to make your styling even more cost-effective.

Try another idea...

Flowers also travel, so if you are having a civil ceremony in a hotel, take the flowers from your altar display through to the reception for the top table. Ensure your florist doesn't bamboozle you with different styles and unnecessary arrangements. You can even try your hand at some aspects yourself, such as the buttonholes: a lovely, simple rose with a little greenery is more than enough for most men and looks very refined and elegant. However, unless you are carrying a single stem, don't attempt anything vital like your own bouquet, as you will be horrified if it goes wrong. And even the most simple country garden bouquet usually has a lot more complexities and scaffolding than us mere mortals will ever understand. Ask the florist about money-saving tricks. For instance, mirrors under a display reflect the flowers and make them seem more bountiful; petals scattered over a white tablecloth look lush and pretty; and one big rose head can cover a standard table easily.

'**Honeymoon: a short period of doting between dating and debting.**'
RAY BANDY

Defining idea...

151

WELL FED

Savings can also be made by making some of the food yourself. If you are having a reasonably small wedding, you should be able to enlist some willing helpers and produce something special between you. The easiest option is a finger buffet, but you can easily make a sit-down meal, too, if you choose your menu wisely – stews and barbeques can be made in large quantities without compromising on taste or quality, and they can all be prepared in advance. You should make sure that some of your food can be frozen so that it can be made a week or two before rather than the day before or you will find yourself too stressed out. Catering equipment, like a very large electric barbeque, outsized pots and pans and refrigerators for the wine, can all be hired. You must have one person in charge on the day, though. Do not make this your mum or another close member of the wedding party, as they won't thank you for missing out on the enjoyment of the day. This could be where you splash out – on a professional chef to oversee the reheating and cooking, and, vitally, the preparation. Make sure they have plenty of helpers and waiting staff at their disposal; anything less is a false economy.

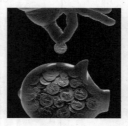
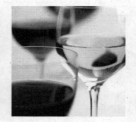
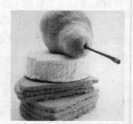

Q **We've got to save wherever we can; we might even have to forget food at the wedding altogether. Is that acceptable?**

How did it go?

A *If that's the only way you can do it, it'll have to be. The best way to handle this is to hold your wedding late in the day, and invite your evening guests at a time that is obviously for dancing, not dining, such as seven-thirty or eight. You will have to consider the needs of your ceremony guests, though – how about stretching to some hearty canapés? Even if your wedding is at six, the guests will probably have been travelling and waiting in the pews for at least a couple of hours; they'll need some kind of sustenance.*

Q **What happens if we can't afford fancy ingredients, let alone a caterer?**

A *Then enlist some friends to make delicious, rustic doorstep sandwiches that you can pile up on huge plates. Place little flags in them to let everyone know what they are, and lay them out on checked table cloths. Make a style virtue of a hearty country offering. It certainly will be appreciated.*

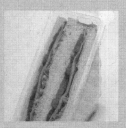 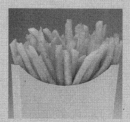

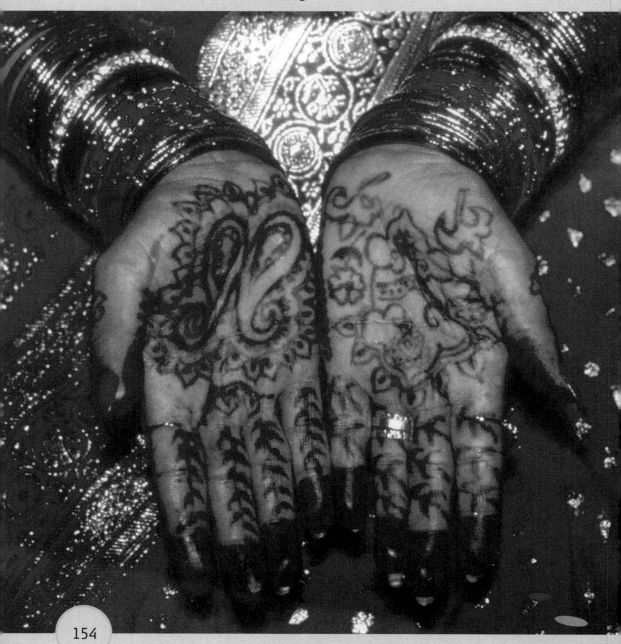

36

Choosing a theme for decoration

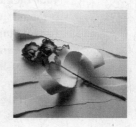

This is much less frightening than you might think. You can take anything for inspiration – a favourite colour, a period from history, even your top film. Be careful, though, not to make your wedding seem like a budget trip to Disneyland.

Whatever theme you want for your wedding, you must research and create it properly. Don't try to go for a medieval look in your local village hall unless you do want it to seem like panto. However, if you have a local banqueting hall in a castle, then you'll have a good chance of pulling it off.

Flowers for the reception, like everything else, should fit your theme. This means more than just choosing blooms that are the right colour. A country themed

Here's an idea for you...

Choose your menu to reflect your theme if you are aiming for maximum effect. Winter formal dinners should offer some hearty, warming fare, ideally using seasonal ingredients. Mint and lemon are fresh flavours for spring weddings. Hot summer days call for light salads, berry sorbets and a classic summer drink, such as elderberry cordial. Consider your presentation. If you are planning a very minimal wedding, white platters in graphic shapes can be used to great effect with sushi. A casual affair in your parents' back garden by the sea could have aluminium buckets (new, of course!) with oysters in ice. Try adding little touches to drinks, such as borage flower heads (or other edible flowers) in your ice cubes so they clink prettily in summer cocktails. Just make sure to use mineral water so that the ice isn't cloudy, spoiling the effect.

wedding will lose its continuity if you plump for graphic, modern arrangements. Try using snowdrops or miniature daffodils planted in little buckets, or large headed, blowsy roses in old-fashioned colours such as dusky pinks and pale lemons. Think about the time of day: if you're having a winter reception, maybe in the evening, a rich, deep colour theme with lots of greenery will add to the drama of the event, whereas pale colours may get lost and are better suited to a sun-drenched marquee.

By choosing the right style and colour scheme, flowers can help transform a stark reception hall into a warm and inviting space. For an especially big space, you can rent small trees to lead into the room, or section off certain areas to create a more intimate feel. Lighting is also vital: make sure you avoid any stark overhead lights; if your room has them, ask if they can be dimmed. Tea lights on mirrors in the centre of the tables create interest and a sparkling focal point. Lanterns can also be used to great effect in marquees – try a mix of pretty pastel-coloured Chinese ones strung from poles.

SOMEWHERE OVER THE RAINBOW

Choosing a unifying colour, or combination of colours, is a great way to give your wedding a coherent theme and will make your efforts more noticeable. However, before you start, think about the bridesmaids. Your favourite colour may be yellow but you need to be careful with the shade – brunettes can look stunning in yellow but few blondes, bar Doris Day, can pull it off. So don't rush off and order hundreds of metres of yellow ribbon before you've thought about how twelve disgruntled maids and flower girls will look if their complexions are indistinguishable from their frocks.

Texture can be just as effective as colour. A seersucker gingham tablecloth with frayed edges is inexpensive to buy and easy to make, and will create a wonderful country feel in a marquee. Tie your table napkins with straw and a single oversized daisy.

Take a look at **IDEA 11**, *Coming up roses*, for more ideas on how to use flowers to their greatest effect.

Try another idea...

'I find that the harder I work, the more luck I seem to have.'
THOMAS JEFFERSON

Defining idea...

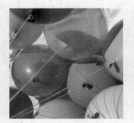
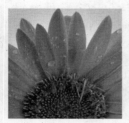

How did it go?

Q **We're holding our wedding and reception in the same venue, and the room looks too big. How can we handle it so we don't all rattle about in it like peas in a drum?**

A *You need to break the space up into more manageable portions. First, check with the venue staff if there's a way of dividing the room (this may be a situation they have had to accommodate before). If not, consider contacting a set-dressing or party organising company to come in with drapes and rigging to make a themed room within the room. Imagine the inside of a maharaja's tent – that's the kind of effect they can create, making the space more intimate and decadent.*

Q **Are there any steps we can take ourselves to cut a cavernous hall down to size so our theme shines through?**

A *Forget about using any top lighting (it will only show how high the ceilings are) and put candelabras on the tables. You can hire (from the catering and events companies that provide things like industrial ovens, chairs and tables) outsized black velvet curtains that have fairy lights embedded throughout them. Use them to divide the room into the desired space and create a walkway into your new, smaller environment. It will add a touch of excitement and feel very glamorous. Just remember to make the solution an improvement on the original rather than a desperate measure.*

37

Get me to the church on time

Want your wedding to run like a well-oiled military machine? Then you need some serious planning and a seamless ceremony schedule. There's more to organise than you might think, unless you want guests napping during yawning breaks and only fifteen minutes to do your hair.

Making sure that you have at least two people with a printed list of all the important contacts, from florist to band, will work like handing out Valium to calm the nerves of all important family members. No one needs to be thumbing frantically through the phone directory trying to remember the name of the missing registrar.

Here's an idea for you...

With so much to consider, it's easy to forget those who cannot attend. Avoid offending anyone or causing confusion by sending announcements cards to any people not invited to the wedding because the number of guests must be limited, or because they live too far away. The cards may also be sent to other acquaintances who, while not being particularly close to the family, might still wish to know of the marriage. Rather than print them up separately, you could always make a more personal gesture by writing letters informing everyone of your plans and news.

ATTENTION TO DETAIL MAKES EVERYONE HAPPY

The best way to guarantee a happy day is to make everything crystal clear to everyone. Don't worry about looking like a control-freak – it's better than having to cope with chaos.

Consider a few extra little tweaks to make things run even more smoothly. Pew cards let special guests and family members know they are to be seated in the reserved section on either the bride's side or the groom's side. You can send them out with invitations and say they should be handed to the ushers on arrival. The ushers can be fully briefed to ensure guests smoothly end up where they should be, and that your stroppy aunt is treated with all due reverence.

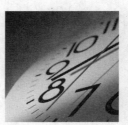 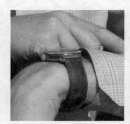

Ceremony programmes are lovely keepsakes of the day. As well as spelling out the sequence of events during the ceremony, they also let everyone know when they are expected to be singing, sitting, listening or crying at the soppy bits. The ushers can hand them out (it's a nice way of greeting people and making them feel welcome) or they can be placed on the pews. Traditionally, they begin with the line 'order of service', and should include the bride and groom's names, the date, entrance music, hymns, prayers, marriage, benediction and any readings. You may also want to use the programmes as an opportunity to make any special announcements or thanks.

Take a look at IDEA 33, *And to your left...*, for tips on creating seating plans to ensure that all the guests are happy and chatty.

Try another idea...

SITTING COMFORTABLY

Seating or place cards let guests know where they should be seated during any formal meal. As well as avoiding an awkward scrum for the table nearest the buffet or bar, it gives you a unique opportunity to ensure that guests meet and mix. As people arrive, you can do one of two things. First, lay name cards out alphabetically by the entrance, and by number, colour or motif, guests should then be able to use the cards to find the corresponding table. Second, you can have a board that lists the names of each guest and shows which table they are supposed to be on. The guests should also have their places marked on the table with a name card. Have your ushers on hand to help any elderly party members find their seats. And bear in mind you may need high chairs and wheelchair access.

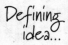

'Meticulous planning will enable everything a man does to appear spontaneous.'
MARK CAINE

Everyone has probably been to a wedding that's run over into mayhem – food nowhere in sight, then children crying and guests eating the table decorations (because they are so drunk on an empty stomach they no longer care). Your toastmaster, whether he is a professional or your best man, should ensure that events keep moving swiftly along in accordance with your planned schedule.

The reception should run in this order (or a close variation of it): the guests arrive at the venue and pass down the receiving line; the meal; the speeches and toasts; the cutting of the cake; the first dance; a big jolly party; the departure of the bride and groom; the departure of the guests. Hopefully.

In the final week before the big day, call all your suppliers and talk through final details. Make sure, for instance, that your florists know where your venues are and what time to arrive for set-up (they should know how long it takes), and that all of your suppliers will have adequate parking (you do not want your caterers circling the block for half an hour unable to unload the ovens because they don't have a resident's parking permit).

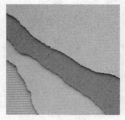

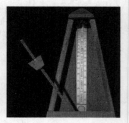

Q **I want to get married in my local church, but the only suitable venue for the reception is a good twenty miles away. Do you think that's a mistake?**

How did it go?

A *Not necessarily, but there are some obvious points to factor in. You should ensure that your ceremony does not end just as the rush hour starts and, ideally, you ought to avoid any trips that would take your convoy through the centre of a busy town.*

Q **Should we make a contingency plan for guests arriving at the reception venue who won't be going to the ceremony?**

A *Yes: make sure that should the worst happen, and you get stuck in traffic, someone will be on hand to greet them and start the festivities. This could be your caterer, who can have staff on hand to welcome guests with a glass of champagne while a harpist plays a gentle refrain. If this happens, you'll even get to make a second grand entrance.*

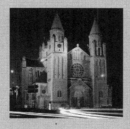 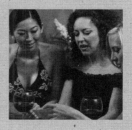

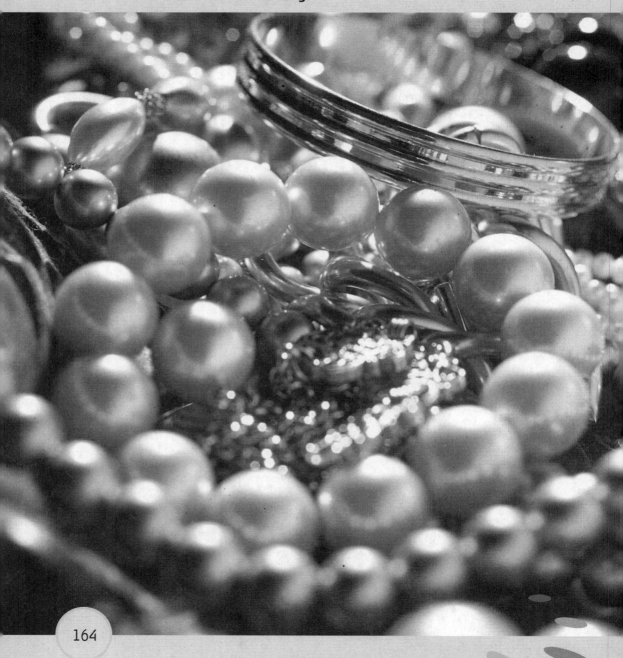

38

Twinkle toes...and other sparkly bits

As well as your dress, there are a few other vital weapons you need in your bridal outfit armoury. Looking effortlessly gorgeous takes a surprising amount of planning.

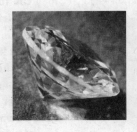

There is more to enhancing your radiance than the jewellery and other accessories on show. Without comfortable underwear and shoes as well, your beaming smile might crack into an expression of pain by the end of the day.

THE FUNDAMENTALS

The most important of all of your wedding accessories will be your 'scaffolding'. The underwear you choose has to operate on several levels – as well as beautiful, it needs to be comfortable and fit like a glove so no lines, lumps or bumps show under your gown.

Here's an idea for you...

Consider the season. Winter may call for gloves, a wrap or even a heavy (but still glamorous) coat. Summer might call for a light wrap or parasol against the sun. If you are having an outdoor reception, remember that when the sun goes down a chill may descend too. If you don't want a wrap or jacket, try a pretty cashmere cardigan in a '50s style. And if you are having an April wedding, don't forget umbrellas – or for a cute, quirky look buy your bridesmaids see-through macs to pop over their pretty frocks if the heavens open.

Your first step is to get yourself measured properly. It has been estimated that around 75 per cent of women in Britain wear the wrong size bra, so go to your local lingerie shop or department store and see a professional. And work out what time of your menstrual cycle you will be in on the day – a lot of women suffer water retention at certain times and can go up as much as a full cup size, which means your slinky lines could be more curvy than you banked on. You may also like the idea of surprising him with the full stockings and suspenders number, but if they are going to show under the dress try lace topped hold-ups instead.

When looking for underwear, remember that skin tone shades are much less likely to show through thin fabrics than white. French knickers can also give a smoother line than briefs or a G-string, so look at all styles, including the ones that you never wear. You'll need the right type of bra, too, especially if you have a strapless dress. It must give you support without digging in. Try on lots until you find the right style for your shape. Some dresses have built-in support, which may be worth considering. If you want to wear a figure-flattering undergarment that tucks in certain parts and flattens others, switch your sexy focus to nightwear instead so you can slope off after the reception and change into your own wedding present for him. That way you save flimsy for later and you won't have to go without support during the day.

SHOES

Take a look at IDEA 5, *The Blushing bride*, for inspiration on getting the right dress to match it all with.

Try another idea...

There are few women who don't relish the idea of a new pair of shoes, but this time there's a lot to take into consideration so look before you leap (in them). You'll be wearing them all day, and that's a long time if you aren't used to wearing heels (and even if you are), especially given that you won't get to sit down for long. You need to choose a pair that are high enough to be flattering, but not so high that you end up staggering from one side of the room to the other. You will also need to dance with them on, so that slinky pair might look great but do they also having staying power?

The best thing to do is find your most comfortable shoes and use them as a model; maybe they have an ankle strap and therefore feel more stable. Whatever you choose, you must make sure that you wear them for a few days to break them in – you don't want to end up with blisters. Make sure the bottoms of the shoes are a little scuffed so that you don't take a tumble during a rumba.

CHOOSING JEWELLERY

When choosing what to wear on your big day, you should first consider the neckline of your dress. A simple neckline can take both simple or very decorative jewellery. A choker is best on a long neck, which also suits a slim strand of pearls at the base of the throat. If you have a short neck, a diamond on a chain might look better, or choose to wear more eye-catching earrings instead. Make sure that all

'*Beauty as we feel it is something indescribable; what it is or what it means can never be said.*'
GEORGE SANTAYANA,
US philosopher

Defining idea...

167

your jewellery works together. You may find that your pearl tiara looks fussy with your gold choker, so try it all on for size. This is often a time that family members could want to step in with 'something old, something new' so if you are going to be presented with your grandmother's drop pearl earrings check they go with your diamante choker. You can always be cheeky and ask in advance if someone has any plans to surprise you.

How did it go?

Q I want a handbag to keep all my little necessaries in. Do you think it's unreasonable to ask my maid of honour to carry it?

A *A compromise would be to share one, but if you definitely want your own then it's fine to ask (or rather, demand) – after all it is your day. Just make sure it is a pretty purse, not a huge sports bag: this is for touch-ups, not rebuilds. (Remember, your maid of honour will have emergency essentials such as tissues, powder, lip gloss or stick, mascara, eye make-up pads (in case you start sobbing), hair spray, and a spare pair of stockings in case you need them.)*

Q What can I do if I just can't find the right shoes to go with my dress?

A *Bear in mind that if you can find the right style but the right colour is eluding you, it's possible to have shoes dyed to match your dress perfectly.*

39

Choosing a morning suit

Grooms: think you're going to get off lightly? Wrong. Your suit will be the most keenly observed and scrutinised outfit you'll ever wear. Get the right one so you'll look like you belong on the catwalk rather than in the litter tray.

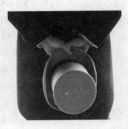

This should be the most expensive tackle you ever buy, so make sure that you don't skimp on the shirt and shoes. And please, please invest in new underwear and socks — you don't want a damper on your wedding night, do you?

It may go against everything you know, but this is a time to bring in a little help. In order of preference, you should choose as your adviser a gay male friend, a stylish woman friend or, finally, your mum. You can't see yourself properly from behind, and you might not be the best person to judge how the fabric goes with your skin tone.

Here's an idea for you...

Get looking for some footwear that's just right. As well as being stylish and a perfect match for your suit, your shoes need to be comfortable. Wear them at least two or three times beforehand to make sure you can get through the day in them. If they have smooth soles, you should consider cross hatching the bottoms so that you won't slide across marble floors as the cameras flash.

BRING OUT YOUR INNER SUPERMODEL

Morning suits are a classic choice for a formal ceremony, black for winter and a lighter more fresh grey for summer weddings. You don't have to do cravats; you can dress it down slightly with a shirt and tie and leave out the top hats if they really make you feel as if you are in fancy dress. A morning suit creates a great sharp line if you feel you have a less than sharp figure. Shine, matt and texture can all be mixed to bring character to a suit, so consider that as a refined way of expressing individuality without going to extremes.

And a key question is how fashionable should you be? You might feel it would be great fun to look back at a wedding that seems incredibly evocative of an era, but then think of a rerun of *Top of the Pops* from the 1970s – hideous. So think of classic images that are both stylish and able to stand the test of time. Is it Prince Edward's grey herringbone and blue tie combination, or perhaps Clarke Gable's dinner jacket? Or maybe it's the Rat Pack cutting a dash through a Vegas landscape. (Just leave the violin case at home.) Then go hunt out your own equivalent.

You can create a bit of extra flash with special coloured lining or a sharp buttonhole. It is the groom's responsibility to provide the buttonholes, so make an effort to choose something with a bit of pizzazz. Your florist should be able to help you choose an arrangement that will reflect the bride's bouquet. Make sure that it works with your tie (and even your socks, to be super smooth).

Do make sure you talk to your best man about his suit. After all, he will be in a lot of the pictures so if he turns up in a suit he picked up in a charity shop the day before, he could be the cause of your first argument. Although your suit and his shouldn't have to match, they should both be the same colour – brown next to navy is not a complementary pairing. Obviously this is less of a problem if you are having a very casual wedding.

Suit's sorted; how about the rest of you? See IDEA 21, *Grooms grooming*, for the finishing touches.

Try another idea…

A STITCH IN TIME

If you have ever wanted your own bespoke suit, now is the one time in your life you can probably justify it but make sure you order in plenty of time. Firstly, you will need to find a reputable tailor: ask snappily dressed friends or colleagues for recommendations. Select a good grade of fabric that will wear well and feel fabulous. Go for the best that you can afford. Choose a style you want: three buttons or four, or a classic suit? You can be as fashionable as you like, but a classic style is the best investment. At this stage, your tailor will take all the required measurements. Now is the time to talk to him about the slightly less than perfect bits you would like to disguise. Tell him how you'd like your suit to fall on your shoulders, waist and shoes. The great thing about a bespoke suit is that you can have it cut to flatter your silhouette. Ask your tailor for all the tips that should work for your frame. You should also consider adding special touches, like a snazzy lining or special buttons. At the final fitting you should be very exacting and demand any little adjustments you feel are needed.

'Just because I have rice on my clothes doesn't mean I've been to a wedding.'
PHYLLIS DILLER

Defining idea…

171

How did
it go?

Q **I can't cope with the pressure of choosing my own suit – my fiancée and her family are such style fascists. What can I do to make sure I don't get it wrong?**

A *Ask her to get a series of images from wedding magazines and clearly mark out what she likes.*

Q **I would have asked her to come along but she wants it to be a surprise. How can I get a clearer idea of what her expectations are?**

A *Ask her to go with you to the tailor's or stores you are thinking of using, and give you a 'definitely not' list. That way you can have some pretence of autonomy when you choose from the rest and you'll know she won't be disappointed.*

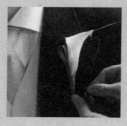
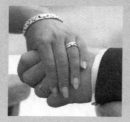

40

Hold a civil ceremony

Holding a civil ceremony is an ideal way of getting the type of wedding you want. Basically, you can have a small registry office marriage and then plan your own second ceremony, which can follow any form you like.

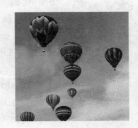

You have to hold the civil ceremony in legally recognised, permanently roofed premises, but you can hold your own blessing afterwards, with your guests and celebrant wherever you like. Let your imagination run riot.

This is a great chance to do something very unique and personal. Think laterally: you could choose anywhere, from an orchard to a little flotilla of boats. You could borrow chairs and make a happy grouping in your back garden, or still have a very formal affair with marquees and an orchestra. It is an ideal way of getting around the restrictions of where and how to marry. (And by 2006 the laws will be changing to include a wider range of locations.)

Here's an idea for you...

If you are having a second ceremony and your civil wedding is simply the 'legal' bit, then be flexible about your timings. Check out availabilities – a Tuesday morning might be an easy slot to get, and you can reserve all your energy and resources for planning your main event exactly when and how you want it.

The vows in a civil wedding tend to be short, although you can add your own readings and hymns. If you are opting for a second wedding ceremony, don't forget to get involved in writing your own vows because you can say whatever you want, however you want.

First stop for a civil ceremony, is the Superintendent Registrar of the district where you wish to marry. You can be married in church, a District Register Office, an army, navy or Air Force chapel, or any building approved by the local authority. For a marriage in the approved premises, you will need to make arrangements at the venue in question and give a formal notice of your marriage to the Superintendent Registrar. Do check with your reception venue if it has a licence for wedding ceremonies – it could simplify your day hugely.

PROPER DOCUMENTATION

Some rules apply to everyone. The minimum legal age for getting married is 16 years old. In England and Wales, the written consent of the parents or guardians is required for persons who have not reached 18 years old and have not been previously married. If either of the persons is below 18 a birth certificate must be produced. You or your partner must attend the register office for the area where you live and give notice of your marriage to the Superintendent Registrar. Each partner must have lived in that district for at least seven days prior to giving notice to the Superintendent Registrar. If you live in different districts then each one of you must give notice in your district. A form giving the couple's names and addresses, ages and location of the ceremony will have to be completed, together with a declaration that there is no legal objection to the marriage. After the Superintendent Registrar has established that he can take notice of marriage, it is entered into a marriage notice book and a statutory form is displayed on a public notice board for fifteen days so that anyone who has any objection to your union can raise it.

A certificate of marriage will then be issued. If notice of marriage is given in two districts, then one should be collected by the couple, as it will have to be produced before the ceremony can go ahead. The certificate of marriage is valid for one year once notice of marriage has been given.

When you visit the Superintendent Registrar to make the formal arrangements you will need to produce certain documents. For example, if you have been married before, a decree absolute of divorce bearing the court's original stamp is needed, or, if your previous spouse has died, a death certificate. Other documents may also be required depending on the circumstances (e.g. the consent of parents to a marriage where one of the partners is under the age of 18 years old).

Take a look at IDEA 17, *Where: choosing a location*, for ideas on choosing the right reception venue to follow your civil ceremony.

Try another idea…

'*A good marriage is like a good trade: each thinks he got the better deal.*'
IVERN BALL

Defining idea…

How did it go?

Q **I'm having a civil ceremony but am unsure about what to wear. Can I wear a wedding dress?**

A *It's your day – you can wear jeans or a bikini or a full 15 ft train. Lots of civil ceremony brides wear a traditional dress. There are a couple of things to consider though. You might want to wear something in which you can travel easily or stay warm in. If so, try a dress with added layers, like a wrap or coat, that you can lose when you get to the reception and start dancing. Think about a snazzy white suit: very Bianca Jagger. If you aren't wearing white, beware hats in case you end up looking like just another guest. Try a headdress with flowers or mini veil. Do carry flowers, even a subtle corsage on the wrist. Make sure you feel like a million dollars, whatever you wear – don't feel the need to play it down just because you may have chosen a registry office. If you are unsure how to get the mix to work for you, why not visit a personal shopper to help you?*

Q **Can I change at the reception?**

A *You can, although it might be nice to enter in your wedding outfit so that your guests can see it, and then disappear to change and make a second entrance.*

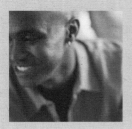
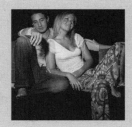

41

Let's do it in a tent

It's a British tradition, in some way embodying that 'spirit of the Blitz' fortitude, that makes a country known for its rain and erratic weather decide to hold dearly cherished social events outdoors in a big tent. Nothing quite says 'English wedding' like a marquee.

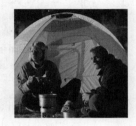

It is basically a style choice to opt for a marquee. If you want all the trimmings, such as flooring and fancy light fittings, flowers, caterers and furniture hire, you can expect it to cost about the same as a hotel reception. However, if you borrowed chairs and tables and did your own catering and decoration, it could be a budget saviour.

When choosing a marquee your first consideration should be space, and you obviously need a garden or field big enough to accommodate it. They come in a

Here's an idea for you...

There will no doubt be a lot of traffic between the marquee and the bathroom. Look into hiring a portable toilet or an industrial-scale cleaner for the trail of mud on your parents' carpets.

variety of sizes and styles, but if you consider that you will need a marquee of roughly 14 by 20 metres for 125 guests having a formal, sit-down meal, that should give you an idea of which ones to start looking at. Go into the garden with a ball of red wool and mark out the size of marquee that you think you would need or like (the wool is red so you can see it in the grass, by the way). Then you need to talk to a marquee hire company about what can be done with the available space. Alternatively, you can tell them how many guests you would like and they can tell you what you will need – they will work out the size from the numbers, so you don't have to. If the tables and chairs will be moved to allow for dancing and the arrival of evening guests, check how many it can hold in that format before you send out invites. After all, you don't want disgruntled guests squeezed out into the cold because you had imagined them happily milling about in the sun.

Don't forget that if you are thinking of having a band, stage, dance floor or buffet tables, say so at the start, as these will need to be added into the equation. If you feel uncertain about your needs, ask for the hire company to make a visit to the site to help you plan. Marquees are usually erected two or three days before the wedding day, which means that if you want to do some of the decoration yourself, you can.

If you are having caterers, they can often be accommodated in a separate or adjoining marquee, or sometimes in the same marquee behind a divider. They will need discreet access in and out of the dining area, and running water and electricity for ovens and preparation. You might want to let them use the kitchen in your home to avoid extra cost but be realistic about the space required and be prepared for the mess.

IDEA 3, *The world and its mother*, can give you pointers on getting the numbers of guests right, so no one is left out in the cold.

Try another idea...

I'M NAKED!

When planning your budget, you need to consider that your marquee will literally be an empty tent and will need lots of styling to give it the atmosphere of a celebration. Sourcing the furniture and decorations is easy – the marquee company can help if you want it fuss-free, or there are many other events companies which can provide you with tables, chairs, lighting etc. Just make sure that all of it will work together – you marquee firm is unlikely to be interested if the lighting doesn't work if it's not their responsibility. Other hidden costs are heaters (in the winter), dance floors and flowers.

'The more you praise and celebrate your life, the more there is in life to celebrate.'
OPRAH WINFREY

Defining idea...

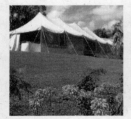
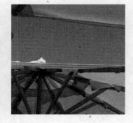

How did
it go?

Q **I really want to have a classic English wedding in a marquee, but I am worried about the space. Are there ways to make the available area stretch further?**

A *If you have French windows, have the marquee joining directly to the house. This means the older guests can retreat inside to sit down and escape from the disco later on. It also means that you don't need to allow space for tables during the reception. Second, empty your garage for the caterers, so that they can use it for ovens, fridges and storage, saving you a bit more garden space. If it's big enough, they may even be able to work from there.*

Q **Our budget is pretty tight. What can we do to make cost savings?**

A *Costs go up as you have a bigger marquee and more guests. You can obviously therefore make savings by inviting fewer people. Anything you can do yourself will also save money. Get some willing friends to help with the decorations. You can also have long tables instead of round ones, in which case ask everyone if they could lend you trestle tables or wallpapering tables and use your own cloths to cover them. Instead of hiring china go for paper plates. A pretty marquee created cheaply but with some thought will be equally as charming as an expensive one decked out to the ceiling with chandeliers and gilt.*

42

Arguing

If you get through the wedding process without arguing it is likely that one of you is either dead or wearing earplugs. Emotions will always run high at times like this. You will have to deal with people and families who are sometimes far from perfect and all of whom have an opinion.

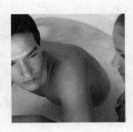

Is his mum interfering far too much for your liking? Before you explode, remember that she's been waiting to see her little boy get hitched since the day he was born, and she'll have imagined it (her way) several times. Everyone must learn to tread with caution.

MAKING IT A HAPPY TIME

People often say that weddings are blissfully happy occasions. The reality is that it can be a very exhausting, stressful and anxious time. It is often the case that happy-go-lucky, loving couples suddenly find themselves arguing, panicking and battling each other over the smallest issues. But by remembering a few tricks, you can get through the worst and still have a good time.

Here's an idea for you...

Stick a photograph of one of your happiest shared times on the fridge door with a note saying 'Why we're getting hitched'. Almost all couples wonder if it's all worth it in the run up to the day. If you've had a rough day and think the world is falling apart because you can't get the hot pink Rolls Royce you wanted, then you need to remember that it's not the point of the day – getting married is.

Firstly, no matter how long you've been together, you will be dealing with issues that you have never worked on before. For a lot of couples, that often boils down to money. Both partners may work and manage their own cash, but they might not have had to deal with shared finances before. It can reveal a lot of unknown personality traits you might not have appreciated before, such as the fact they hide their bank statements in their sock drawer and never open them. Don't imagine these problems will go away. Use this as an opportunity to discuss how things will work in the future, and if you feel unsure get some professional advice, such as from a financial adviser, who can create a sensible impartial plan for you to follow.

STAYING FOCUSED

Always defend each other to your parents, or anyone else chipping in their opinions, over the big issues. Discuss anything that might cause problems. If your fiancé's mum is adding to the guest list until it looks like a modern-day version of the Domesday Book, talk it through before you tackle her about it. Although it might be tempting to earn some in-law points by sympathising with them on a one-to-one basis, you will only store up problems for later when it's used against you with your beloved. Agree on a policy together and stick to it, even if you have private reservations. And no matter how irresistible it is to sound off, be careful who you talk to. While you think you are just letting off steam, others may have longer memories.

SPLITTING UP AND GETTING BACK TOGETHER

IDEA 14, *How to say 'I don't' and 'you do'*, will show you how to get some extra help to save your nerves.

Try another idea...

At times like this you need to make sure that you plan enough time into your schedule to have some completely 'non-wedding' time. That means you should go to a film, have a country walk or just go out clubbing; whatever it was that you enjoyed doing before you decided to get hitched. That will put you back in touch with your real-life relationship. Make sure you don't talk about the wedding or arrangements at all, or you may find that after the wedding you've forgotten what you did before and have nothing else to talk about. (And remember, every bow and posy may be fascinating to you, but most people can only take so much wedding-speak. Be self-aware and don't turn into a 'big day' bore.)

This 'non-wedding' time should also work hand in hand with some time on your own. The reality is, no matter how much we would like to think that the battle of the sexes is over, weddings often illustrate that it's really just having an amnesty; the female partner is usually the one doing most of the planning and organising. If this is the case, then make sure that you have some quality time for you. Plan a regular facial or massage. Try to delegate tasks and find something you enjoy that is totally unrelated to the stress of planning – and make it more than just talking to your friend over a glass of wine (although you can do that too), as she may be a bridesmaid with whom you are also arguing about dresses. Exercise is a great stress reliever, as is dancing, painting or learning any other new skill.

'I'd like to have engraved inside every wedding ring, "be kind to one another" – this is the Golden Rule of marriage and secret of making love last through the years.'
RANDOLPH RAY

Defining idea...

How did it go?

Q **I really wanted to get married but suddenly everything seems to be falling apart. My partner won't get involved in any of the planning and seems to think it's all my responsibility. It doesn't bode well. Should I call it off?**

A *Almost every couple you meet will have a similar tale to tell. It often ends up with the bride being responsible for the majority of the planning, so the best way to avoid this is to play to your combined strengths. Write a list of all the chores and divide them up. Maybe your partner is great at finances, in which case he can be made to be responsible for paying deposits and managing the money. Rather than repeatedly having to ask for help, make sure he's got the list and understands what his chores are. Then leave him to it.*

Q **How can I make sure he does do the tasks on his part of the list?**

A *Make sure all the chores have a deadline, and that you both know them. Give yourself plenty of safety time so that if things aren't done you still have time to rescue things. Try not to chase him up until the deadline has arrived – if you harass him, he'll become resentful. If he really can't be relied upon to take some responsibility, you have one of two choices. You can accept it and ask friends for help instead, or call it off.*

43

The future is here...

So you got married and it was a wonderful day; you've even got the pictures to prove it. But what happens after you've found the last of the confetti and everyone has seen the video? Your life together begins in earnest, and it can be tough at first.

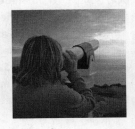

Lots of people find that they feel a bit flat after the wedding. It's a completely natural sensation after having been the focus of attention for months, sometimes even years. To go from being the golden couple to being just like everyone else can be a bit strange.

THE FALLOUT

As well as falling back to earth, you can also suffer from 'marriage movies'. Even people who have happily lived together for years suddenly find they are in conflict. This is often because they have conscious or unconscious ideas about how being married works, like a film playing somewhere in their heads of every marriage

Here's an idea for you...

Most people like to remember their wedding day and why they got married by celebrating their wedding anniversaries. Traditionally, certain materials are associated with particular years of marriage, the theory being that they will replace the wedding gifts as they wear out. Good spouses never forget an anniversary. So, here's a list of the transitional gifts. Add it to your diary so you'll have no excuse for forgetting...first, cotton; second, paper; third, leather or straw; fourth, silk or flowers; fifth, wood; sixth, iron or sugar; seventh, wool or copper; eighth, bronze; ninth, pottery; tenth, tin; eleventh, steel; twelfth, silk and fine linen; thirteenth, lace; fourteenth, ivory; fifteenth, crystal; twentieth, china; twenty-fifth, silver; thirtieth, pearl; thirty-fifth, coral; fortieth, ruby; forty-fifth, sapphire; fiftieth, golden; fifty-fifth, emerald; sixtieth, diamond; seventy-fifth, second diamond

model they have seen from Doris Day films to their own parents. Even if you think this isn't the case with you, you should talk through how you expect things to change. Most people find they have new expectations, as they wouldn't have chosen marriage if they didn't expect it to transform their situation in some way. It can be as simple as feeling more committed, in which case maybe you expect your partner to reorder their priorities.

Hopefully, you have discussed all the key issues before now, but, even so, you should have a good chat about your expectations. Are you going to keep your joint wedding account? How will you divide your assets as a married couple? (Lots of people have their own homes before they marry nowadays; will you put them in joint names?) Do you want children? Do you even have a time frame for having children and is it the same?

WAYS TO KEEP IT GOING

Everyone has their own ideas on how to keep love alive, but there are some techniques that most experts agree on. Make sure that you keep your own friends and pastimes so that you have new things to bring to the relationship; it may be tempting to spend all your time together but for most people that becomes more difficult as time goes on. Everyone needs to have somewhere to let off steam.

Many couples feel that avoiding arguments is a sign of success, for others a screaming match where anything goes can be an everyday occurrence. Both can be harmful in their own way, from storing up resentments to making spiteful accusations, but the main key for any couple is finding a way to express themselves, that both are comfortable with, when dealing with conflict. Part of being close means that you can say things to each other that you couldn't to other people, but this sometimes means that courtesy can slide – 'please', 'thank you' and 'can I make you a cup of tea?' will go a long way to keep you both feeling appreciated. And keep reminding yourselves that there's more to taking care of each other than just stopping the joint account from becoming overdrawn.

What else makes your relationship different to the others in your life? Your sex life. This can often suffer in the run up to the wedding as you have so much else going on and can often be too stressed or exhausted, but it is one of the key factors that makes your relationship special. Your honeymoon can be a great opportunity to reconnect on this level before you get back to your normal life.

IDEA 42, *Arguing*, helps you navigate the choppy waters of conflict before the big day. The same principles hold after you've got back from the honeymoon and your new life stretches ahead of you.

Try another idea...

'*A wedding anniversary is the celebration of love, trust, partnership, tolerance and tenacity. The order varies for any given year.*'
PAUL SWEENEY

Defining idea...

187

CHANGE – THE BIG CHALLENGE

Hopefully, you will spend the next 50 years in a state of bliss. A big part of this is allowing each other to change. Be realistic: the disco monster you married can't always be relied upon to get the party started when they've had little sleep thanks to your new baby. Don't tie people into the person they were at twenty, unless you can guarantee that you haven't changed a jot since you met; not even your underwear. (Which, in itself, could be grounds for divorce.)

How did it go?

Q   Sometimes I do worry that my partner and I might not change together. How can I help make that happen?

A   *Make sure that you re-evaluate your situation regularly, and keep questioning how things are working. That's why anniversaries are so important.*

Q   Aren't anniversaries just a chance to get some nice pressies and celebrate?

A   *Only if you don't use them properly. Book a nice restaurant and have a good old chinwag. It might seem a bit contrived at first, but it is a good time to reflect and recall all the good (and slightly dodgy) things about marriage during the past year, to take stock of the relationship and check that you are still heading in the same direction.*

188

44

The soundtrack to your life

Choosing the musical accompaniment to your wedding can be tricky, but if you get it right it can also unify your whole day *and* the congregation. You may love a bit of thrash metal when you're riding your Harley, but consider whether you'll want to dance to it when you're celebrating your twenty-fifth anniversary.

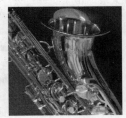

Spend plenty of time planning the music, and make sure you look beyond the boundaries of your normal tastes. Not everybody likes thrash metal! Your choice has to span generations and provide an atmosphere of good cheer. And make sure it is something that both of you really respond to.

PRACTICAL STUFF

Not sure where to start? There are lots of options, from string quartets, harpists, solo singers, jazz bands, and even a full choir. You will probably need ceremony music, reception music (as guests arrive), and band and/or a DJ.

Here's an idea for you... **Want to make sure that your first dance is memorable and super sleek? Book some dance lessons so that you can cut a dash. It will also give you a chance to relax together and escape the stressful bits of wedding work for a while, and have some fun.**

First, when you visit the locations consider their size and acoustics. The hotel manager, vicar or marquee provider should be able to give you some direction about what you need in terms of size, power and also, importantly, space. Also think about your surroundings: a spring church wedding might call for a string quartet whereas a night-time winter wedding might better suit a classical pianist.

Plan your requirements carefully with your musicians; don't just expect them to turn up and play as the guests are being seated. Ask them for recommendations – they will have lots of experience and might have some great suggestions. Make sure they get plenty of breaks and have ample space in which to play.

MUSIC FOR THE CEREMONY

There is more music for the ceremony than you might imagine. Firstly, you have the prelude, what the guests will hear as they are seated and wait for the proceedings to begin. This can be played by your harpist, classical quartet, organist or even on CD. Next, you have the bit everyone knows – processional music plays as you and your wedding party make your grand entrance. The classic wedding march music is 'The Bridal March' by Wagner. Other popular choices are 'Arrival of the Queen of Sheeba', Handel, 'Grand March' from Verdi's *Aida*, Vivaldi's 'Spring' from *The Four Seasons*. As well as thinking of the arrival music, you need to think of the recessional music (the piece played as you depart) and how they work together.

Don't be frightened of doing something a little off the wall – this is a buoyant time, everyone is happy and about to go and celebrate, so something equally cheery and happy should be played here. There are also 'interludes' during the ceremony, such as the signing of the register, when you may want music playing. Bear in mind you might also want hymns here too. There is also something called a postlude, which is the musical backdrop played as the guests mill out after your departure for the reception. This can stop things from feeling 'flat' if the church is suddenly empty and silent after you leave.

Make sure the DJ gets your party going by checking out IDEA 52, *All night long*, and making sure you give him the best direction.

Try another idea...

RECEPTION REVELLING

When selecting a band for the reception, ask them to give you a recording of their music or tell you where you can see them live. Some bands will only do their own set – and not play requests – so you need to be certain they will suit the occasion. It is common practice to pay the balance of the band's fee on the night (having paid a deposit to secure the date). The best man should have the money with him and deal with this. Even if you have a band, it is also common to have a DJ as well. With a carefully thought out play-list, you'll have the music you want.

'Life is like music: it must be composed by ear, feeling, and instinct, not by rule.'
SAMUEL BUTLER

Defining idea...

THE FIRST DANCE

What should your first dance be? It may be the first song that you danced to, or your favourite snogging song. Whatever you choose, you should be able to dance to it. If you don't have an obvious contender, maybe opt for an old classic that you could have a waltz to, or the popular song you hear everywhere that summer and that will always remind you of your happy day.

How did it go?

Q **My future wife is as wonderful a woman as she is terrible a dancer. I know she's dreading the idea of the first dance. Can we just forget that part?**

A *You can do whatever you want, but it's a nice tradition that adds another special touch to the day. If you do decide to drop the dance you should get your toastmaster or DJ to let all the guests know that you want everyone to do the first dance as a joint effort. Make sure they're not waiting for you to take a twirl or you could have a very empty dance floor. But are you sure you can't persuade her?*

Q **She really has no sense of timing so what sort of dance could I suggest that might persuade her to try?**

A *You could always try a waltz. A few lessons should teach her at least what her feet are meant to do, and then you can clamp her close to your body and take the lead. You'll look all manly and protective while stopping her from knocking over tables.*

45

Religious ceremonies

For many couples a religious ceremony is a vital part of making their matrimonial pledges. It is an essential part of how they see their commitment not just to each other, but also as part of their wider faith. Such ceremonies can add an extra layer of formality, though, so check what it would mean for you.

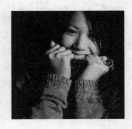

To avoid disappointment, talk at length with your selected celebrant about restrictions. For example, some houses of worship have limitations on the music that can be played (such as Wagner), the timing of readings and minimum church attendance by the couple. There are also simple factors, such as whether or not you can use confetti — some allow only biodegradable, some none at all.

Here's an idea for you...

If you want to be spontaneous start investigating how you can get a 'special licence'. This requires that one of you has lived in the registration district for at least 15 days prior to giving notice at the registry office. This is a more expensive option but it then allows a marriage to take place after only one clear day of giving notice (excluding a Sunday, Christmas Day or Good Friday). Be ready to provide certain documents to show the Superintendent Registrar – these may include a passport or some other form of identification. If either of you is divorced, you will need to show the original decree absolute of your divorce.

Some rules apply to everyone getting married in the UK, regardless of their faith: the minimum legal age for marriage is sixteen years old; in England and Wales, the written consent of the parents or guardians is required for those under eighteen who have not previously been married; and if either of them is below eighteen, a birth certificate must be produced.

A religious ceremony takes place in a venue that has been formally registered by the Registrar General for marriages. Some insist that you attend 'marriage lessons' and services, so do check with your desired church right from the outset. The first step should be to speak to your minister, who will talk you through all of the requirements.

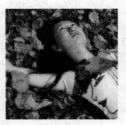

THE MAIN RELIGIOUS REQUIREMENTS

For Roman Catholic weddings you need to be baptised and confirmed, and you will also have to obtain a licence to marry. You must also be a regular attendee of the church or attend mass at least six weeks before the big day.

Although Jewish weddings are usually held in a synagogue, they can also be held in other locations. Talk to your rabbi about your specific requirements. Remember that you cannot marry on the Sabbath.

For Church of England ceremonies, generally you or your spouse-to-be have to live in the parish but you can ask to make a request with some other specific church. You need to get the approval of the vicar, who can facilitate this in one of two ways. He can either add you to the parish electoral role and you can be considered a regular worshipper, or you can apply for a special licence. If he is able to marry you he will arrange for the banns to be read on three Sundays before the day of the ceremony or for a common licence to be issued. These have to be posted to allow anyone to raise oppositions to the union. The vicar can also register the marriage so you do not need to get a licence as well.

Try another idea...

If you want to add some special personal touches to your ceremony, take a look at IDEA 6, *Getting readings right*, which outlines the ways you can use the readings to express yourselves more fully.

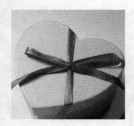

Defining idea...

'*All marriages are mixed marriages.*'
CHANTAL SAPERSTEIN

In the Church of Scotland, it is the celebrant that needs to be authorised, not the location, and there is no residency requirement, although you must still register at least 15 days before. Other religions in Scotland still have to meet with certain restrictions.

MIXED FAITH CEREMONIES

When mixed faiths are marrying, you need to find ways of bringing different aspects of your ceremonies together. One way of doing it is to get married in a civil service at a registry office and then create your own ceremony incorporating the most important aspects from both faiths. Alternatively, you can have your ceremony at one church, say a Catholic church, and ask a minister from a different religion to come and take part. The ceremony will be recognised as Catholic, however, and must be completed in full.

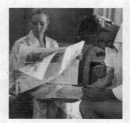
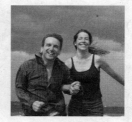

Q **My partner is Catholic, but I'm not. What does that mean about us getting married in church?**

How did it go?

A *You will probably need to have permission from the local bishop, and this can be arranged by your parish priest, who can also tell you how long it will take. (Leave plenty of time.) As a couple, you do have to make some commitments to the Church – you will both be expected to have wedding lessons on the Catholic idea of marriage, and your partner must promise to bring any children up as Catholics. (Don't fret if you can't promise this; it's your partner's responsibility as the Catholic parent.)*

Q **Can my sister – who isn't a Catholic either – do a reading?**

A *Yes, she can, and you can even include non-religious readings – just check with the priest before you cast any plans in stone.*

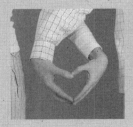 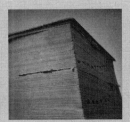

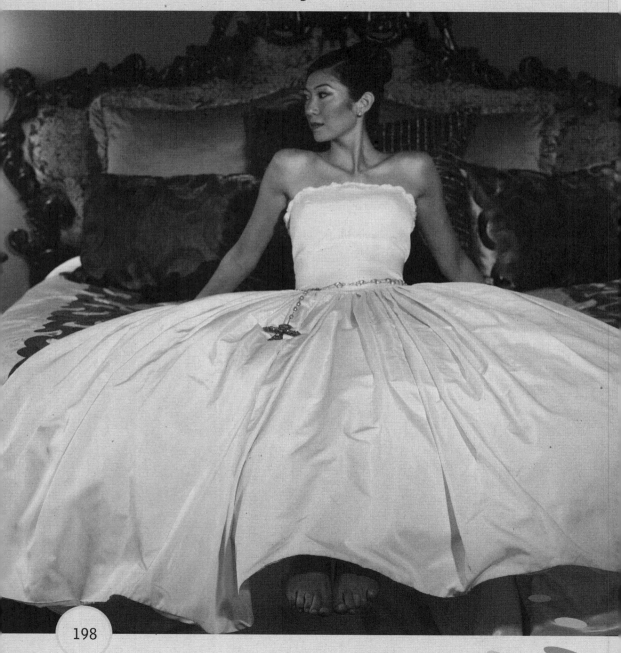

46

Seconds out

Second (or seventh) time around? Can you wear white? Do you have to invite ex-spouses? There are a few additional things to think about if this won't be your first time. Don't worry, though – with your experience and maturity, you'll breeze through them all.

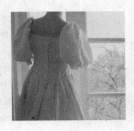

Legally, there is no limit to the number of marriages you can enter into, providing you are free to do so (meaning that you are widowed or divorced and can produce an original death certificate or decree absolute with the original court seal). However, the options can be more limited if it's not your first wedding.

There are, of course, restrictions to the kind of marriages that you can have second (or more) time around. You may be prevented from having a religious ceremony, although you can have a blessing by your minister. Only some denominations will allow second marriages in church. Start by speaking to your local church or synagogue about the options.

Here's an idea for you...

Ushers, bridesmaids, flower girls, ring bearers, best men and pages are all great roles for the various family members you would like to honour. Make a list of those people and see if you can find ways for them all to take part in a special way. You can always ask family members to do readings or even host tables so that they are all given a sense of place and importance. Having soon-to-be-step-sisters as bridesmaids can be a great way for them to get to know one another without the focus being on them.

ALL CONCERNED

Getting hitched more than once is not unusual these days, and despite the fact that everyone will probably be very happy for you, you will most likely need to tread with caution. The first important task is to tell all closely interested parties, so you don't run the risk of them hearing it elsewhere. Children from previous marriages or relationships should be the first to hear, to ensure that they feel special – after all, this will be a new family in their lives. Regardless of your relationship with the ex-partners, they should know as quickly as possible too. Even if things are strained, it is not fair for your children to deal with the fallout of spreading the news. When you make your announcement to them, you should already have an idea of how the future will look – where you all will live, what effects it will have on the others' daily life, how you envisage the children's relationship working with their new step-parent. It is natural for them to have a mix of fear and excitement, so give them enough warning to get used to the idea; not just the week before the wedding!

GETTING YOUR GUEST LIST TOGETHER

Another major issue is deciding who gets invited. You may have a very close relationship with your former in-laws, and want them to be there; or your partner's children may really want their mum or dad present. The Americans have a tradition called the rehearsal dinner, which usually takes place the night before the event. You could hold your own version of this some time before the wedding to introduce all key parties to one another – they shouldn't all be meeting for the first time on the big day. This should calm any initial anxieties and, with luck, leave you free to concentrate on your arrangements. Make sure you allow for partners and friends to accompany and support those who might find things a bit awkward.

Worried about where to put everyone? IDEA 33, *And to your left...*, will help you understand how seating plans work.

Try another idea...

WHAT DO I LOOK LIKE?

Again, here you'll need a little sensitivity. Don't drone on to your partner about what your last do was like – this is meant to be a fresh start for all of you. A lot of couples will also be paying for their second weddings themselves, so that might have a big influence on style. However, there are no restrictions here. As far as wearing white goes, do whatever you prefer: there are few people who adhere to the original implication that it represents purity, even those getting married for the first time.

'You can make those promises with just as much passion the second time around. Such is the regenerative power of the human heart.'
MARION WINK, *O Magazine*, 2003

Defining idea...

201

Do, however, consider your environment. If you are having a civil wedding, make sure that you dress suitably, and differently from the first time around. A second wedding is a great opportunity to do something that radiates your personality and how the two of you see yourselves living in the future. A big white wedding might have seemed right in your twenties, but in your forties you will probably have changed a lot. Maybe you've become an aficionado of salsa dancing in recent years and fancy a garden barbeque with a dance-off and hay bales for seating.

How did it go?

Q **We're planning our honeymoon and I really want my kids to come along, but my partner wants me to leave them at home. Who's being unreasonable here?**

A *As your married life will be about being a family, you really should acknowledge your partner's desire to spend your honeymoon purely as a couple. This will give you a good grounding for heading home and hitting the realities of your new family life.*

Q **What if the kids are too small to be left with grandparents for a whole two weeks?**

A *There's no point in going away if you will spend all the time making long-distance phone calls and fretting. Why not try a compromise? Perhaps you could arrange a short break so you can enjoy some quality time together as a couple in the aftermath of the wedding and then do something with the children.*

47

Tied to a lamp-post in Germany

Stag and hen nights are increasingly more elaborate and expensive, so how do you choose the one that's right for you? Here's how to get them right – basically, photocopy this and give it to your maid of honour and best man.

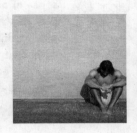

Traditionally these evenings were for each of the couple to say goodbye to their old lives with their old friends. However, some couples nowadays do a joint weekend of stags and hens. Just make sure you head off in the right direction when you set the wheels in motion.

MONEY, MONEY, MONEY

It's not easy to get the balance right, but do think about everyone you would potentially like to include. You may want a week in Ibiza clubbing and getting nice

Here's an idea for you... **Plan a dress code to give a sense of occasion, even if you plan to stay in. A load of men playing poker in dinner jackets will boost your glamour factor, as will a pampered hen in a tiara and dressing gown.**

and brown, but is it affordable for everyone else? (Think time as well as money.) You also won't be able to expect your beloved great aunt Agnes to mix it up in a club all night on her walking frame. If you are sure you want to do something big, be prepared to accept gracefully if people can't come, and resist the temptation to apply emotional blackmail.

There are ways, however, to make the large-scale ideas more affordable, such as hiring a villa or country cottage, which can make a trip away seem much more affordable. When it comes to making the finances add up, your best man and chief bridesmaid should be charged with the organising.

GETTING THE RIGHT RIOT

Listen, best men and chief bridesmaids, your idea of the perfect stag/hen night might not be the same as your guest of honour's. The fact of the matter is that opposites attract, and that includes friends as well as lovers. So don't plan something that they will find offensive or dull. Most brides and grooms expect their good humour to be stretched, but don't go so far that you alienate them.

Think laterally when planning your do. Dragging a drunk and motley crew around the streets isn't the only option. For sports buffs, a trip to a match, the dogs or horseracing can all provide entertainment as well as the hospitality that your guests might be expecting. More active sports buffs should consider a round of golf or a day on the dry ski slopes, kayaking or a spot of surfing. For any novices, signing them up to a surf or ski school for the day should cater for their skills deficit and make sure they get something out of it. Make sure you plan this in advance so no one is left out. Those feeling brave can even take it one step further and try a spot of camping; just don't combine pitching your tent on a cliff and a lot of booze. Alternatively, you can do something entirely regenerating, like a whole day in a spa.

Worried about what your role should be? Take a look at IDEA 26, *The supporting cast*, to let you know what is expected from your role in the proceedings.

Try another idea...

Any kind of activity that people can do together and gives a focus is ideal. Remember that you won't know everyone that your guest of honour does, so you may have to unify a fairly disparate group, including non-drinkers and older members of the party. Be sensitive when making plans. You can always start the evening with a nice dinner, which moves onto more raucous entertainment, so that people can bale out at different stages when they've had their fill.

HOW FAR IS TOO FAR?

Shaving bits, leaving someone stuck in another country and buying them sex with strangers are probably all going a bit too far.

'Everything is funny as long as it is happening to Somebody Else.'
WILL ROGERS, *Warning to Jokers: lay off the prince*

Defining idea...

205

PLANNING: A GUIDE FOR YOUR BEST MAN AND CHIEF BRIDESMAID

Ask the bride and groom what they want, but remember that you don't necessarily have to stick to it. It will give you an idea if they expect everyone to head off for a week in Bali or just pop along to the local pub. You will also get an idea if they want their parents invited (some do, you know), and if there are any people you should be inviting that you don't know about, such as long-lost school friends. Make sure you get all the contact details in one go so you don't have to worry about bugging them and letting things slip. Agree on a date too, as they may have something else planned. Let all the invitees know the date as soon as possible, even if you haven't confirmed the activities. Make sure it's *not* the night before if you have anything huge planned – no one will thank you for wedding photographs that look like the happy couple have been dug up.

You will need to think about transport, and making sure everyone gets about safely. If you are partying abroad, ask your hotel to help. And let everyone get an idea of cost beforehand. The guest of honour shouldn't pay for anything so the others need to chip in for their share. If you have an itinerary, copy it and give it to everyone in case you get lost. Have the requisite silly hats, plastic teeth and embarrassing outfits all ready before you take the first drink, or you may end up being lumbered with hundreds of penis shaped balloons in the kitchen drawer.

Q **I want to do a proper hen night the night before the wedding but I don't want to look like the bride of Dracula and stink like a chemistry set the next day. Any suggestions?**

How did it go?

A *Stay in.*

Q **OK, if I stay in the night before, what can I do that'll make it up to my bridesmaids?**

A *I said stay in, not go to bed. A great way to have your hen night the night before the wedding and look even buffer, rather than rougher, the following morning is to have a big pampering night in. Everyone gets a massage, facial or manicure, depending on how skilled you all are. Of course, you could always get a professional in – a masseuse or beautician that can make house calls to help with any tricky bits. Just don't let a drunk bridesmaid loose with some hair removal wax if she isn't too keen on the frock you've made her wear.*

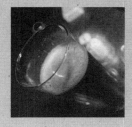 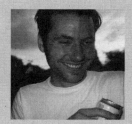 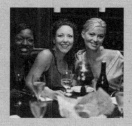

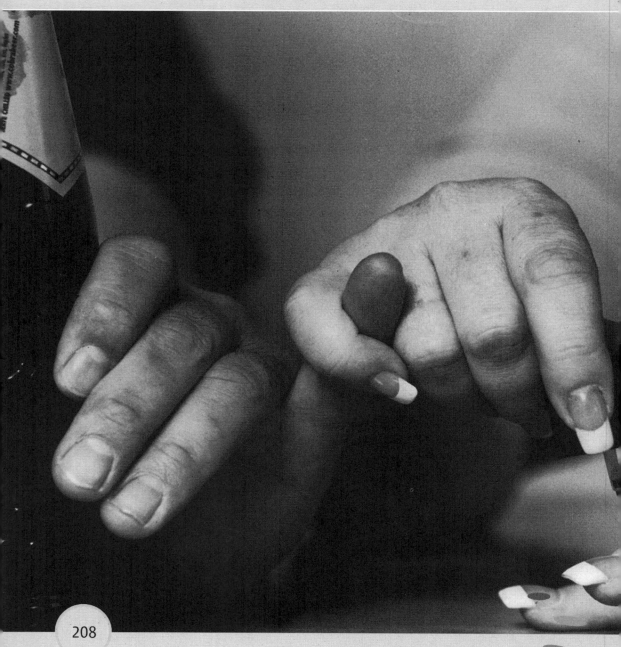

48

Commitment ceremonies

Not everyone can, or wants to, make a religious or legal commitment. Instead you could have a commitment ceremony, which allows you to signify your love for each other in front of your nearest and dearest. It can be as moving and memorable as a regular wedding.

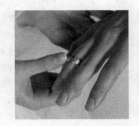

If you want guests to take your commitment ceremony seriously, you should select an officiant they can respect. Do not leave it just to your 'hilarious' best friend who can't resist limericks.

A religious celebrant, or some other person affiliated with a respected group, can get you started by giving you an example of typical ceremony wording from which to work. If you are religious and can't have a traditional wedding (such as a same sex marriage) you might have a sympathetic rabbi or vicar who is happy to come along and do a reading or take part in some other way. If not, you can have a friend or respected non-religious figure take the role of officiant.

Here's an idea for you...

Unfortunately, same sex weddings are not yet legal or recognised in many countries or religions, so a commitment ceremony is by far the best alternative. A same sex wedding does, however, bring up its own set of problems. Weddings, like all major life events, can bring up lots of feelings and issues for people, not all of them pleasant. Check with family members and friends that they are willing to acknowledge such a union. You may discover that they aren't comfortable taking part in such a major public ceremony, even though they seem to be happy with your relationship normally. If you encounter criticism, make sure you have other important but supportive figures in your life a phone call away, to remind you of how exciting it all really is.

SAYING 'I DO'

A commitment ceremony gives you a chance to write any kind of vows that you like. You can, of course, run it along the lines of a traditional ceremony to give it a sense of *gravitas*.

Start your ceremony by getting your celebrant to express your intentions. This will let everyone know what you believe your commitment means. As well as your vows to each other, consider including other traditional elements such as the exchanging of rings, having a friend or family member recite readings, and of course, the best bit, the kiss.

If you are opting not to make a legally binding commitment, you will not be protected by the rules of law (although common law rights can apply after a certain period of cohabiting). You may, therefore, want to make some other changes to your situation. Doing this is also a great way of starting a dialogue about what you will expect from each other, and your relationship, as a result of this ceremony.

Financially, you may want to open a joint account and change the names on your mortgage. If you want to protect your partner's future interests, you need to draw up wills to include each other, and make him or her the official recipient of any insurance policies. They will not automatically receive the benefits, regardless of your living situation. Make sure you are listed as the nearest of kin in passports and on medical records to protect your right to information in case something happens. Speak to a financial adviser or solicitor to clarify things. Your situation will be slightly different if you have children so you need to seek advice if you are concerned.

Want to plan a big do? IDEA 17, *Where: choosing a location,* will give you some ideas.

Try another idea...

HAVING IT ALL

Just because you haven't gone down the traditional route, it doesn't mean that you should miss out on the nice bits, such as fabulous outfits, big party, a wedding list and lots of flouncy bridesmaids.

When deciding what to wear, you can do exactly what you want, and follow tradition or do something completely different and have everyone in fairy wings and jeans. Make sure that your guests know what to expect, though – no one wants to turn up in an evening gown to a Hawaiian barbeque. Make sure that everybody know what to call you, too – will you still be 'partners' or are you two 'wives'?

'Intimacy is what makes a marriage, not a ceremony, not a piece of paper from the state.'
KATHLEEN NORRIS, writer

Defining idea...

How did
it go?

Q   **We want a commitment ceremony rather than a traditional wedding because we want a pagan union. Is it fair that we miss out on the perks other married couples get when they book their honeymoon?**

A   *Of course not, but you need to remember that hotels and airlines need to make sure that every couple claiming special treatment actually are wed, or they'd be handing out privileges and upgrades all over the shop, which is why they usually require the marriage certificate. You can try either booking a honeymoon package (you might have to explain the situation to your travel agent) or speaking to the airlines and hotels themselves. It will be up to their discretion, but you may be pleasantly surprised.*

Q   **Is there an easy way to ensure we don't miss out on the perks enjoyed by regular couples?**

A   *You could always avoid all the major hassles by holding your ceremony abroad. The specialist wedding departments of travel agents should be able to organise all the usual flowers, cake and dinners, but without the official legal bit. That way you are guaranteed the special treatment.*

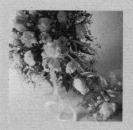 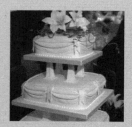

49

Have a great wedding night

So much thought goes into the wedding day it's easy to forget the wedding night. After all, surely those things take care of themselves. In reality, you'd be shocked to discover how many wedding nights end in disaster, or, more accurately, a chaste lump in a hotel four-poster. Make sure yours doesn't.

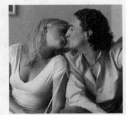

So, what's the wedding night all about? Well, the key ingredients are privacy, intimacy and, of course, a little sweet lovin'...

The honeymoon, which starts with your wedding night, has its roots (or one of them) in the Norse word 'hjunottsmanathr', which relates to the time when a bride was kidnapped from a neighbouring village, and then was hidden by the future husband. Their location was unknown, and when her family gave up searching for her, they could return from 'hiding', which is what the word means. In Ireland, the 'month of honey' relates to the strong honey brew mead, which they drank at the wedding and was meant to promote fertility. These explanations sum up the sentiment. So how do you make it live up to the expectations?

Here's an idea for you...

Your libido can be depleted or suppressed by being overtired and stressed, both of which are likely to happen to you in the run up to the wedding. Schedule in some decent rest in the month before your wedding, to make sure you are relaxed, happy and ready to roll, rather than strung out and desperate to turn out the lights.

RECONNECTING

It is not uncommon for couples to have spent time apart as the wedding day approaches, with hen and stag nights and last-minute plans all taking their toll. Consequently, you can't expect just to launch yourself into a love fest the minute you close the hotel door behind you. Intimacy doesn't just reappear without some effort. Take some time to refocus your minds back onto each other. Have a glass of champagne and enjoy the view from your hotel window, or take a bath together.

ALL IN THE TIMING

Most weddings are lengthy affairs nowadays, so you need to be realistic about your stamina. Don't party till three in the morning and then expect the performance of the century, as you will simply be too tired. If you really want a special night on the romance front, then why not consider leaving early? Make a proper exit while the party is still in full swing, then create your own. A good way of putting the party behind you is to book a first-night hotel, away from the reception. It will remove the temptation to go back downstairs for one last dance, and stop the best man and ushers from filling the bed with sausage rolls. Make sure that the hotel knows it is your wedding night, and be clear about any special requirements you have. Give them an estimated time of arrival and ask them to get the room ready. Low lamp light instead of glaring overhead light, champagne chilling on ice and petals across the bed will all create a wonderfully seductive mood as you enter. Call the hotel, or ask one of your attendants to, on the morning of the wedding to make sure they don't forget.

If you want to feel your desirable best, take a look at IDEA 20, *The body beautiful*, for hints on making sure you are as buff as you can be.

Try another idea...

DRINKING TOO MUCH AND PUTTING ON YOUR GLAD RAGS

This is one of the classic enemies of seduction, be it your wedding night or standard Saturday night. You should try to pace yourself and have a glass of water for every second drink. If you can't bear the thought of keeping your hands off the bubbles on your special day, then ask your bartender to mix you up a champagne cocktail with fruit and ice to keep you hydrated and the alcohol content slightly lower.

Slinky underwear is also a vital seduction tool, but don't feel that you have to wear something uncomfortable all day just because you want to be a sex goddess. You may also need to choose something special to wear under your dress if it is clingy or low cut. So you can always be a bit of a '50s siren and buy a special negligee for the occasion, making an entrance from the bathroom when you've slithered into it. For men, usually anything clean and new will suffice.

'If sex is such a natural phenomenon, how come there are so many books on how to?'
BETTE MIDLER

Defining idea...

How did it go?

Q **I've been with my partner for ten years and I'm afraid our wedding night is just going to be like any other – a ready meal and TV! Even fancy underwear seems passé nowadays. What can I do to spice things up?**

A *Think about learning a little sexy dancing, such as stripping or a hot tango. You might think you'd be embarrassed, but that's exactly the point of the class, to make you feel differently about your body, build some confidence and help you see yourself in a different light. Try it. You might like it.*

Q **I'm worried that we'll be so emotionally drained that we won't be in the right mood for anything much on our wedding night. Any ideas on how we could get a fruity feel to the evening?**

A *You will have a powerful sense of relief, maybe loss, that it's all behind you but this is the chance for you to relax. While you're sipping champagne, why not get the mood right by playing some erotic games as you wind down? There are many saucy books out there that could get your imaginations going.*

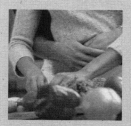
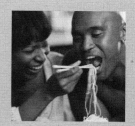

50

Time lines

There are lots of ways to organise a wedding, and plenty of different types of weddings to organise. Here's a plan of attack for you, based on the average wedding in the UK.

In some faiths you may be expected to attend 'wedding lessons' (a series of meetings to discuss the expectations you have of marriage) and a Catholic marrying a non-Catholic will usually need special permission from the bishop, which may take a little time. These sorts of requirements need to be planned for well in advance.

A year to the day before the event, you will need to book your wedding and reception venues. You should also meet with your celebrant to talk about the type of ceremony you would like and whether there are any conditions you must fulfil. At this point, you should also start meeting caterers to ensure that you get them for the date that you want.

Here's an idea for you...

Finding it all too much to handle? Get a professional in to do the work for you. A wedding organiser can take the pressure off and manage all the chasing and arranging. If they are good, they'll do all this with a huge book of contacts containing all the best suppliers in the business. If you are doing the planning yourselves, make sure that both of you read these pages and get a clear idea of the work involved and when it needs to be done. Many wedding stress complaints come from partners who feel they are doing all the work themselves, so divide the responsibilities up early in the planning.

Around this time, you should also start creating your guest list, as should your partner and close family members, to give you a reasonable idea of the numbers to work with. It will also give you a good idea of budget expectations and help you make decisions about sit-down meals versus buffets.

At ten months, you should book your photographer and/or videographer, musicians and/or band, and order your wedding cake. Suppliers who can only be booked for one job a day need to be booked up first.

At eight months you can start the more fun bits, such as choosing your attendants, best man and ushers. You can then get them to help you decide on the tough stuff like wedding dress, suits and their outfits. Remember, it can take at least four months for a made-to-measure dress to be created, and even some off-the-peg dresses need to be ordered from abroad.

This is also a time when you need to start confirming things. You need to plan flowers, and order them with your florist if you want something complex or out of season. Take a look at honeymoon brochures, and investigate wedding lists. You will need to register before you send out your invitations.

At seven months, plan your ceremony and whether or not you will need musicians. Visit your stationer's and order your invites, cake boxes (if you intend to send them out), reception cards and place cards, and the printing of the order of ceremony. If you want special cars or transport, book them now. Make sure anyone doing a reading has the relevant pieces.

At six months, we get another dose of fun stuff. You can plan your going away and honeymoon clothes, and any hired formal wear needs to be booked. You might also want to send out 'save the date' cards if you have a particularly popular weekend in summer planned for your nuptials.

At four months, you should tie up any outstanding bookings, such as the first-night hotel and confirming the DJ or band. You might also want to think about changing your passport, driving licence, insurance, doctor – all the things that you need to have your new married name on. This will give you plenty of time to make sure the name on your passport matches the one on your ticket. Check if you need any immunisations or visas for your honeymoon. Choose your wedding rings.

You should now be entering a more peaceful period, one that allows you to spend time working out seating plans and making up your gift list. It is customary to send out the invites at least six weeks before the wedding, but do it as soon as you feel comfortable – you can then start making a list of acceptances to finalise the catering arrangements. Don't forget to include your gift list cards.

Want to get started on the planning? Have a look at IDEA 2, When: date and time, on choosing the right time of year to say 'I do'.

Try another idea...

'Marriage is that relationship between man and woman in which the independence is equal, the dependence mutual, and the obligation reciprocal.'
LOUIS K. ANSPACHER

Defining idea...

219

At two months to go, make sure you have any missing pieces of your outfit, such as shoes, underwear or jewellery. You should also be able to start confirming numbers with your caterer. Purchase attendants' gifts and make sure that you have them engraved straightaway if necessary.

In the final month, arrange a rehearsal, learn any readings or lines, make sure the rings are ready, enjoy your hen and stag nights and get your luggage ready to send to your first-night hotel. Give yourself a pampering treat to get into the spirit of celebration and excitement, and to ease the stress of it all. It's fun from here onwards.

How did it go?

Q **I've just got a job abroad and so we've had to bring our wedding date forward by two months! Am I going to have to kiss my glam wedding goodbye?**

A *Not necessarily. If you are now marrying in the less popular winter months, you may be able to get the church and reception room you originally wanted (allowing for Christmas parties of course). These are the hardest parts to rearrange. And there are often cancellations for various reasons (such as yours), so do bother to check.*

Q **What's the best idea if we can't get the church on the right day?**

A *Then have a quiet, legal civil wedding early in the week and find a grand venue for the day you wanted. Have a celebrant present so you can do your vows again, as you would like them.*

51

When things go wrong

Sometimes the best intentions in the world aren't enough, and things go wrong. Here's what to do if you think you've come to the end of the road.

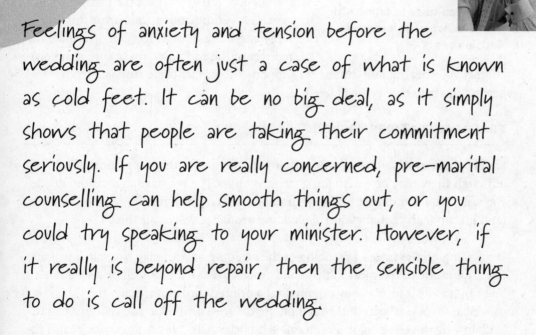

Feelings of anxiety and tension before the wedding are often just a case of what is known as cold feet. It can be no big deal, as it simply shows that people are taking their commitment seriously. If you are really concerned, pre-marital counselling can help smooth things out, or you could try speaking to your minister. However, if it really is beyond repair, then the sensible thing to do is call off the wedding.

Don't be frightened: if you need help, ask for it. Your whole present and your planned future life have changed in a heartbeat, which no one can be expected to cope with on their own. A counsellor will be able to help you come to terms with the news, whether it was your decision or not.

BREAKING IT OFF

The place to start is to talk to your partner, although you may want to talk to a close family member or friend beforehand to help you choose the correct wording or gain confidence. You can expect the usual fallout of pain and recriminations, unless you are very lucky and it is a mutual decision. If you are the receiver of the bad news, make sure that you contact your nearest and dearest for support – do not let pride stop you from getting the help that you will need.

PRACTICAL CONSIDERATIONS

Ideally, the person calling off the wedding should deal with the practicalities, although there may be extenuating circumstances. If it is a mutual decision, divide the task. You must expect to lose your deposits on most, if not all, of your bookings (and it is unlikely that any kind of wedding insurance will cover this).

Depending on the stage of planning of the wedding, invites may have already gone out. This is one of the most difficult and emotional parts of cancelling a wedding. You can handle it formally by sending out a printed card announcing the cancellation, or deal with it through phone calls or emails. You may not want to explain why the wedding has been called off, in which case ask family or friends to deal with this and give them an official line.

You should always try to return gifts, although it is not always possible. At the very least, a thank you card should be sent. Gifts not yet delivered from your wedding list should be easy to cancel, but your list service may demand a fee for refunding payments – check their small print.

Find yourself overwhelmed by the wedding plans but unsure how to change your situation? Don't let things get on top of you: see IDEA 14, *How to say 'I don't' and 'you do'*, for pointers on getting help.

Try another idea...

LIGHTENING THE FINANCIAL BURDEN

It will be up to you to decide who has to carry the financial burden, and whether it is shared or not. Be careful that you are fair to people who have not hurt you, such as family members who have offered to pay for parts of the wedding. You can try to minimise the financial fallout from this situation by checking all of the cancellation policies. For some there could be a cut-off date after which you have to pay the full fee. At a stressed time like this it may be hard to pay attention to such details, but remember that it could save you from paying for the cancellation for years to come.

If you are having the wedding dress made, you might be able to pay for work done so far. Your shop will expect payment but they may be prepared to try to sell the dress on for you. You can also choose to give it to charity.

'When you make a mistake, don't look back at it long. Take the reason of the thing into your mind and then look forward. Mistakes are the lessons of wisdom. The past cannot be changed. The future is yet in your power.'
HUGH WHITE

Defining idea...

223

WHO GETS TO KEEP THE ENGAGEMENT RING?

As with deciding who has to make the phone calls, what happens to the ring is up for some debate. You may simply want to reclaim as much money as possible from the wedding costs and decide to sell it, or you may want to hold onto it as a keepsake. As a rule of thumb, the person calling off the wedding should be led by the wishes of the second party, all things being equal. However, the wedding may be called off due to unreasonable behaviour, in which case the rules change again. Once again, think of the other people involved – a family heirloom should be returned to the family it came from, regardless of why the wedding was cancelled. Let your conscience be your guide and do think carefully. After all, do you really want to keep a ring from a wedding that didn't happen?

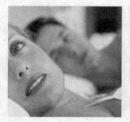 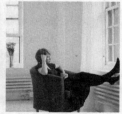

Q **Unfortunately, I decided to call off my wedding. After all of the stress of the planning and upset of cancelling it, I want to go away. The honeymoon destination is my dream ticket. Is it ethical for me to ask if I can take the trip?**

How did it go?

A *You'd need to approach this with supreme caution, and expect some bitterness. If your ex-partner agrees, you need to cover the full cost of the trip yourself. You will also need to have his name changed on the tickets and this will probably cost you extra.*

Q **What if he says no?**

A *Accept gracefully and check if you can reclaim some of the costs from your travel insurance.*

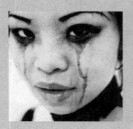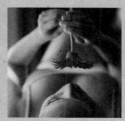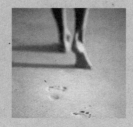

225

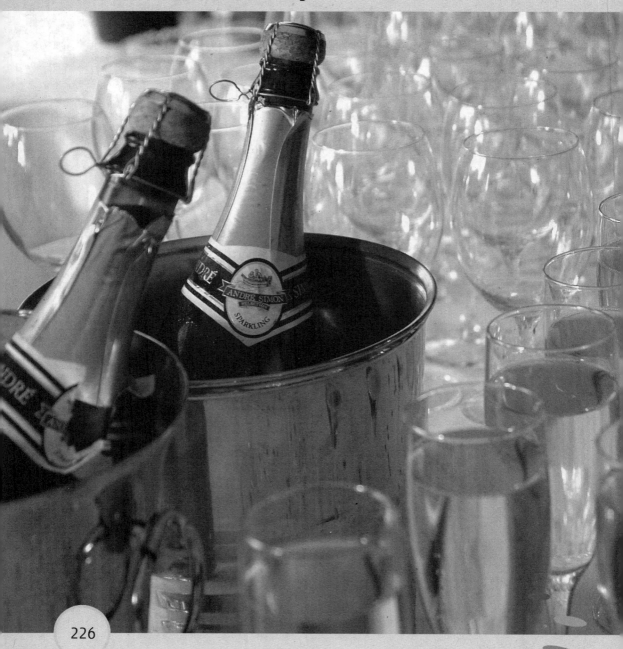

All night long

There's a knack to throwing a party, and if you don't want everyone to end up in the kitchen – or in this case, the bar – you need to follow this guide to get (and keep) the party going.

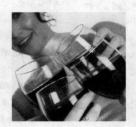

Good parties don't come easy, and the more you plan the better chance you have of enjoying it yourself.

The first step is to have a designated party handler. If you have a schedule to stick to, you will want to be sure someone else is in charge of monitoring it, and you won't want to be trying to help the DJ find an extra plug for his amp. The best man is a good candidate. Unlike any other party you will ever throw, it shouldn't be your responsibility.

When planning the schedule, allow for the fact that not all guests will be arriving at the same time. You shouldn't expect guests to hit the dance floor immediately; they will want to arrive, mingle with friends and warm up into the party spirit gradually. If you want your evening guests to witness your first dance, make sure that you allow enough time for the stragglers to arrive. A good way to make sure that

Make a track list of the songs you would like to have played. Give it to the DJ in advance; it will ensure that you are not disappointed on the night when you discover the last record he bought was purchased in the year you were born. Make CD copies of these favourites, or ones that you feel are most evocative, and give them to guests as wedding favours.

weddings keep moving along is to keep people informed, so get someone to act as toastmaster. They can welcome the evening guests, announce the running order for the celebrations and introduce the first dance.

Think about the length of your wedding and make sure that you cater properly, with enough nibbles and drinks for each phase. A dry wedding would equal a complete disaster in most people's eyes but ensure that among the alcohol you have a great mix of soft drinks that are a little more enticing than warm cola. You don't want people passing out from either boredom or alcohol poisoning.

Some people aren't comfortable with children being at a wedding reception, so think this through beforehand and decide on a policy. If they do come, make it clear that the parents must be responsible for their good behaviour. Watching little Joey slide across the dance floor, toppling bridesmaids as he goes, very quickly loses its charm and nobody will thank you for their broken ankle.

LIGHTING

This is one of the key factors when planning a good party. A room with naked light bulbs hanging grimly over the dance floor will certainly not guarantee any kind of swinging mood. What you need to make people feel ready to shake their funky stuff is a touch of low-level anonymity. Talk to your hotel or marquee hire company about the effect you want to create. You can have lanterns or candlelight on the tables, or something a bit more flashy if you want to create a '70s disco feel. Also talk to your DJ about any lighting he usually provides. He might be able to save you money, or you may want to stop him bringing his lights if they clash with your theme.

IDEA 25, *Drink and be merry,* **will help you organise that other party essential – the bar.**

Try another idea...

GET INTO THE GROOVE

Choosing the right music is essential for setting a great tone for dancing. You and your partner may have met in the flickering lights of a techno rave, but not everyone is going to thank you if you book the same DJ for old time's sake. You have many different age groups and tastes to consider, so give it some serious thought. You will want to see all your favourite family members and friends hitting the dance floor, so a range of styles from different eras is most appropriate.

Don't forget that some guests won't want to dance. You need to make sure there are places for them to sit and relax. Don't have the music too loud in the early part of the evening, as some guests will want to chat and catch up with arriving friends; they won't appreciate blaring music.

PIMP OUT THE USHERS

Ask your ushers to keep an eye out for ladies of all ages, from five to ninety-five, and see that they get a dance. It's a great way to make sure that they feel taken care of and included, and it gets people chatting and mixing.

'Dance is the hidden language of the soul.'
MARTHA GRAHAM, US modern dancer and choreographer

Defining idea...

229

How did
it go?

Q **I want a proper DJ at my wedding that my friends will really enjoy but I don't want to alienate my older relatives. What can I do to keep everyone happy?**

A *One option is to have a separate marquee for dancing that leaves other guests free to stay chatting and mingling in the main marquee. That way people can come and go as they please.*

Q **What's an option if we haven't got enough space for a separate dance tent?**

A *You could have a live band earlier in the evening dedicated to old classics by the likes of Cole Porter and Ella Fitzgerald. That gives a chance to those who want to dance to something traditional and refined. Then you start the hardcore dancers off a little later after the relatives have had their turn around the floor.*

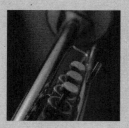
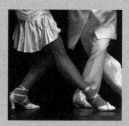

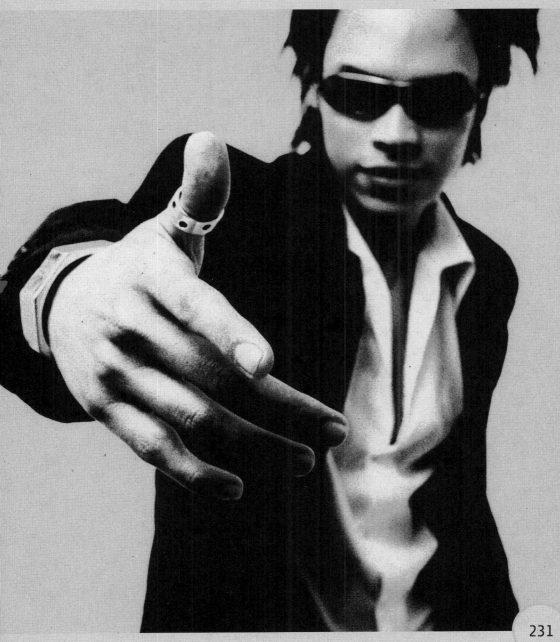

The end...

Or is it a new beginning?

We hope that the ideas in this book will have inspired you to go for your fantasy wedding.

So, why not let *us* know how you got on? What did it for you – what helped you get hitched without a hitch? Maybe you've got some tips of your own that you'd like to share. If you liked this book you may find we have more brilliant ideas for other areas that could help change your life for the better. You'll find us, and a host of other brilliant ideas, online at www.infideas.com.

If you prefer to write, then send your letters to:
Perfect weddings
The Infinite Ideas Company Ltd
36 St Giles, Oxford OX1 3LD, United Kingdom

We want to know what you think, because we're all working on making our lives better too. Give us your feedback and you could win a copy of another *52 Brilliant Ideas* book of your choice. Or maybe get a crack at writing your own.

Good luck. Be brilliant.

Offer one

CASH IN YOUR IDEAS

We hope you enjoy this book. We hope it inspires, amuses and educates you.
But we don't assume that you're a novice, or that this is the first book that you've
bought on the subject. You've got ideas of your own. Maybe our author has missed
an idea that you use successfully. If so, why not send it to info@infideas.com, and if
we like it we'll post it on our bulletin board. Better still, if your idea makes it into
print we'll send you £50 and you'll be fully credited so that everyone knows you've
had another Brilliant Idea.

Offer two

HOW COULD YOU REFUSE?

Amazing discounts on bulk quantities of Infinite Ideas books are available to
corporations, professional associations and other organizations.

For details call us on:
+44 (0)1865 514888
or e-mail: info@infideas.com

Where it's at...

Lose weight and stay slim

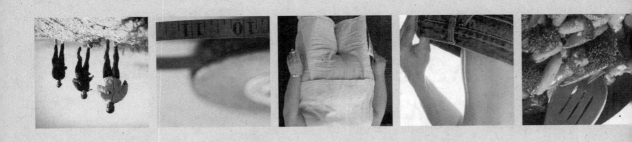

Eve Cameron

Secrets of fad-free dieting

Lose weight and stay slim

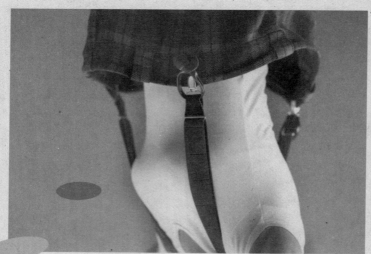

52 brilliantideas
one good idea can change your life...

First published in 2008 by
The Infinite Ideas Company Limited
36 St Giles
Oxford
OX1 3LD
United Kingdom
www.infideas.com

A CIP catalogue record for this book is available from the British Library.

ISBN 978-1-905940-34-9

Previously published as *Perfect weddings* (978-1-904902-25-6) and *Lose weight and stay slim* (978-1-904902-22-5).

Brand and product names are trademarks or registered trademarks of their respective owners.

Text designed and typeset by Baseline Arts Ltd, Oxford
Cover designed by Cylinder
Printed and bound in India

Brilliant ideas

Brilliant features

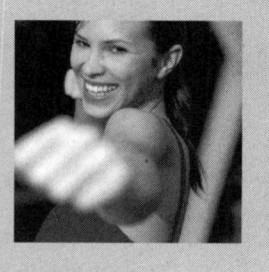

Each chapter of this book is designed to provide you with an inspirational idea that you can read quickly and put into practice straight away.

Throughout you'll find four features that will help you to get right to the heart of the idea:

■ *Try another idea* If this idea looks like a life-changer then there's no time to lose. *Try another idea* will point you straight to a related tip to expand and enhance the first.

■ *Here's an idea for you* Give it a go – right here, right now – and get an idea of how well you're doing so far.

■ *Defining ideas* Words of wisdom from masters and mistresses of the art, plus some interesting hangers-on.

■ *How did it go?* If at first you do succeed try to hide your amazement. If, on the other hand, you don't this is where you'll find a Q and A that highlights common problems and how to get over them.

Introduction

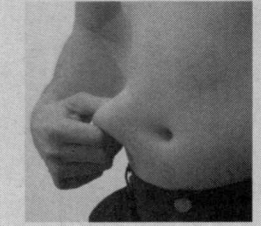

I swear it appeared overnight. That spare tyre around my middle was not there when I was thirty-four. But on my thirty-fifth birthday I saw it hanging over my jeans.

I tried holding my tummy in. I tried walking taller. I tried on a different pair of jeans. But there it sat, like a hideous unwanted gift that you haven't got the receipt for, so can't take back. I knew perfectly well how it had got there though. Despite being a regular exerciser, I was also a big eater. As well as consuming large portions of food, I had, and still have actually, a Very Sweet Tooth, so I'd have lots of sweet things as snacks too. At some point, the calories in must have overtaken the calories out, which is how I, and in fact how anyone, puts on weight. Yes, there may be other reasons (medications and medical conditions for example) but mostly you gain weight because you eat too much and don't move enough. So, the solution is quite obviously to eat less and move more. But of course that's easier said than done. Still, there's plenty of help out there. Isn't there?

Does the world really need another diet book I asked myself when I first spoke to Infinite Ideas. If it didn't, we decided, we'd all be slim, healthy and happy, because all those other diet books would have answered our questions, given us all the advice and tips we need and the motivation and success tools to help us lose weight and, importantly, keep it off. So, what's different about this book? First, there's the fabulous format. The chapters, or ideas, as we prefer to call them, are nice, manageable chunks, that are self-contained, yet link to other ideas. Each also has a section that answers the questions you might have on a given subject. This format means you can dip in and out as you please, though if you want to read the whole book in one go, do feel free.

Content-wise, rather than being the sort of diet book that tells you to have 50 g of pineapple for lunch, or to do fifty press ups before breakfast, you'll find that this is a more holistic guide to losing weight. It deals with motivation, body shape, healthy eating, decoding food labels, fitness and examines popular diets and much more! In short, it's packed with everything that could possibly be relevant to you and losing weight.

Throughout the book, you'll find some recurring themes, which I think are the key issues of successful weight loss. And because they're key issues, I'm going to tell you what they are here (but I hope you still read the rest of the book).

Diets are not something to be jumped on and off like buses. That's why most diets don't work. A special diet may be fine (unless you get really bored by day three) until you go back to eating normally and then you pile the pounds back on. The only way to lose weight permanently is to change your eating habits for good. That doesn't mean denial either (most diets are about denial by the way) – it's about eating healthily, consuming a variety of foods, some in moderation and keeping a check on your portion sizes. Small changes and a long-term view are more successful than short-term bursts of enthusiasm.

Physical activity is a must. That doesn't mean that you have to work out at a gym with muscle-bound Vin Diesel look-alikes every night of the week. But what it does mean is getting at least half an hour's moderate exercise five times a week. It could be gym-based, studio classes, sports, dancing, running, walking – anything really to get your heart rate up and work those muscles. As well as burning up calories and toning your body, exercise has so many health benefits, it's worth making time for it. And if you have kids, make activity part of their lives too, for fun, but also for their future health and wellbeing.

Realistic goals are essential for motivation and success. There are tools in this book to help you work out whether you really are overweight and by how much. But it's important to be realistic in your goals. A small, apple-shaped person can never be a tall pear-shaped person and vice versa. Aim to be in the best possible shape you can be. If you set yourself achievable targets you'll get there. Goals that are impossible to reach just make you miserable. Equally, be realistic about the speed at which you'll lose weight. Crash diets (which are faddy diets or very low calorie ones) cause rapid weight loss, but it's mostly water and lean tissue, rather than fat. Eating sensibly and losing just a pound or two a week is preferable – it's easier for one thing, not to mention healthier for your body and most important of all is sustainable, i.e. you won't suddenly return to your former weight the minute you so much as look at a doughnut. Remember, the tortoise won the race, not the hare!

So those are the big learning points, but this book gives you all the knowledge, tips and ideas you'll need in bite-sized chunks that will get you to where you want to be. And if there's one other suggestion I could make, it's cook, or learn to cook! Most experts now agree that part of our burgeoning obesity problem is due to the fact that we rely on junk food, takeaways and processed, ready-made meals. Home-made food tends to be lower in fat, salt and sugar (and of course contains fewer additives). I found myself agreeing with Prince Charles recently, who was saying how he thought domestic science should be reintroduced to schools. Most kids I know don't have a clue how to boil an egg. In fact, lots of grown ups I know don't know how to boil an egg! The truth is it takes the same amount of time to whip up a tasty, healthy, weight-loss-friendly meal as it does to reheat a ready meal or get a takeaway. The price isn't that different either. The only difference is to your waistline. Do you think the world could use another cookbook?

Here's to your success!

Eve

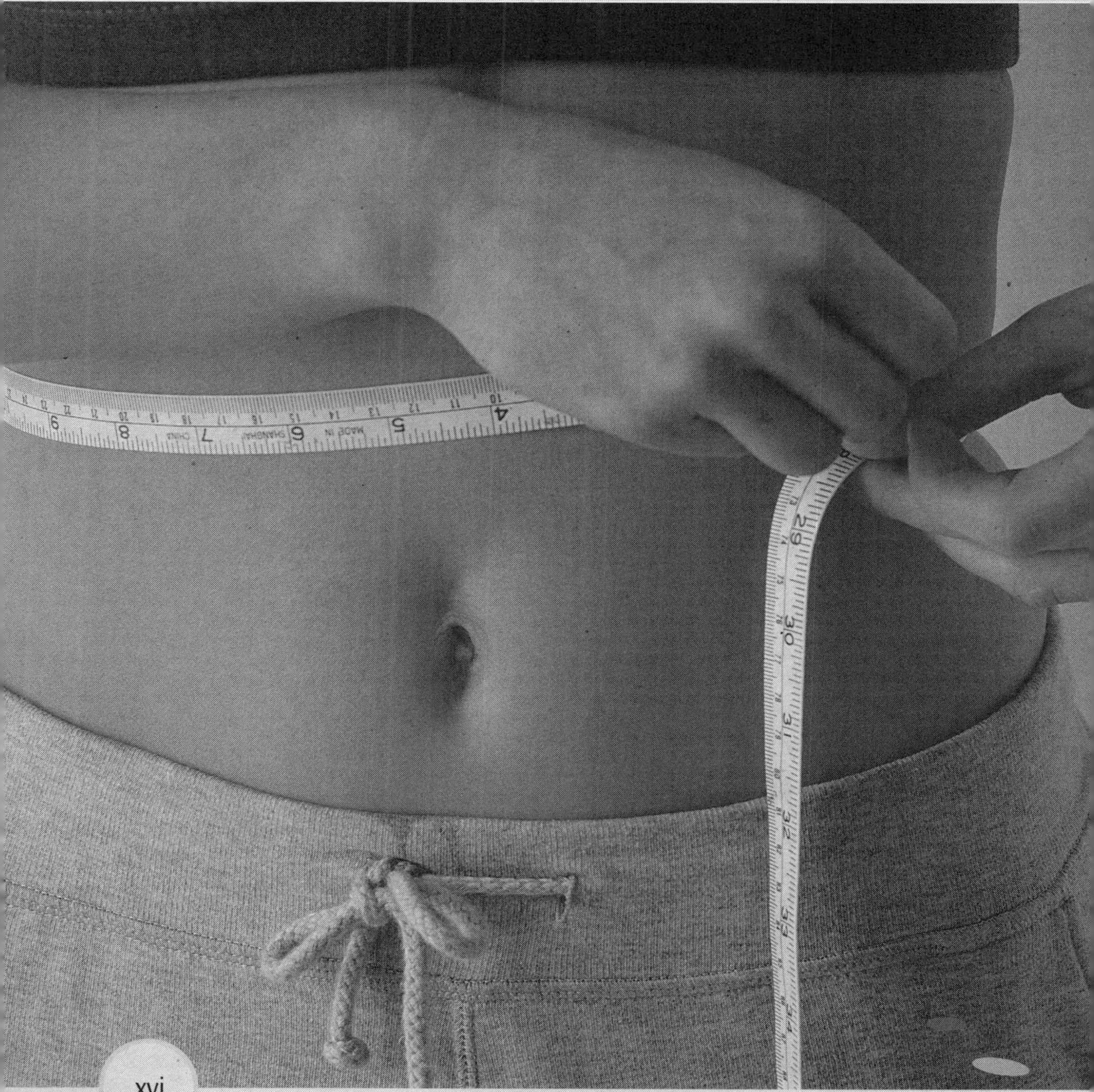

1

A weighty issue
(or, a weighty question)

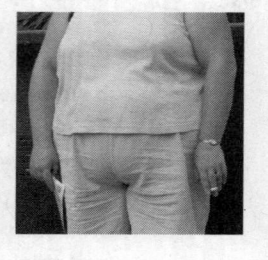

Have your waistbands been feeling a little tighter recently? Or are kaftans the only clothes you really feel comfortable in now? Here's how to work out roughly the right weight for you, plus some news you can use about body shape.

Judging by the newspaper headlines screaming about some new statistic or research about obesity, you'd think there was a moral obligation to be thin.

Often the subtext is that fat people get sick and are a burden on our medical resources. And then there are the images of super-slim models and celebrities that confront us in magazines and on our TV and movie screens. The underlying message here is that this is the way you're supposed to look, especially if you want to be happy and successful, not to mention being sexually attractive. Yet half the world is starving. It's enough to make you choke on your chocolate bar, isn't it?

Here's an idea for you...

Measure your waist and hips. Many experts are now saying that abdominal fat is the killer, with apple-shaped people who have relatively slim hips and a larger waist being more at risk from developing heart disease than the pear-shaped – those who carry their fat on their hips and thighs. The ideal waist measurement for men is less than 95 cm (37 inches) and less than 80 cm (32 inches) for women. Over 100 cm (40 inches) for a man and over 90 cm (35 inches) for a woman indicates the greatest risk to health.

Obesity is undeniably a growing problem in the Western world, due mainly to the over-consumption of the wrong kinds of foods and decreased activity levels. Experts warn of the host of health dangers to which carrying too much weight exposes you, including heart disease, diabetes, high blood pressure and, for women in particular (though not exclusively), fertility problems. It's not guaranteed that you'll develop these kinds of health problems – obesity just heightens your risk, which is of course why most of us just carry on regardless – until something goes wrong. The chances are that if you're already suffering any of the conditions mentioned, your doctor has grilled you on your diet and suggested losing weight.

For the majority of us, slimming down is more of a preventative health measure or something we want to do for cosmetic reasons: i.e. we just don't like the way we look. This is fine, as long as it isn't interfering with daily life and manifesting itself as disordered eating (anorexia, bulimia, faddy eating and so on). If that is the case for you, please seek help through a doctor or therapist. Life is too short and too precious not to enjoy it to the full.

Working out if you're really overweight is easily done using the Body Mass Index calculation. I have to point out that this method is not without its critics (partly because if you're quite well-muscled, you'll be heavy, not fat, because muscle

weighs more than fat) but my feeling is you have to start somewhere! All you have to do is weigh yourself and record the result in kilograms. Then measure your height in metres. Then do the following sum:

If you're doubtful or put off by the idea of more physical activity, turn to IDEA 12, *Why exercise makes you feel on top of the world.*

Try another idea...

weight in kilograms divided by (height in metres × height in metres) = BMI

Example:
You weigh 70 kg and you are 1.6 metres tall

$$70 \div (1.6 \times 1.6) =$$
$$70 \div 2.56 = 27.34$$
$$BMI = 27.34$$

'*I'm not overweight. I'm just nine inches too short.*'
SHELLEY WINTERS

Defining idea...

Check your own result against the ranges below

BMI for men	BMI for women	
Under 20	under 19	underweight
20–24.9	19–24.9	normal
25–29.9	25–29.9	overweight
30 plus	30 plus	obese

I fall into the upper level of normal weight, which is fine from a fatness perspective, but I know that I've crept up two dress sizes in the past decade and so estimate that losing three kilos (and keeping it off!) would take me where I want to be. That's my weight-loss mission; now work out yours.

How did it go?

Q   But I come from a fat family. I don't stand a chance...do I?

A   *We can blame our parents for lots of things, including a tendency to gain weight. However, much of 'hereditary' weight gain can also be explained by learned behaviour. For instance, if you come from a family that loves food, over-eating may be part of your lifestyle, but habits can be unlearned.*

Q   Could my weight gain be a result of a slow metabolism?

A   *Your BMR, or basal metabolic rate, is the number of calories your body needs to maintain its vital functions. This is partly to do with genetic inheritance. A friend who is a similar height and weight to you may well be able to eat more than you and not gain weight. This is very annoying, but you're probably better at other things than he or she is. There are two things to remember. First, if you have less body fat and more muscle, your metabolism will be higher, as muscle burns up more calories than fat. That's why including exercise in your weight loss plan really works. Second, don't try to cut calories drastically, as your metabolic rate will slow to adjust – and you'll just feel hungry all the time. Eating less but eating well is the key to long-term weight loss.*

Q   Why is it that men can eat more than women?

A   *The reason is that they are mostly bigger than women, so they use more energy for day-to-day maintenance. They also tend to have more lean muscle tissue than women – muscle tissue is more metabolically active than fat tissue, which means it uses up more energy (calories) to exist. Women tend to have more fat tissue.*

2

Food accountancy
made simple

You can eat them, count them or ignore them, but here's why knowing your calories from your onions is the key to losing weight.

Many books make calories unnecessarily hard to understand, but the concept is really quite simple. Once you have grasped what calories mean, you have a powerful tool to help you control your weight.

Put simply, calories are just the basic units by which both the energy values of food and the energy needs of the body are measured.

You may be familiar with diets that advocate counting your daily calorie intake. It's now seen as a rather old-fashioned way to slim, not least because you have to weigh things obsessively and eating anywhere but at home becomes a nightmare. It can also make you very boring to be around as you proceed to tot up the number of calories on everyone's plate. You may find that friends stop returning your calls!

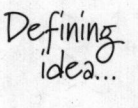

Include soya products in your diet. A particular isoflavone in soya may hold the key to improving the rate at which your cells burn up fat. It also boosts your metabolism slightly and reduces your appetite. From a looks perspective, I have it on good authority that soya helps to make your nails grow too!

However, it is really important to have some general knowledge about the calorific value of foods so you can make the best choices about what you're going to eat.

Most foods are a combination of protein, fat and carbohydrate in different ratios depending on the food. Gram for gram, fat contains 9 calories, protein and carbohydrates 4 calories and alcohol, if you're interested, 7 calories.

Basically if you eat anything in excess, there's the potential that it will be more than your body needs in terms of energy or calories and will end up stored as fat. Of course it's easier to reach your maximum calorie needs quickly if you cram in lots of high-fat foods, as they have the most calories. Also, the most nutritious choices may not always be available, especially when you are away from home.

HOW MANY CALORIES DO YOU NEED?

I'm going to give you a basic formula to work this out (calculators at the ready!) but it will only be an approximate calculation. It should still be enlightening, though. The reason it is only an approximation is because if we were going to be really scientific, we would have to factor in other information. Your gym or local health centre can probably help you with these calculations if you want to be more precise.

Defining idea...

'Two out of every three men in the UK are now classed as overweight or obese.'
THE BRITISH DIETETIC ASSOCIATION

One of the factors that makes a difference is your age, because your calorie needs diminish as you get older. By the way, this is for adults only,

so please don't try this on your kids. Your sex is important too. As men have more muscle than women and muscle burns up more calories than fat, men need more calories just to exist.

Understanding the nutritional values of what you eat is vital. Wise up with IDEA 30, *What does it say on the label?*

Try another idea...

Now let's play with some numbers:

First work out your *basal metabolic rate* (BMR) which tells you the energy you need to stay alive. Multiply your weight in pounds by 10 if you're a woman, or 11 if you're a man. (If you're a metric sort of person, first multiply your weight in kilos by 2.2 to get the poundage.) Next, factor in how active you are by multiplying the sum above by 0.2 if you only do very light activities, by 0.3 if you do a little more formal exercise such as walking as well as housework, by 0.4 if you are moderately active and you rarely sit still or by 0.5 if your job involves manual labour or you play lots of sports. The result is the number of calories you need on top of your BMR.

'If you are going to lose weight and avoid gaining it, eating less is more effective than exercise alone... Doing both is the most effective combination.'
Sir JOHN KREBS, Chair of the Food Standards Agency

Defining idea...

Eating and digesting food uses up around 10% of your calorie needs, so, after adding your BMR and the extra calories you worked out for your activity levels together, work out what 10% is. Now add all three of those figures together and you'll have the number of your total calorie needs per day.

To lose half a kilo (a pound) a week, you need to cut your daily calories by 500 (or cut fewer than that and make up the difference with exercise), which is a safe amount to aim for. Although this might not sound a lot, it's easier to achieve in the

long term and easier to sustain. If you lose lots of weight very quickly, you're more likely to put it back on and get into that yo-yo dieting spiral.

OK, end of accountancy lesson. Who'd have thought that playing with numbers could be such fun!

How did it go?

Q   Couldn't I just cut my calories to make the weight fall off?

A   *You could, but it's not a smart thing to do. This kind of crash dieting means that water and protein are lost from the body rather than fat. Your metabolic rate will also slow to conserve calories. As soon as you eat normally, you'll gain weight. For this reason, you really shouldn't go below 1200 calories a day. If you take the long-term view and lose weight slowly, you'll still lose water to begin with, but you'll soon start making a dent in your fat reserves, which is what you really want. Losing weight slowly with an accompanying change in lifestyle is the recipe for long-term success.*

Q   Surely if I eat high calorie foods, I could just burn off the excess with exercise?

A   *In principle I suppose you could eat rubbish and run it off. The trouble is that you could end up malnourished if this is your long-term diet tactic. Many high-fat foods don't offer enough of a nutritional balance to subsist on. Equally, even if you ran off the calories from, say, a daily ham, egg and cheese quiche, the saturated fat could still have an effect on your cholesterol levels. So, it's better to have a balanced diet with plenty of variety for your health and weight.*

8

3

Setting goals (without always having to move the goalposts)

Master the art of goal-setting to turn your dream of losing weight into reality. Most of us don't do it, but planning really works!

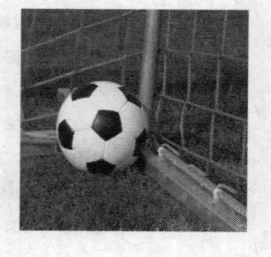

A well-known study of a group of US students in the 1950s found that only three per cent of the graduates wrote a set of goals for their lives.

A follow-up survey some twenty years later discovered that the goal-setting students were worth more financially than the other 97% put together. You may say, well, life's not all about money. No, it's not – but the goal setters were also healthier and happier in their relationships than the others.

Goal-setting is as relevant to weight loss as it is to life plans, but it's not always as straightforward as it seems. Simply saying 'I want to lose weight' may well be true and seem to be a goal, but it won't get you very far. Why? Because goals need to be SMART:

Here's an
idea for
you...

Write your goals down and pin them up in a place where you will see them every day, like the fridge door. When you look at them, repeat them to yourself and visualise how you will look and feel when you have achieved them. This will keep your goals real and alive.

that's Specific, Measurable, Attainable, Realistic and Time-framed. Put simply, by analysing how to reach your end goal, you increase your chances of achieving it.

OK, let's do it. Get some paper and a pen and start writing.

Be Specific – Write down how much weight you want to lose. Is there also a particular reason you want to lose this amount, for a special occasion, or is it for health reasons? Perhaps you've always been overweight and really want to do something about it. It's important to think around the reasons you want to slim down as part of the 'why' of your goal. Once it's clear in your head, you'll be in control and focused.

Measurable – How will you measure you weight loss? By weighing yourself regularly or by dropping a clothing size? Or will you just go by the way you look or feel? How often will you take stock of your achievements? There's no right or wrong answer here – it's just about what works for you.

Attainable – Question yourself as to whether this goal is really what you want. You could think about it in terms of your commitment and enthusiasm. If you're not 100% happy about your goal, maybe you need to revisit the specifics to review whether it is too ambitious or too challenging for you to feel confident about it. A goal does have to stretch you, but if it seems unattainable you'll become downhearted pretty quickly. Of course, we all have different definitions of what's attainable and what isn't – it depends on factors such as your personality, confidence and experience.

Realistic – With the best will in the world, if you are 165 cm (5 ft 5 in) and pear-shaped, no diet is going to turn you into Aussie model/actress/business woman Elle McPherson – especially if you're a man! Make sure your goal is realistic. Think about your goal in terms of being the best you can be.

Setting goals is a major step in slimming successfully. You can take it further by developing it like a formal business plan. Turn to IDEA 5, *Learn to act like the chief executive of You Inc.* for inspiration.

Try another idea...

Time-framed – A time frame keeps your goal on track. Set a start point, such as 'I will start my healthy eating weight loss plan on Thursday' and give yourself an end time too, such as 'I will lose five kilos by my summer holiday.' I think it also makes sense to include a couple of time frames in your overall goal representing short and longer term achievements. This helps with motivation. So you could add 'I will start exercising three times a week on Mondays, Wednesdays and Saturdays from next week' and so on. Use positive goal-getting language when writing down what you're going to achieve. There's no room here for 'might' and 'ought to'.

By now your goal should be looking so clear that you can reach out and touch it. I hope you feel all revved up and ready to go. One other thing: do remember to congratulate yourself every step of the way, whether it is with little (non-fattening) rewards or simply a mental pat on the back.

'To begin with the end in mind means to start with a clear understanding of your destination.'
STEPHEN COVEY

Defining idea...

11

How did it go?

Q   My goals seem a bit confused. How can I make them clearer?

A   *Maybe you're just very good at listing what you don't want in life! You may need to work a bit harder on identifying what you really do want. You need to be clear about this in order to make it happen.*

Q   What if I mess up and don't achieve my goals?

A   *Come on, do you know anyone who does everything perfectly all the time? Everyone messes up. Learn from your mistakes, move on and try again.*

Q   How much weight could I aim to lose per week?

A   *The ideal weight-loss pattern needs to be long-term and sustainable. If you crash diet, by dramatically reducing the number of calories you take in, you will lose more weight initially (though this won't all be fat), but you will soon plateau, as your body slows down to cope with what it sees as starvation. The end result is that you will be terribly hungry most of the time and as soon as you start to eat normally you will put weight back on. To lose half a kilo (a pound) a week, you need to shed 500 calories a day on average. That means eating a bit less and/or exercising more. And that's not really too hard. Trust me!*

Pyramid selling

What's a healthy balance of foods? Get to grips with the basics and you're halfway to being slim – eating better becomes much easier when you are clear about this.

One of the cleverest tools to help you to keep to a balanced diet has to be the food guide pyramid, first conceived in the USA.

The food guide pyramid is a simple way of visualising the kinds of foods to eat and the proportions in which we need them for a healthy diet. The pyramid is a standard for health, and it is incredibly useful for dieters as you can still use its principles, but just eat less. An added bonus is that the more you know about food, the greater your chances of slimming successfully.

It's important to be reminded that eating a variety of foods is considered essential for optimum health. By eating as the pyramid suggests, you should get your protein, vitamins, minerals and fibre, without overdoing the fat, cholesterol, sugars, salt and calories! Each group in the pyramid has a suggested amount of servings attached to it, with the lowest number intended for people consuming 1600 calories a day, such as sedentary women, while the highest number is intended for people

Here's an idea for you... **If you're not keen on pyramid shapes, try a circle, split into the following segments, as suggested by the UK Food Standards Agency: 30% fruit and veg, 30% bread, pasta, rice and potatoes, 15% dairy, 15% meat and fish, and 10% fat and sugary foods. These are the proportions you need for a balanced diet.**

needing around 2800 calories a day, such as male manual labourers. The large differences in calorie needs have confused some people, so right now the Americans are working on making it clearer. As long as you remember to look to the lower levels, you'll be doing well!

The food pyramid works like this. At the bottom of the pyramid, the wide base, you'll find the bread, cereal, rice and pasta group, of which the recommended intake is 6–11 servings. Moving up a layer are the fruits and vegetables, with a little more emphasis on vegetables, with 3–5 servings recommended and 2–4 of fruit. The next layer of the pyramid is for milk, yoghurt and cheese (dairy products), but excluding butter and cream and, sharing the space on this tier, is the group featuring meat, fish, dry beans, eggs and nuts. You should aim for 2–3 servings per day from each of these groups. Then at the top, in the tiny space at the pyramid's summit, is the fats, oils and sweets group, with the caution 'use sparingly'.

As an exercise, compare the pyramid with your daily or weekly food intake. How does your diet shape up? The vast majority of people in the Western world have diets that turn the pyramid on its head, with fats and sugars making up the bulk of their food consumption.

By this point you may feel as though your head is exploding, but I have to tell you one more thing: within each of the groups there are healthier and more diet-friendly choices to be made. For example, in the cereals group, choose wholemeal, brown or unrefined products because they give you more fibre, vitamins and minerals. In principle cakes such as muffins and croissants belong in this group, but they bring more fat and sugar to the party than anything really nutritionally interesting.

You can't go far wrong with fruit and vegetables, apart from serving them up with cream, butter or deep-frying them! Frozen and canned fruit and vegetables count too, but with canned produce check that what you're buying doesn't contain added sugar or salt. Wherever possible choose lower fat versions of dairy products and watch out for creamy dishes. With meats, look for lean cuts or trim off any visible fat; for example, chicken is much less fatty if you remove the skin. Avoid processed meat products as far as possible, as they tend to be very fatty. Fish is mostly lean, apart from oily fish such as fresh tuna, mackerel and salmon. However these contain the omega-3 essential fatty acids which have great health benefits, such as reducing the risk of death from heart disease. You should definitely aim for two portions of oily fish a week.

As well as what you eat, how you prepare it counts too. See IDEA 23, *Make your kitchen more diet-friendly*.

Try another idea...

'I do not like broccoli. And I haven't liked it since I was a little kid and my mother made me eat it. And I'm President of the United States and I'm not going to eat any more broccoli.'
GEORGE BUSH, SENIOR

Defining idea...

15

How did it go?

Q **I'm not keen on meat. Is there a vegetarian pyramid?**

A *Yes and it's pretty similar to the original. Soya, nuts, seeds and legumes replace meat and are actually a great alternative to meat for carnivores who want to ring the changes. The wide base of the pyramid is a mix of fruit and vegetables, whole grains and legumes. These should be eaten at every meal. You have to watch getting overly dependent on eggs and hard cheese, because as well as being a source of protein they are high in fat and should only be eaten occasionally. Nuts and seeds should be eaten daily as they are highly nutritious, but only in very small quantities (a small handful) as they are fat-rich too.*

Q **What group does something like a burger fall into?**

A *If it's between two bits of roll and has salad added, it contains meat, cereal and vegetable. Many dishes are a combination of the food groups.*

Q **I don't eat much fish, but I do eat canned tuna – does that count as oily fish?**

A *Fresh tuna counts as oily fish but canned tuna does not. In the canning process, the omega-3 benefits are lost. However, canned tuna is still a good source of protein. Make sure you buy it in spring water though, to avoid adding extra fat in the form of oils used in canning or salt, which is added when it is canned in brine.*

Learn to act like the chief executive of You Inc.

You wouldn't run a business or a household without a plan, especially if big changes were looming. As the person in charge of your mind and body, try this life coaching technique to develop your successful slimming strategy.

I first got interested in life coaching when I wasn't happy in my life, but wasn't sure what was really wrong. Going on a coaching course helped me to focus my thoughts with amazing clarity.

I ended up quitting my job as a magazine editor and became a freelance editor and writer, reinventing and rediscovering my life along the way. But enough about me! My point to you is that wanting to lose weight is a serious business and like any of life's challenges, it can be fraught with confusion, doubts, false starts and questions. A proper game plan can iron out many issues you'll face along the way, hence this introduction to a really useful life coaching exercise (and at a fraction of the price of a course!).

There's nothing like a declutter to rev up your energy and motivation levels. Try one or all of these for your fresh start:

- **Clean out your fridge and cupboards and get rid of diet saboteurs such as the deep fat fryer and the biscuit tin.**

- **Go through your wardrobe and bag up all the clothes you haven't worn for a year and are unlikely to wear again.**

- **Give yourself a new haircut or a beauty/grooming treatment. Make yourself feel good.**

The GROW model stands for Goals, Reality, Options and Will. Grab a piece of paper and write those headings down leaving enough space to add your thoughts and answers beneath them:

Goals – I know that you are reading this book because your goal is to lose weight, but you need to break that goal down to make it achievable. Go for specifics, such as 'I want to lose three kilos by my wedding day' or 'I want to be my target weight by my holiday'. As well as making your goal realistic and positive, give it a time frame. Also, write down why you want lose weight. Is it for health reasons, for instance? Or is it about your self-esteem? Reminding yourself why you want to lose weight reinforces that goal.

Reality – Think about your weight now. How much control do you have over reducing it? What are the main obstacles you see that could prevent you from losing weight? What resources do you have that will help you? Maybe you have inner resources, such as a determination to succeed that you've demonstrated in your career, or perhaps you have a great municipal leisure centre near you or a corporate gym membership through your workplace. Think about what else could help you achieve your goal and who else you could ask for help.

Options – OK, now you really have to free up your mind to think laterally and creatively! Write down all the ways you think you could approach your weight loss (following the ideas in this book should be on your list, but add your own thoughts) When you've come to the end of your list, write down some more ideas, even if they seem silly or far-fetched. If you're stuck, think about what you might advise a friend if he or she wanted to slim down. If time and money were unlimited, what might you do then? Do you know anyone who has recently lost weight? How did they do it? How would you feel if you didn't lose weight?

Positive encouragement from friends, family and fellow dieters will help you to stay motivated and make the process easier. Why not join a slimming club? See IDEA 28, Members only.

Try another idea...

Will – Looking at your options, write down the ones that appeal to you and which could take you part or all of the way to your final goal. Think about the obstacles you could face if you chose any of those options. Here's another hard bit. When are you going start? Are you fully committed to seeing this through? Give yourself a mark on a scale of 1–10.

'If you can dream it, you can do it.'
WALT DISNEY

Defining idea...

Well done! You've completed your self-coaching exercise and should have a clearer framework about what you want to achieve and how you're going to get there. May be it threw up other areas in your life which need attention, in which case, follow the same process through, substituting the issue. All for no extra charge!

'Imagination is more important than knowledge.'
ALBERT EINSTEIN

Defining idea...

19

How did it go?

Q I've tried losing weight before and just can't seem to do it. How can I make it different this time?

A *Have you ever heard of a self-fulfilling prophecy? What you think is what you get, so work on your beliefs about what you can achieve, rather than what you think you can't. Use positive self-talk. You could start by rephrasing the negative attitude above to say, 'I have tried losing weight before and have learned a lot about how not to do it.'*

Q I have so many responsibilities in my life that I usually come last on the list. How can I find the time?

A *Go back to the reality section of the GROW model exercise and make a list of all the obstacles and all those other responsibilities in your life that may prevent you achieving your goal of weight loss. There are always solutions to issues, whether that means rethinking your childcare arrangements, working different hours, going to bed earlier so you can wake up earlier to go to the gym, preparing yourself a healthy packed lunch, asking your partner to do more around the house and so on. Think hard, think long, think laterally and ask someone else to help think with you. You could also probably learn to say 'no' more often. Don't be a martyr.*

6

Get the write habit

Why keeping a diary helps you lose weight.

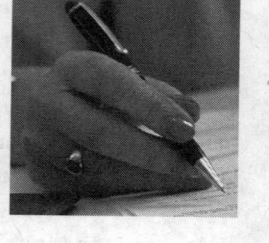

Noting down what you are eating may give you some surprises. It will definitely help you to identify the changes you need to make to help you to lose weight.

All too often we're not realistic about what and how much we really eat. Sometimes we truly forget. Check how often you're eating, too.

Sometimes we're in denial and it's simply easier to forget, to assuage feelings of guilt, self-loathing or defeatism (all common negative attitudes when you're trying to lose weight). Keeping a record of your food and drink consumption is an invaluable tool when you're starting out on a weight loss plan, as it gives you a real insight into the kinds of foods you usually eat and the quantity and frequency of meals and snacks. Unless you know where you're going wrong, how can you put things right? The food diary doesn't lie – unless you cheat, of course. All you have to do is record faithfully everything you eat and drink for a week. That includes the 'I

Here's an idea for you...

Visualisation techniques are used by high achievers in many demanding fields such as sport and business. It is a proven psychological method of helping you to attain your goals. For a few minutes every day, picture yourself achieving your goals and how you'll feel and look when you've achieved them. Don't laugh – it works for Olympic gold medal winners!

nibbled such a small piece of cheese that I'm sure it doesn't count' snacks and the croissant (so full of fat!) that you grabbed on your way to work. If you ate it while you were walking, it doesn't mean you didn't eat it. Equally, don't try to change your eating habits temporarily to appear more virtuous, as you'll miss the benefits of the exercise.

At the end of the week, take time to really study your diary and ask yourself the following questions:

■ Am I eating regularly (breakfast, lunch and dinner)?

Skipping proper meals is not a good way to lose weight. You'll probably compensate by over-eating at the next one or indulging in high-calorie, fat-laden, quick-fix snacks when you're suddenly ravenous.

■ How often am I eating between meals and what am I grazing on?

This could be because you are skipping meals, or are you are snacking a lot as well as eating regular meals? If those in-between snacks are fundamentally healthy, such as fruit or low-fat yoghurt, then that's OK, but if they are more likely to be crisps and bars of chocolate or an entire packet of biscuits (hey, I've done it!), you'll simply be taking in more calories than you need. The result? Weight gain.

- Is my diet sufficiently varied? Does your diary tell you that you're eating the same foods day in, day out? And what types of food are they?

We need a variety of foods for optimum health as well as keeping our taste buds interested. Check the mix in your meals. Do they include a variety of different food groups on a daily basis? Very broadly, we need proteins (meat, fish, eggs, pulses, beans) carbohydrates (bread, cereal, pasta, rice, potatoes) and plenty of fruit and vegetables, plus some fats and dairy produce.

- Do I rely on junk food, take-aways and ready-prepared meals?

Our lives are busy, but if you eat this way all the time, weight gain is inevitable due to the high fat and calorie content of these types of food. You can improve on convenience and fast foods by serving your own vegetables or salads as an accompaniment. Cooking from scratch gives you the ultimate control over exactly what goes in to your food. It doesn't have to be expensive, difficult or time-consuming. Buy yourself a low-fat cook book and impress yourself.

Try another idea...

Make notes in your food diary of what you're feeling when you eat. It could be that sometimes you're eating because you're bored or feeling unhappy. If this sounds familiar, try reading IDEA 14, *Are you an emotional eater?*

Defining idea...

'My doctor told me to stop having intimate dinners for four. Unless there are three other people.'
ORSON WELLES

23

■ What am I drinking?

Consider your alcohol consumption. If you drink it, are you within the recommended health guidelines? The recommended maximum is 21 units of alcohol a week for a man and 14 units for a woman Seen from a dieting perspective, alcohol is just empty calories. Do you drink lots of fizzy drinks? Some contain up to seven teaspoons of sugar. Fruit juice, although 'natural' and seemingly good for you, also contains lots of sugars which, if you're downing a litre a day, adds up to a lot of extra calories too. Are you drinking enough water? Are you drinking any water at all? Our bodies need water to help the absorption of nutrients from food. When you're properly hydrated, you'll feel and see other benefits too.

Now make a list of what you could change and how you'll do it. Start with the simplest changes and implement them quickly so you'll feel encouraged.

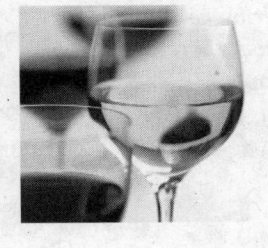
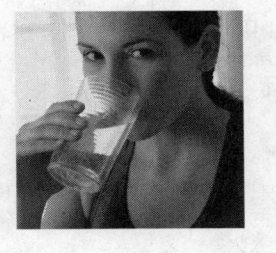
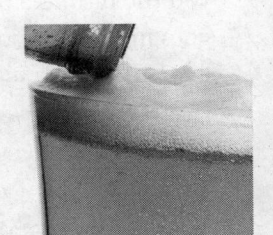

How did it go?

Q **I'm too busy to write things down and besides at the end of the day I can't remember what I've had. How am I going to keep my food diary up to date?**

A *The idea of a food diary may seem pedantic, but research shows that people who keep these records are more likely to lose weight. Rather than trying to recall everything at the end of the day, get a little notebook and write details as you go. If you whip your diary out before you consume something, it gives you a moment to really consider your food choices too.*

Q **In my job I have to eat out a lot. How can you expect me to control my diet, let alone keep a diary?**

A *That's a great excuse! The occasional meal out and eating what you fancy is fine, and if you do have to eat out a lot, you need to make the best choices from what is available. That means saying no to creamy sauces and anything fried. Choose a salad as a starter with a light vinaigrette rather than heavy dressings like Thousand Island or mayonnaise. Choose a fruit salad for dessert, not a sticky toffee pudding with extra cream. Say yes to grills and anything steamed and keep sauces and dressings on the side so you can control how much you add, which will be just a spoonful or two, won't it?*

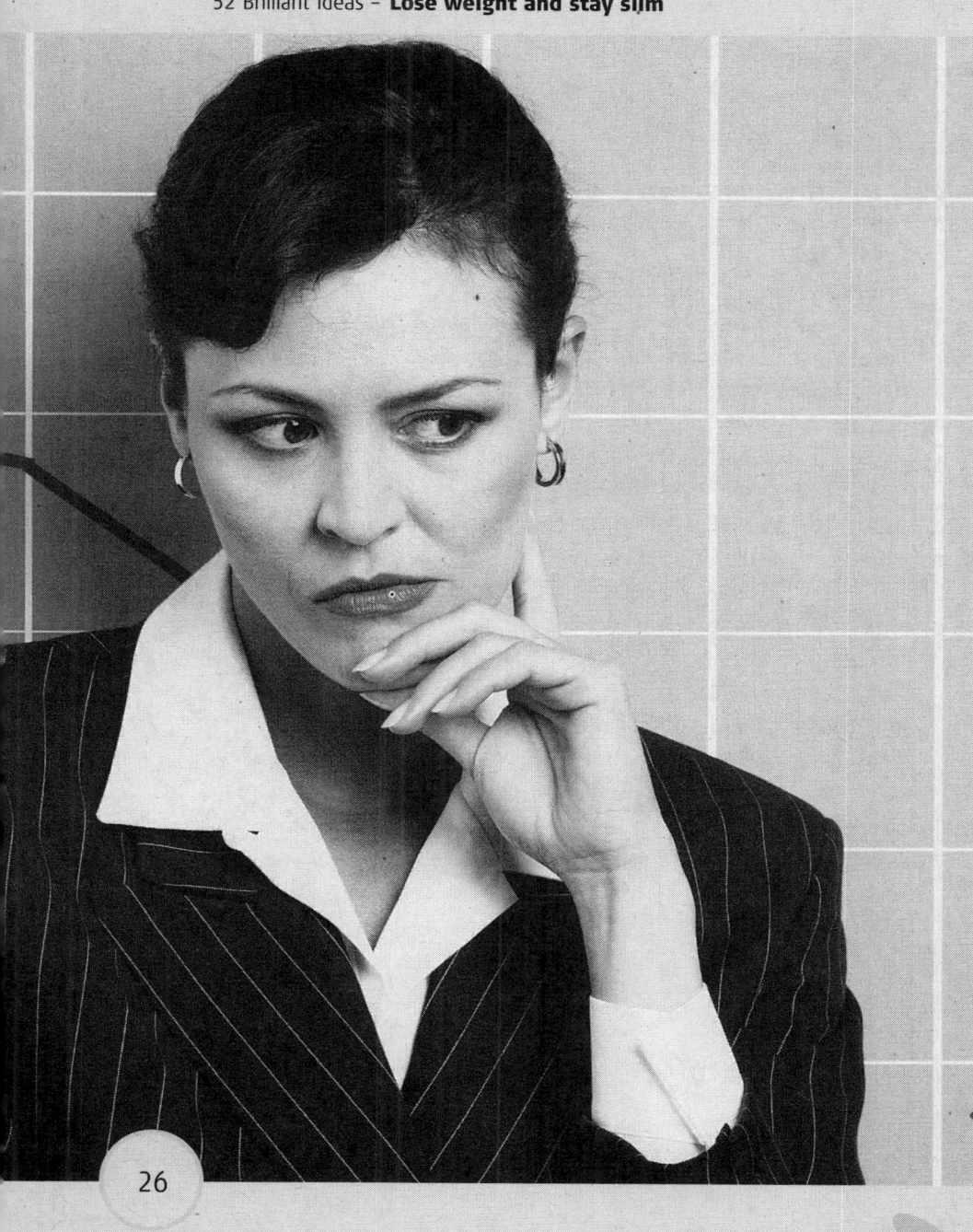

7

It's never too late to change your mind

Have you been on diets before, lost weight, then regained it and lost motivation? Change your attitude to dieting and use your mind to get ahead.

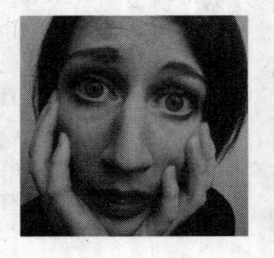

I have a friend who's been on every kind of diet going: cabbage soup, high protein, eating for your blood type, meal replacements and all the rest. The trouble is, she hasn't changed her poor mental attitude to dieting.

She uses diets like buses, jumping on and off. If she's just missed one, well, there will be another along in a minute, won't there? Has she lost weight? Yes, she has and then she's gained it, until the next period of dieting when the cycle repeats itself.

Why is it that most diets only seem to work temporarily? In my opinion the main reason is that they don't teach you much about healthy eating or help you learn a healthy attitude to food. All too often, entire food groups are banned, which,

Here's an idea for you...

Drink fruit juice not cola. According to new research from the American Diabetes Association, just one regular can of a fizzy drink a day is enough to increase your risk of diabetes by 85%. A can a day could also lead to a weight gain of around a stone in four years.

depending on the group, can be unhealthy or even dangerous if you follow it for a long time. Meal replacements, although designed nowadays to be nutritionally safe, don't really give the average dieter any idea of what a healthy meal looks like. If a diet promises you rapid weight loss, you can bet it will be due to consuming significantly less calories. It won't be because of some magical fat-burning enzyme found in the bongo-bongo fruit or whatever the angle is! Besides, you'll just lose water and lean muscle mass anyway, so it won't necessarily be sustainable.

Diets can be as dull as ditchwater, particularly if they are very strict about what you can and can't eat. Not only do you feel bored and start fantasising about bathing in jelly and custard (mmm, with some chocolate sprinkles too), but they can make eating out difficult, especially when you visit friends' houses. You have to be very good company indeed to make up for your inconvenient food requests. Let's face it, a diet can simply be hard to fit into your life, particularly when you also have a family to feed or if you work long or unusual hours. And then there's the hunger, the growling stomach and the faintness-inducing pangs that all too often lead to a binge. Then you feel guilty – and move on to another diet in the hope that it will be better.

Many people who sincerely want to lose weight are failing to stick to their diet regimes. So what does work? There isn't one single way to lose weight successfully. You need to develop a combination of tricks that work for you, and an acceptance

of certain key points. The first is that you will probably need to change your idea of what a diet and losing weight is all about. The kinds of diets mentioned above are not going to help you. To lose weight and keep it off, you have to change your eating habits and lifestyle

Still hankering after a quick-fix? What about the beauty creams that claim to help you lose inches? See IDEA 27, *Can beauty products help you slim*?

Try another idea…

permanently. Before you shriek that this sounds even scarier than a wasp-chewing diet, remember that losing weight is about the long haul, not dieting in short four-week bursts. There are no quick fixes, but if you make small changes over a period of time, they will add up to big results.

Next, you have to realistic about your weight-loss goals. Aim to be in the best shape you can be, which is to be healthy, not to look like a stick insect. Eat a balanced selection of foods with plenty of fruit and vegetables, protein and carbohydrate and a little fat. A balanced diet is essential for good health, keeps things interesting for you and ensures you won't suffer endless cravings because you're denying yourself certain foods. Remember that you do need to keep a check on the portion sizes. You'll also be doing yourself a big favour if you become more physically active. Exercise makes you feel and look good, helps to control your appetite and, in conjunction with sensible eating, helps you lose weight faster. Using these guidelines, weight should come off slowly but surely, without you feeling as though you've put your entire life on hold to accommodate a short-term diet. You might just enjoy yourself too!

'*I never worry about diets. The only carrots that interest me are the number you get in a diamond.*'
MAE WEST

Defining idea…

How did
it go?

Q   **If I'm not following a strict diet where certain foods are forbidden, can I eat junk food and whatever else I like?**

A   *Whoa! Steady on. There's a big difference between having a bit of what you fancy and winning an award for being the most regular customer at the burger bar. The key is to make fattening, less healthy foods an occasional treat rather than your regular diet and to choose small portions. That way, you don't feel deprived. Be flexible in your approach. If you eat sensibly most of the time, the odd blow-out really isn't going to make much difference.*

Q   **How can I stop feeling hungry all the time?**

A   *Try using this mental trick to manipulate your appetite: visualise a dial that represents your hunger, on a scale from zero to ten. Eight to ten is ravenous, five to seven is hungry, below five is not very hungry. At the moment, where does the dial have to be for you to eat? Perhaps it's hovering around four, in which case you need to set it a little higher, so you're only eating when you're really hungry. Reset your dial in your imagination, perhaps to six to begin with. Every time you're about to eat something, see your dial and stop to ask yourself where you are on it hunger-wise. Over a period of time, you'll find that you've stopped eating when the dial is under five. Think before you eat and only eat when you're hungry!*

I'll have a 21, 34 and 52 please...oh and a large portion of 15

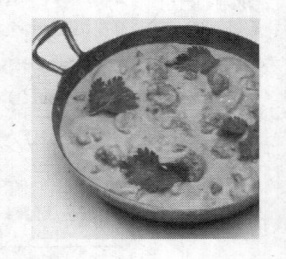

The road to Fatville is paved with fast food and takeaways, but you don't have to cut them out of your life completely – it's just a balancing act.

Eating takeaways and other fast foods is the norm for many of us. With little or no washing up to do, no shopping and cooking, this way of eating can feel like a life-saver for busy people.

The trouble is that when you eat fast food you have no idea what you're really consuming in terms of fat, calories, hidden salt and additives, which is bad news for your health and diet. For example, sometimes a chicken nugget is only distantly related to chickens and what you're really eating is just a load of old filler. A beefburger, fries and cola drink are one of the cultural icons of the free world, but they are also a symbol of today's fat world and can easily add up to over a thousand calories with colossal amounts of saturated fat thrown in.

Here's an idea for you... **Why not choose soup as a starter? All that liquid fills you up and means there's less room for the temptation of garlic bread with cheese and bacon or 'Death by Chocolate' fudge cake.**

It's fine to eat takeaways and fast food occasionally, but you can always make healthier less fattening choices. I think that sometimes we just get lazy about food – here are some tips for lazy people about three popular junk food staples:

FISH AND CHIPS

- The good bits: high in protein, vitamins B6 and B12, plus a few minerals.

- The bad bits: high in fat, low on fibre. If it's a big portion, you could quite easily be consuming half the daily recommended fat levels in one sitting.

- Try this: balance out your other meal of the day with a vitamin-packed salad and some low-fat protein, such as cottage cheese, skinless chicken or tuna. Or make your own fish and chips. How hard is it to stick a piece of fish under the grill? Use prepared oven chips, rather than deep-frying your own, or make potato wedges and roast them.

PIZZA

- The good bits: cheese and tomato offers protein, calcium and some vitamins.

- The bad bits: if you go for pepperoni and extra cheese, you're piling on fat.

- Try this: balance out the pizza at your next meal with a chicken casserole and lots of vegetables for low-fat protein and plenty of fibre and vitamins. Or make

your own pizza using a ready-made base. My life seems too short to make my own, but if you can, feel free. Award yourself extra points if you use wholemeal flour, which gives you more fibre and other nutrients. Top it with heaps of vegetables, a little protein (for example, chicken, turkey, lean beef, tuna or tofu). Add grated cheese, which is better than lumps, for a bit of flavour and less fat.

BEEFBURGER, FRIES AND A MILKSHAKE

- The good bits: high in protein, carbohydrates and calcium, plus some vitamin A, B12 and riboflavin.

- The bad bits: high in saturated fat and sodium, low in fibre, and often a good sprinkling of additives.

- Try this: redress the balance with another meal of wholemeal pasta and vegetables for fibre and vitamins. A home-made burger is easily made with lean mince. Serve it with potato wedges and salad and either leave out the bap or use half a wholemeal roll. Make a more slimming milkshake by using skimmed milk and flavoured powder.

Try another idea...

Is it small, medium or large? Check your sense of portion control with IDEA 10, *Why size matters.*

Defining idea...

'We were taken to a fast food café where our order was fed into a computer. Our hamburgers, made from the flesh of chemically impregnated cattle had been broiled over counterfeit charcoal and placed between slices of artificially flavoured cardboard and served by recycled juvenile delinquents.'
JEAN MICHEL CHAPEREAU, French author

When you order a take-away to eat at home, follow the advice above plus the following tips for cutting down on calories and fat overload:

■ Avoid anything fried and choose grilled, steamed, broiled or baked foods without cheese and creamy sauce.

■ Say no to all creamy and buttery sauces. Choose tomato-based ones.

■ Watch out for coconut. It seems innocuous, but it's full of saturated fat.

■ If you're having a side order of rice, ask for it plain boiled.

■ Leave out the side orders of garlic bread or bread and butter. If you must have bread, do as the Continentals do and have it plain.

Here's a final thought: Stop eating when you're full!

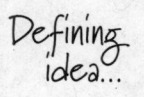
Defining idea...

'The journey of a thousand pounds begins with a single burger.'
CHRIS O'BRIEN, writer

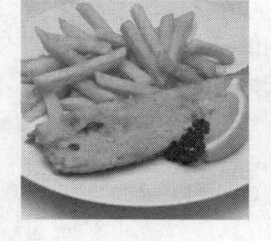
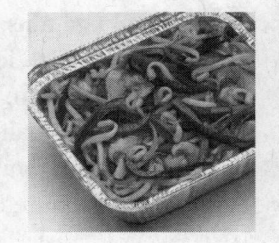

Q   **I love eating out and getting takeaways. How can I stop forgetting my good intentions and ending up hating myself?**

How did it go?

A   *If you do pig out, just get back to your sensible ways the next day. Try these points as a strategy and see if they help: skip bread or whatever snacky treat is on the table and order a couple of starters rather than a starter and a main course. You could also try sharing a dessert. Avoid anything that is described as breaded, battered, tempura, en croute or creamed and don't order dishes with fatty sauces such as béchamel, Bearnaise and Hollandaise.*

Q   **My partner and I go for an Indian or Chinese meal once a week. What are the best choices?**

A   *It's hard to avoid ghee (clarified butter) in Indian dishes, but one tip is to avoid as much sauce as you can. Creamy kormas and fried starters such as samosas and bhajis are very high in fat too, so they are best avoided. Wiser choices include tandoori chicken and prawns, grilled chicken kebabs, chicken or prawn Madras, vegetable curries, plain rice, chapattis and raita.*

At Chinese restaurants, watch out for the fattening battered or crispy dishes, such as crispy duck, prawn toast and spring rolls. Go for stir-fried and steamed food as much as possible.

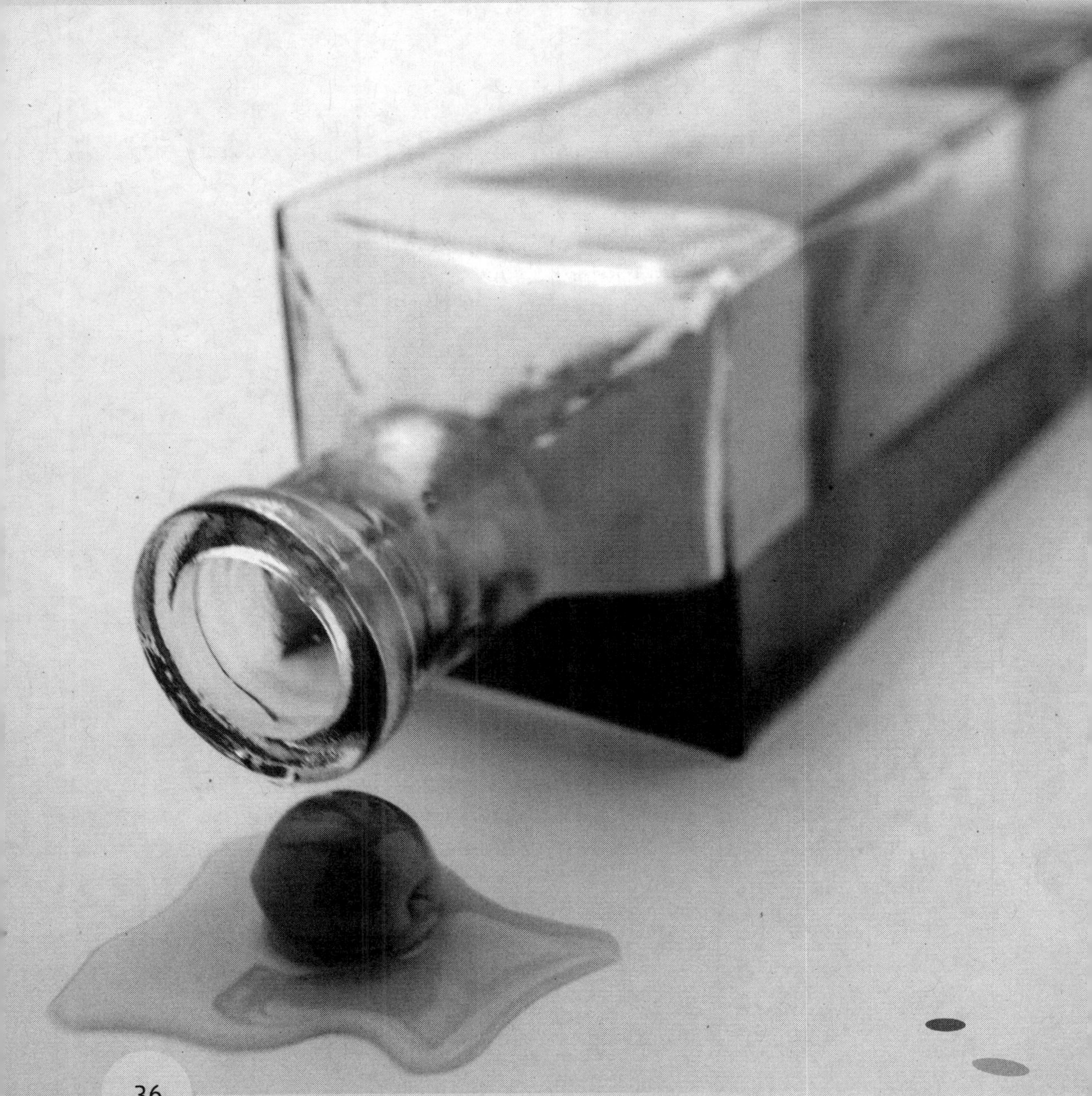

Fats: the good, the bad and the downright ugly

Fat friends and foes.

Eating too much of certain fats is definitely harmful to both your waistline and your health, so here are some handy hints on how to perform a bit of liposuction on your diet.

You need to know about fat in food because it's a rich source of calories. In fact, it contains more than twice as many calories, weight for weight, as carbohydrates and proteins.

As well as being a major cause of weight gain, a high-fat diet, particularly one that is high in saturated fats, can also increase your risk of heart disease and breast and bowel cancers.

Fat isn't all bad; our bodies need it. It delivers vitamins A, D, E and K and aids their absorption. It helps to regulate a variety of bodily functions. It makes food taste

Here's an idea for you...

Reach for your extra virgin. A drizzle a day might keep the doctor away. I use olive oil in just about everything. The trouble is that I tend to use lots of it. Yes, it's a healthy oil, but if you eat a lot of it you are just adding unnecessary calories. The key is to measure it. A tablespoon is usually enough for everything.

delicious and gives it a creamy, more-ish texture. The thing is not all fats are created equal and we typically consume too much of the wrong kind of fat and not enough of the good stuff. We should all know our rights from our wrongs for the sake of our health, but there's even more reason to get clued up when there's weight to be lost. So here are the big fat facts to chew on:

- **Saturated fats** – Foods with high levels of saturated fatty acids include butter, lard, whole milk, hard cheeses, cream, meat and meat products, palm oil and coconut oil. These are the diet wreckers and you should aim to have only a very small amount of them in your daily diet. You can reduce your intake of these kinds of fats by buying leaner cuts of meat and chopping off visible fat. Grilling, baking or steaming foods is a more slimming way to cook than smothering everything in butter and cream.

- **Trans fats** – These are found in processed foods such as crisps, cakes, biscuits and pies and also in many brands of margarine. Cross the street to avoid them. Check food labels for these fats – they'll be listed as 'hydrogenated'.

- **Unsaturated fats** – These break down into monounsaturates and polyunsaturates. Monounsaturates are found in olive oil, nut oils, avocados and seeds, which have health benefits for your heart and so are a better choice than saturated fats. But they're still fattening, so use them sparingly. Polyunsaturates

pop up in most vegetable oils (corn, sunflower, safflower), fish oils and oily fish. They are generally a good thing, particularly if you consume them in place of saturated fats, although they are still calorific.

Could your lunch be piling on the pounds? Chew on IDEA 13, *Let's do lunch*.

Try another idea...

Overall, fats should make up about a third of your total daily calorie intake, with saturated fats making up less than 10% of all the calories you consume. This rule is just for general health, but as most of us consume too much fat, it should help you lose a couple of kilos. It is quite safe to cut your total intake of all types of fat to about 20% of your daily calories. To reduce the fat you eat, you will probably need to play with the balance of fats in your diet. In the western world, especially in the UK and US, we generally consume a lot of saturated fat. People who live in southern Europe tend to have a better fat balance as they generally eat less dairy, more fish, more plant oils and much more fruit. Think of your favourite region of the Mediterranean and imagine being a local there. How do they eat? French, Italian and Spanish people who live in the countryside tend to eat well-balanced meals prepared from fresh ingredients, avoiding processed foods. If you must drink a lot of milk, try choosing skimmed or half-fat instead of whole milk.

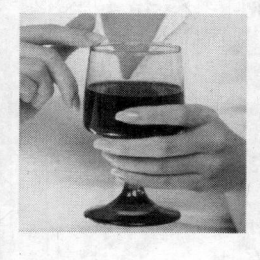

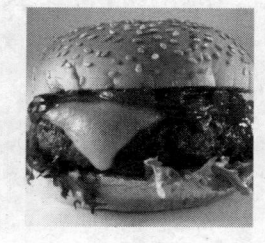

'Except for the vine, there is no plant which bears a fruit of as great importance as the olive.'
PLINY

Defining idea...

How did it go?

Q   **If I buy foods marked 'low fat' or 'lite', will I reduce my fat intake?**

A   *If something is low in fat, it may still be high in calories, so you could still be consuming too many calories to lose weight. Compare the label on a low fat product with the standard version of the product.*

Q   **How many grams of fat should we eat a day?**

A   *For average adults of a healthy weight, women should aim for 70 g and men 95 g. When you're trying to lose weight you should be aiming lower. For example, if you are eating around 1800 calories a day, you should go for around 63 g of fat in your diet.*

Q   **I've read about a slimming pill with a fatty acid in it. Does it work?**

A   *Conjugated linoleic acid (CLA) is a fatty acid found naturally in many foods, including dairy products and beef. Back in the early 1990s some researchers found that CLA plays a role in keeping body fat levels low and helping lean muscle tissue to develop. Other studies have since found that CLA can improve the body's muscle-to-fat ratio. A pill containing CLA is not a miracle cure, but there does seem to be enough evidence to give it a try. Remember, though, that you will still have to eat less and increase your level of physical activity. Think of CLA as the icing on the cake, not as an excuse to go back to old bad habits!*

10

Why size matters

It's not just what you eat that counts on the road to losing weight, it's about how much you eat too. How does your sense of portion control measure up?

What do you think a portion size of say, breakfast cereal or meat should be? I hope you're sitting down because it will probably be a shock. I know it is to me every time I see this particular truth in black and white!

According to healthy eating guidelines, a serving of breakfast cereal should be one ounce and a serving of meat should be two to three ounces. Cereal belongs to the food group of which we can have 6–11 servings a day, but it could be very easy to eat all of it at breakfast alone. The meat group, which also includes fish, dry beans, eggs and nuts, should be contributing 2–3 servings a day to our diet. Again, it's astonishing how quickly that can add up.

Here's an idea for you...

Squeeze a lemon. Citrus fruits are a great source of vitamin C and also a phytonutrient called limonoids, which can help to lower cholesterol. These phytonutrients are concentrated in the rind, so try to incorporate the zest of citrus fruits into your cooking. They work especially well in sauces and garnishes.

The simple fact is that most us eat too much and have lost all idea of what a portion size should be. This is due to a variety of reasons but the most significant is that food is so readily available in our affluent society. We don't have to go and hunt for it – we can just gather it at the supermarket. When eating out or buying takeaways we demand value for money. What better way to appear to offer good value than with enormous portion sizes? At home we'll cook a meal which could serve four or six people, but it's often eaten by just two or four.

Portion control is essential to weight loss. You could be eating all the right things and still gain weight because you're overeating.

Here's a checklist of the sorts of foods we should be eating for a healthy balance of nutrients. It gives a range for the number of daily serving (e.g. 6–11 servings). The upper end of range really intended only for a very active man; most of us, especially sedentary women, should look to the lower end. There are also a few handy little visual ideas of what that amount looks like. It helps to get good at estimating these by eye because you can't carry around a set of scales everywhere you go. Well, you could, but it would look a little obsessive.

...and another

To take your mind off how much smaller your portions may have to be from now on, try a nice swim. It will stop you from eating and thinking about food.

Bread, cereal, rice and pasta – 6–11 servings

A serving is:
1 slice of bread (the size of an audio cassette tape)
1 small bread roll
2 heaped tablespoons of boiled rice
3 heaped tablespoons of boiled pasta
2 crispbreads
2 egg-sized potatoes
3 tablespoons of dry porridge oats

Fruit and vegetables – 2–4 servings of the former, 3–5 servings of the latter

This is based on US recommendations. In the UK, the suggested amount of fruit and vegetables is 'at least 5' a day.

A serving is:

2–3 small pieces of fruit, such as plums
1 heaped tablespoon of dried fruit such as raisins
1 medium-sized piece of fresh fruit such as half of a grapefruit or a melon
1 side salad, the size of a cereal bowl
3 heaped tablespoons of cooked vegetables such as carrots

Try another idea…

Swimming burns off some calories, and you can easily turn it into a workout for even more benefits. See IDEA 26, *Fancy a calorie-free dip?*

Defining idea…

'A fat person lives shorter, but eats longer.'
STANISLOW LEC, Polish poet and satirist

43

Meat, fish, eggs, nuts, dry beans – 2–3 servings a day

A serving is:
60–90 g (2–3 ounces) of cooked lean meat, poultry or fish. This the size of a deck of cards or the palm of your hand.
150 g (5 ounces) of white fish (or three fish fingers)
120 g (4 ounces) of soya, tofu or quorn
5 tablespoons of baked beans
2 tablespoons of nuts and nut products

Milk, yoghurt and cheese – 2–3 servings a day

A serving is:

200 ml milk
1 small pot of yoghurt
90 g (3 ounces) of cottage cheese
30 g (1 ounce) of cheddar or other hard cheese. This is roughly the size of matchbox.

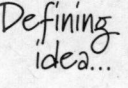

Defining idea...

'*Never eat what you can't lift.*'
MISS PIGGY

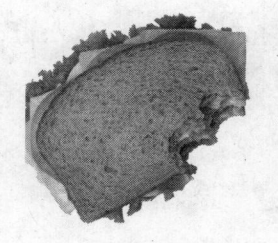 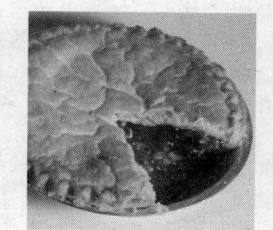

Q How do you expect me to eat such tiny portions?

A Try drinking lots of water. We often mistake thirst for hunger, and most of us don't drink enough water, so this is not just to fill up your stomach. Space out your food by snacking healthily between meals so you never feel ravenous. Don't forget that you can pile up the vegetables – they do fill you up, I promise.

Q Are all vegetables equally good?

A The majority of vegetables are mostly water (as well as all those lovely vitamins, minerals and fibre), but some are starchy and have more calories. Opt for fewer starchy vegetables and more watery ones. Starchy vegetables include potatoes, peas, corn, squash and turnips. Most of the others, from asparagus to zucchini (courgettes) are watery.

Q The only beans I use are tinned baked beans. How can I make good meals out of beans and pulses?

A You're not alone! Beans can go into casseroles and chilli sauces, just like meat. Beans and lentils are great in salads and can form the basis for the meal. Ethnic food makes good use of pulses: think of dhal at the Indian restaurant. Tofu, made from soya beans, is often used in Chinese food. There are lots of delicious recipes available. If you're not used to cooking with them, buy ready-cooked beans and pulses in a tin – otherwise you have to cook them for ages and if you don't do it properly you can get an upset stomach.

How did
it go?

45

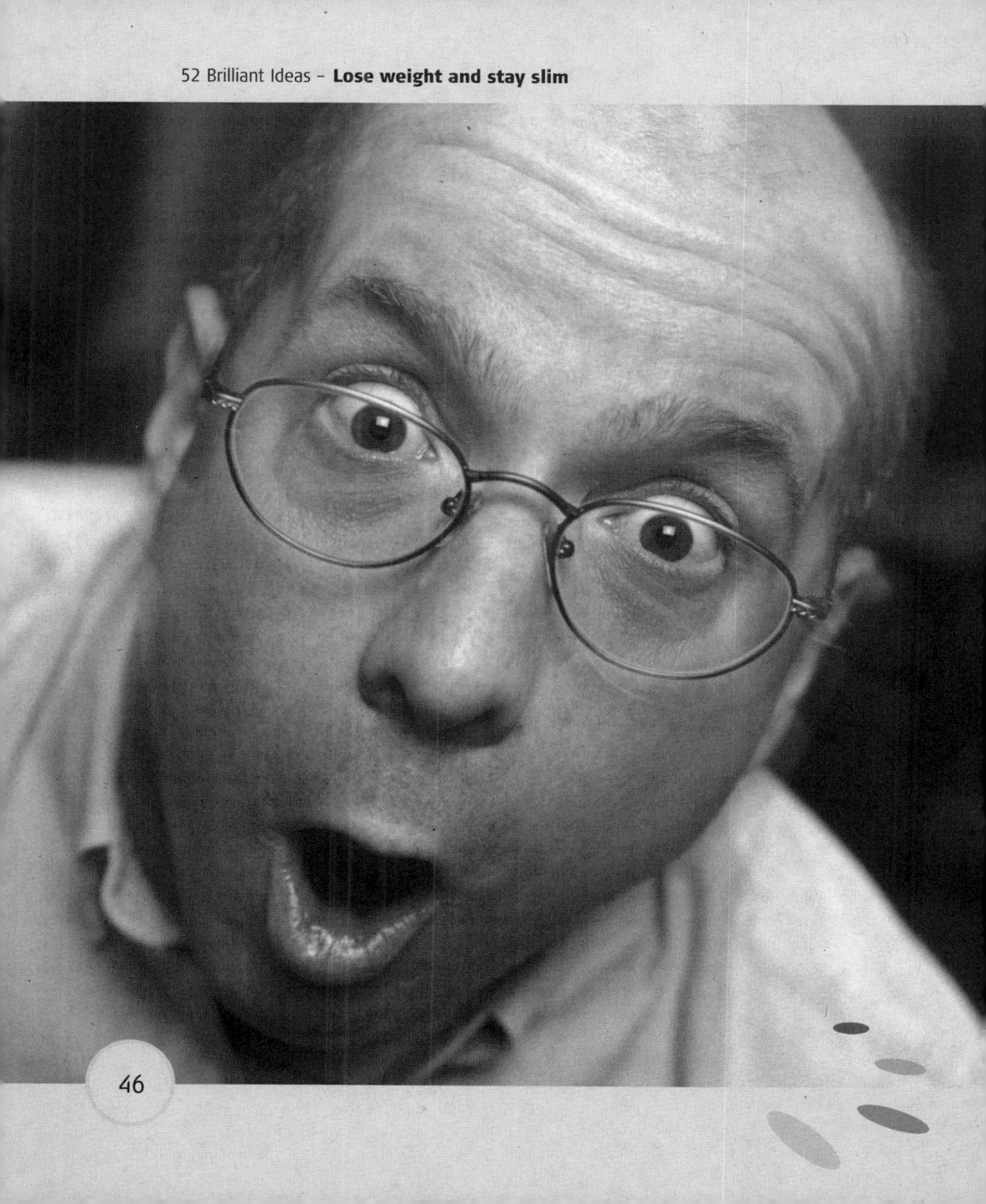

With friends like you, who needs enemies?

How do you feel about your body? Having a poor body image is a surefire way to sabotage your diet, so shape up with a little self-love.

I know a man who looks like the nerd from central casting. He's overweight, has comedy ginger hair and wears rather thick spectacles, but he truly believes he's a love god.

He really does do rather well with the ladies because he is a fabulous man. He is kind, funny and clever. The point is that he has no problems with his body image. Conversely, in my years as a journalist I have met many of the world's most beautiful women and they have all expressed negative feelings about their bodies, complaining about bellies, cellulite, feeling gawky, ugly and many other 'flaws'. It's not simply a female affliction either – just as many gorgeous men worry about their flabby bellies and 'man breasts'. No one is immune from disliking their shape and looks, but some people seem to manage to get over the problem more readily.

Here's an idea for you... **Dieters often wear black from head to toe because it is 'slimming', but adding touches of colour can really lift your mood. Use red is for energy, blue for communication, green for emotional encounters, yellow for intellectual sharpness and purple when you want to appear calm.**

This is not easy in a society that prizes slimness and makes negative judgements about people who are overweight. It's a prejudice that finds its way into the workplace and relationships, eating right into your self-esteem. The issue intensifies if hating the way you look turns into a negative view of your personality and character. 'I'm fat and stupid' or 'I'm not worth anything, no one likes me' are examples of this kind of dangerous auto-suggestion.

If you don't like yourself, it is going to be really hard to make the lifestyle changes that will help you lose weight. Often these sorts of thoughts are coupled with the habit of comparing yourself with others, especially with images in the media of celebrities and models. The truth is that these people's lives depend on how they look and they have the time and money to spend on an array of products, services and people who will keep them looking fabulous. What's more, the images you see are often 'improved' – for example, photos of models are often airbrushed to remove 'flaws'. For most of us, comparing ourselves to the thin and famous is just going to be a recipe for misery. That's rule number one: don't do it.

You need to develop a more realistic picture of how you would like to look: to look like you, but in better shape. Once you have done that, you can try some other self-esteem boosting tricks. Try writing down all the things you like about yourself, then turning them into positive statements and saying them to yourself every day like a mantra. If that seems too hard, ask your friends or family to write down what they love about you. You never know, you might finish up discovering things you had never even dreamt of that will warm the cockles of your heart.

Next, if someone pays you a compliment, accept it without putting yourself down. Avoid conversations like this:

Friend: 'You look really well.'

You: 'Yes, but I really need to lose some weight because hardly any of my clothes fit anymore.'

Instead, try something like:

'Thanks. I feel great, too. How are you?'

Focusing on being a healthy weight is a realistic goal. For more on weight and shape, turn to IDEA 1, *A weighty issue (or, a weighty question).*

Try another idea...

Exercise is good for your self image. Not only will you see physical results, but you'll feel benefits, from the satisfaction of doing something positive for yourself to a greater sense of wellbeing. Exercise has been proven to stave off depression.

Finally, rather than seeing your body as a collection of parts that you think are awful or could use improvement, focus on it as a whole and think of the wonderful things you have done or will do with it. Cuddle someone, run a marathon, give birth, climb trees, build something, help old ladies across the road.... it's your list, you finish it.

'God made a very obvious choice when he made me voluptuous: why would I go against what he decided for me? My limbs work, so I'm not going to complain about the way my body is shaped.'
DREW BARRYMORE

Defining idea...

How did it go?

Q   **I'm very self-conscious about my weight and dread meeting new people. What can I do?**

A   *Meeting new people is daunting for most of us. Studies show that everyone thinks they look worse than they do! The solution is to use the kind of body language that says to others that you're confident and interesting. Rather than avoiding eye contact and slouching away, stand up straight, shake their hand and look them in the eye. If you're sitting at a table try leaning in towards someone: it gives them the signal that you're really interested in what they have to say.*

Q   **My poor self-image has a knock-on effect to other areas of my life. Sometimes I feel down about everything. How can I change?**

A   *Try the Wheel of Life exercise, which is one of my favourite life coaching techniques. Draw a circle and divide it into eight segments. Give each of those segments a label that represents an area of your life, such as looks/weight, health, money, work, love and so on. Taking the middle of the circle as 0, or satisfied, and the outer edge as 10, completely dissatisfied, make a cross on each spoke to rank your feelings about each area. When you've finished, join up the crosses. The lowest three scores are the areas you really need to focus on. If you really do feel down more often than up, do go to see your doctor for professional help. There are plenty of things your doctor can suggest, so don't just suffer – make an effort to find a solution.*

12

Why exercise makes you feel on top of the world

You may hate the idea of it, but taking exercise is life-changing and has real benefits for dieters. Once you get into the exercise habit, you won't want to stop.

I think the reason that so many of us are put off formal exercise as adults is a hangover from childhood. I detested Physical Education at school because I was useless at most sports.

At school there was cross country running on a cold winter's morning, followed by a cold shower. As I got older, however, I discovered exercise I liked. For me it was aerobic dance classes in the wake of Jane Fonda's 'feel the burn' trend. I couldn't wait to get into my leotard, leg warmers and head band and leap around like crazy for an hour. That was over twenty years ago and I still go to the gym four or five times a week.

That's the key to incorporating exercise into your life – it has to be something you enjoy. I do believe there's something for everyone. Some of us love swimming. For others, it's running or tennis. These days gyms have a huge variety of classes on

Here's an idea for you... **Keep a log of your TV viewing time over a week. If you watch TV for more than four hours a day, you'll consume more calories than you need to because you'll have more opportunity to snack and you'll burn fewer calories while you are still.**

offer, ranging from the highly choreographed to gentle classes featuring very simple moves. There's no excuse for at least not trying some of them out. If you really don't like gyms, there is walking, which is a very good exercise indeed. It is easy to get into the habit of taking regular walks. Just one foot in front of the other, walk out of your door and keep going.

Why bother to exercise? I'll give you seven compelling reasons:

- Exercise uses up calories. You will lose weight by cutting down on the calories you consume, but if you're active too, your weight loss will be faster. I love food and working out means I can eat more. It also means that I don't end up losing any weight, but just maintain the weight I am. When you exercise you build up muscle, which gives you shape; even thin people can use muscle tone. Muscle burns up more energy than fat tissue.

- Exercise gives you a buzz. You've probably heard of the runner's high, that happy, almost euphoric feeling during an exercise session. Experts put it down to a combination of factors – a release of endorphins, hormones that mask pain and produce a feeling of wellbeing; the secretion of neurotransmitters in the brain that control our mood and emotions and a plain old sense of achievement. Whatever gives you the high, there's no doubting the feel-good glow it gives you.

- Exercise boosts your confidence. Every time you work out or play a sport, you're doing something positive for yourself, which is mood-enhancing in itself. When

you start to see the results in the mirror, your self-esteem rockets. As soon as you see results, you will find it easier to stick to your weight loss plan too.

Could a detox diet be a short cut to weight loss? See IDEA 20, *Detox diets – con or cure?*

Try another idea...

- Exercise reduces your appetite. As well as being a good distraction from the allure of the fridge, exercise slows the movement of food through your digestive system, so it takes longer for you to feel hungry.

- Exercise helps you keep weight off. The trouble with only tackling your weight loss from a dietary perspective is that it is usually quite hard to maintain your weight loss in the long term. Once you have reached your goal and are a little less strict with yourself, the weight can begin to come back. Studies have shown that people who have successfully lost weight by taking exercise as well as a sensible approach to food are better at keeping their weight stable long-term.

- Exercise really can be fun. Depending on what you choose to do, you could discover a whole new social circle. I know a few people who met their partners on the Stairmaster at their gym! Don't imagine that everyone else at the gym will be gorgeous. Only the very expensive gyms are stocked with beautiful, thin and rich people – the heaviest weights they lift are their Louis Vuitton bags. Avoid them unless you're looking for someone beautiful, thin and rich.

- According to studies at the New England Research Institute, regular, vigorous exercise can be effective at lowering men's risk of impotence.

'If you think it's hard to meet new people, try picking up the wrong golf ball.'
JACK LEMMON

Defining idea...

How did it go?

Q   **I am thinking of taking up yoga. Will it help me to lose weight?**

A   *Yoga and other mind/body exercises involving stretching are wonderful for flexibility and toning. They are also fantastic for teaching you an awareness of your body's strengths and weaknesses and help you to manage stress. They won't do much for your weight loss plan, however. To burn a significant amount of energy you need to do exercise which will get you moving fast, raise your heart rate and make you sweat, such as walking and aerobics classes. Swimming and cycling are good too, but as your body weight is supported, they burn fewer calories – but you may prefer them because this kind of exercise is less stressful on the body. Good, fast sports like basketball, football and rugby are all great alternatives to gym and studio-based workouts, but more sedate activities, such as golf, don't really cut the mustard. If golf is your thing though, don't give it up; any activity is better than nothing, and if you enjoy something you tend to do more of it.*

Q   **Is housework a way to get fit?**

A   *Compared with a gym class or running session, housework does not burn a lot of energy. You would need a big house to clean, too! It's not a sport, but housework does count as activity, and some chores count more than others. Ironing, dusting and washing up are light activity, equivalent to walking along slowly at about 4km/hour and don't count towards fitness targets. Window cleaning, vacuuming and mowing the lawn are classed as moderate exercise, equivalent to brisk walking and doubles tennis, and will help to burn up calories faster.*

13

Let's do lunch

If the weight's not shifting, chew on this: your lunch could be making you fat. But a healthy midday meal is easy when you know how.

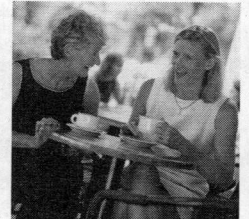

In a perfect world, we'd all have a leisurely lunch, lovingly prepared by a diet-savvy chef. Afterwards it would be time for a little siesta while someone else cleared up.

In a perfect world we'd all look like Kate Moss and George Clooney and have a few million tucked away in a Swiss bank account too. Back in the real world, whether we're at home, on the move or stuck at our desks at work, we tend either to bolt down something large and fattening that we grabbed at the shop, or we eat standing at the open fridge because we have no time to prepare a meal. Do you ever delay or miss lunch altogether? I do. Then I make up for it with a yummy chocolate bar and fancy coffee to wake me up mid-afternoon, which is very bad news indeed. The trouble with skipping meals is that you get tired and hungry later, and are likely to make unwise snacking choices. By the way, a large coffee with whipped cream tots up to around 500 calories. Learn to love it black or with skimmed milk for the sake of your waistline!

Here's an idea for you...

Make your own sandwiches – it's the only way to be sure what you're eating. Many ready-made sandwiches contain more than 6 g of salt, which is the total intake recommended per day. Reducing our salt intake from the average 10 g we consume to 6 g could prevent thousands of strokes and heart attacks. Salt is also linked to water retention which makes you feel bloated and loads heavier.

For most of us, a sandwich is often the simplest way to do lunch, but it can contain an astonishing amount of fat and calories. A popular classic is a chicken and salad sandwich – a white bap or roll filled with chicken, mayonnaise, avocado and a lettuce leaf or two. Let's examine each of these elements:

- White bread doesn't fill you up or sustain you as well as brown and can often leave you craving more carbohydrates.

- Mayonnaise really clocks up the calories – 100 g is around 700 calories and 70 g of fat. Even a lighter, reduced calorie version can contain 275 calories and around 25 g of fat.

- Avocado, whilst providing the healthier mono and polyunsaturated fats, plus vitamin E, is a rich source of calories too.

This shows how easy it is to blow the diet without even realising it! Other lunch date baddies include fatty meats, such as sausage and bacon, which are loaded with saturated fats, big wedges of hard cheeses and lashings of butter for the same reason and the rather innocent looking pickle-type relishes which can contain considerable amounts of sugar and salt.

So what does a healthy slimming sandwich look like? It's on brown bread, contains a lean protein-rich filling such as tuna, chicken, ham, brie or cottage cheese and is stuffed full of salad and vegetables for volume, crunch and vitamins. It doesn't contain mayonnaise. In a shop there may be no alternative to mayo, but at home you could try making your own creamy dressing with low-fat yoghurt and chives or other herbs and spices.

It does get boring having a sandwich every day for lunch and perhaps you're not a sandwich person at all. A big salad featuring lots of tomatoes, peppers and other vegetables, plus low fat protein is always a good alternative midday choice. Just watch the dressing. A vinaigrette swimming pool around your salad will pile on the pounds, so a light drizzle is better. Better still, you can substitute it with some lemon juice and herbs for flavour. A baked potato with some low fat protein and salad is great, too – filling, healthy and diet-friendly. Remember to watch out for ready-prepared fillers as they may be heavy on the mayonnaise. Dessert? Fruit wins every time.

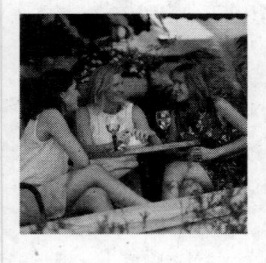

If this has got you thinking, turn to IDEA 18, *Rise and dine*, which is all about breakfast. Did you know that people who eat breakfast are generally slimmer than those who skip it?

Try another idea...

'Luncheon: as much food as one's hand can hold.'
SAMUEL JOHNSON

Defining idea...

How did it go?

Q   I eat out for lunch quite often. What should I choose that is light but won't make me look like a diet bore?

A   *Choose grilled meats or fish and steamed dishes, and pile up the vegetables. Opt for tomato-based sauces where possible as they're always less fattening than creamy ones.*

Q   How can I stop the mid-afternoon slump?

A   *Lunches that are high in carbohydrates can make you feel slow by four o'clock. Try balancing your meal with some low-fat protein. The theory is that increasing the protein to carbohydrate ratio will inhibit the release of serotonin in the brain, which, in large amounts, can make you feel sleepy. Try chicken and salad or a ham and salad open sandwich.*

Q   Is it OK if I just drink a large smoothie for my lunch sometimes?

A   *That brings new meaning to the idea of a liquid lunch! It is fine every now and then, but you could get a better nutritional balance by eating proper food. Smoothies can have a high calorie content. I looked at a litre bottle of an orange, mango and banana smoothie recently and saw it contained 600 calories. If you're thinking of a smoothie as a slimming substitute for food, think again.*

Are you an emotional eater?

If you find that you often eat without being truly hungry, perhaps it's time to work out what's eating you instead.

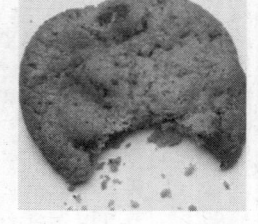

On a physical level food is simply fuel for the body, yet our relationship with it is complex. It is a story filled with love and hate.

We read books about food, watch TV programmes about it and pay lots of money to go and eat what someone else cooks for us at restaurants. Over the years we learn habits and behaviours around food that can become inappropriate. These are often rooted in well-meaning parenting. How many of us polish off every last morsel from our plates because mum told us that the poor kids in Africa are starving or that in her generation all they got was bread, potatoes and water? How many of us will have a sweet treat in response to physical or emotional pain, recalling being soothed with confectionary after a childhood fall? We even give foods a moral value – some are bad or sinful, while others are good and virtuous.

Here's an idea for you... **Eat more slowly. It takes 20 minutes for 'I'm full' signals to reach the brain. Work with your body by giving it the time it needs to respond.**

It's a rollercoaster of a relationship, which is fine if you don't have any issues with weight. If you do, and food seems to be controlling you, remember you are not alone. Thousands of us are stuck in this kind of one-way relationship. You need to work out why you are feeding your emotions and what you will do about it.

The desire to eat is masterminded in the brain and involves more than twenty different chemical messengers in your body. Eating anything will stave off hunger, but not overwhelming cravings for a particular type of food. If you are hungry you have to eat, but when you want to eat for any other reason, you need to develop coping strategies that don't involve food. It is usually the negative emotions that drive us to munch more – unhappiness, stress and boredom, for instance. Different approaches work for different people; coping tactics could include talking to a friend, doing some physical exercise, confronting a situation at work that is troubling you or scheduling in some 'me time', such as a fun shopping trip, a facial or a game of golf. The point is to identify the where, when and how of your emotionally reactive eating and deal with that rather than continuing the behaviour that's holding your diet to ransom.

Another trigger can be tiredness. Again, you need to get to the root cause. Are you exhausted because of work pressure or certain relationships? Or is it because night after night you go to bed too late? Tiredness lowers your mood, which makes you want to eat and perk yourself up, and it also makes your body send hunger signals because it is looking for more energy to get you through the day.

My downfall is boredom and procrastination. I often look for the answers to life in the fridge. I can also spend a long time seeking inspiration in a slice of cheesecake, especially the lovely crunchy bit at the bottom. The cure is to do something more interesting than the thing you're putting off. Alternatively, set yourself mini goals; for example, if you finish a task in one hour you will then reward yourself (not with food) before tackling the next task.

You don't have to finish up everything on your plate. You could try ordering or cooking a smaller portion to begin with. If you need to assuage guilty feelings, pledge some money to charity for every kilo of weight you lose.

Not hungry? Not feeling over-emotional either, yet feeling absolutely desperate for a BLT sandwich? It sound as if you have cravings you need get under control. Flip to IDEA 22, *I want it and I want it now.*

Try another idea...

'Stressed spelled backwards is desserts. Coincidence? I don't think so.'
ANONYMOUS

Defining idea...

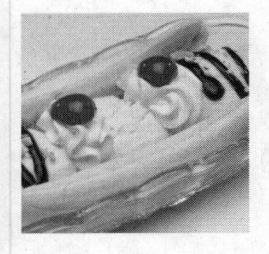
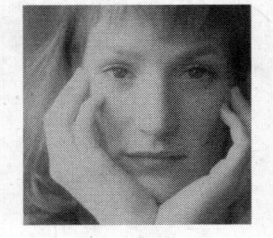
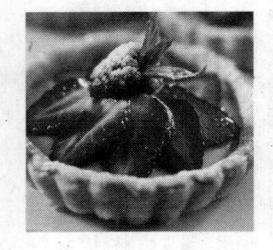

Q I've been trying to consume more good foods since I've been dieting, but I'm not finding them very satisfying. Can you help?

A When you say good foods, do you mean those classic diet type foods such as rice cakes, celery, cottage cheese and so on? Have you ever liked those things? If not, don't bother. They are not going to fill you up and make you happy. Go for something you do like, but make it a small portion if it's high in fat. Try buying a low fat/reduced calorie alternative.

We all tend to perceive some foods as 'good' or 'bad', but I think it is a habit that should be unlearned. Food is just food. Some of it happens to be less calorific or more nutritious. Taking away those sinful/saintly associations gives you a healthier attitude to food, which is the route to weight loss.

Q When I'm unhappy why do I easily devour an entire tub of ice-cream on my own?

A Fatty foods don't send such strong satiety messages to the brain as carbohydrate or protein-rich foods. A meal with a carbohydrate and protein mix will fill you up for longer, while a high-fat meal or snack will leave you feeling unsatisfied. As a solution to the tub of ice-cream situation, if your diversionary tactics don't work, serve yourself a small portion in a bowl and eat it very slowly.

Water works

We can't live without water, yet most of us live in a state of dehydration most of the time. Discover the myriad benefits of drinking more water for your diet, energy levels, skin and more.

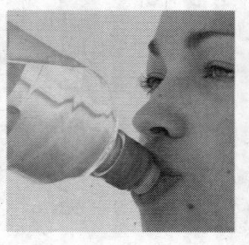

Look through the pages of magazines at the celebrity shots and you'll see that they often carry a bottle of mineral water or have one close by.

It is not because they are being paid a fortune by some water company to endorse their product. They are drinking water because they know it makes their skin glow, look health-conscious and stops them from over-eating. Water is a little miracle. We can't live without it for more than two to five days, but in extremes we can live without food for about a month.

YOUR BASIC BIOLOGY LESSON

Did you know that approximately 60% of an adult's weight is water? Or that two thirds of the water present in the human body is contained within your 50,000

Buy some softly coloured plates as your crockery could be influencing your appetite. A US study revealed that bold, bright patterns stimulate your hunger, while pastel hues decrease it. Strange, but true.

billion cells? Water is important. It's not a nutrient in itself, but it is the main component of cells, tissues and blood and is needed for many bodily functions including assisting the absorption of nutrients from food, the regulation of body temperature, the lubrication of our joints and eyes and the elimination of toxins from the body. We lose roughly half a pint of water a day just through breathing.

TELL ME MORE

About a third of daily fluid intake comes from food, not from liquid. Fruit and vegetables generally supply the most water – for instance, salad leaves are mostly water. Our bodies also get water by burning fats and carbohydrates. Experts reckon that we need one and a half litres of fluid a day to stay healthy and more if it's hot or if you're losing extra water through sweating. It is hard to drink too much water, but it is quite easy to not drink enough. Drinking too little water for an extended period can lead to urinary tract infections, kidney and gall stones. You might also find that you suffer headaches, lack energy and have poor concentration. Research suggests that water also plays a role in keeping the skin moisturised and healthy-looking and helps to regulate emotions. So, if you have poor skin and feel cranky and tired, just try drinking more water!

Defining idea...

'It is astounding how quickly skin responds if you drink three pints of water a day. This water cure helps clear impurities from the system feeding the skin.'
HELENA RUBINSTEIN

A feeling of thirst indicates that you are already dehydrated. Thirst is a signal that there is a water deficiency in the cells. Often we interpret this feeling as hunger, so we eat rather than drink. This leads quite easily to an unnecessary intake of calories! A large glass or two of water containing zero calories will sort out those 'am I hungry?' feelings. It's important to remember the dehydration spiral: you haven't drunk enough water so you feel hungry and tired, so you snack, but it doesn't make you feel better because you're thirsty, so you eat more before realising you need fluids. Then you feel guilty because you've been snacking, so you snack some more. It's a spiral into more guilt and bad food choices. Break the spiral by drinking frequently, whether or not you think you're thirsty. Eight glasses of water a day is a good target. Take one before and after every meal, and one mid-morning and mid-afternoon.

Going abroad soon? Find your way around foreign menus with IDEA 24, *Trip ups.*

Try another idea...

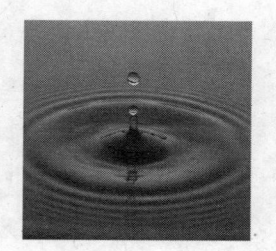

Defining idea...

'*Individuals often find that drinking more water increases the energy levels and can reduce the risk of conditions such as headaches and constipation. However, there is also evidence that a good intake of water is associated with a reduced risk of chronic health conditions.*'
Dr JOHN BRIFFA, quoted on www.naturalmineralwater.org

How did
it go?

Q   Does the temperature of the water you drink make a difference?

A   *No. There is a rumour that if you drink iced water, your body needs to work harder to absorb it and hence burns up more calories in the process. Most experts think this is nonsense. Drink it at room temperature, iced or warm – whatever your personal preference.*

Q   Should I drink tap, spring or mineral water?

A   *I think you should drink whatever you think tastes nicest and whatever best suits your pocket. Tap water is perfectly safe to drink, but is subject to treatment so it may have chlorine or fluoride added which you may be able to taste and not be partial to. Spring water comes from an underground source, but may be treated to remove impurities too. Natural mineral water has to come from an identified underground source and be bottled at source, with nothing added or removed except perhaps carbon dioxide to make it fizzy. It must have its mineral analysis on its bottle. Depending on the minerals and their quantity, mineral water may not be suitable for people with kidney problems or for babies to drink. It is fine for everyone else, so if you want to spend the money, feel free to enjoy it.*

Metabolism masterclass

Think of your metabolism as your inner energy thermostat. If you turn it up, you will use calories faster, but first you need to understand how it works.

Everyone knows someone who's skinny as a rake and yet could represent their country if eating were an Olympic sport. Meanwhile, a salad seems to go straight to your hips.

We may put this down to having a faster or slower metabolism, but is this really true and if so, can you do anything about it? First you need to get to grips with the science – but there won't be an exam at the end.

Each day your body uses up calories or energy in three main ways. First, there is your basal metabolic rate (BMR), sometimes also known as your resting metabolic rate. This is the number of calories your body would use up if you just lay around all day. The BMR is what your body needs to carry out essential bodily functions, such as keeping your heart beating and breathing. It accounts for 60–75% of your total energy expenditure. *Thermogenesis* is the energy you use to digest food and keep

Here's an idea for you...

For the next week, keep a diary of what and when you eat. Adjusting the frequency of your feeding might give you a boost. Some experts say that eating little and often will boost your metabolic rate because your metabolism is raised by about 10% for a couple of hours after you eat. Others disagree but concede that leaving long gaps between meals can leave you nutritionally deficient.

warm, which accounts for around 10% of energy expenditure. The last part of the equation is movement, which covers everything from daily activity to sport. This can be from 15 to 30% of energy expenditure.

There are different ways to work out your metabolic rate, which tells you how many calories you use up in an average day. Here's one:

Take your body weight in kilograms (remember 1 kg = 2.2 lb), then, if you are between 18 and 30, multiply your weight by 14.7 and then add 496. This gives you an idea of your BMR. If you are 31–60, multiply your weight by 8.7 and then add 829. With these numbers, think about how active you are. If you take no exercise and mostly sit or stand during the day, multiply your BMR figure above by 1.4. Multiply it by 1.7 if in addition to sitting or standing all day, you also take some exercise, such as brisk walking. If you're very active, moving around a lot during the day and taking regularly exercise, multiply that figure by 2. The final number is the approximate amount of calories you're using each day.

Now back to the BMR. Your genes can play a part in it – some people are born more revved up than others. But you can't change your genes. Your overall body weight makes a difference too. The larger you are, the more calories your body needs for its basic

Are you achieving your weight loss goals? Get on target with IDEA 3, *Setting goals (without always having to move the goalposts).*

Try another idea...

maintenance. If you lose a dramatic amount of weight very quickly, your BMR will slow, which will ultimately disrupt your long-term efforts at weight control. The best solution lies in building muscle, which burns more calories than fat. Some experts say that an increase in lean body mass can increase energy expenditure by as much as 8–14%. Half a kilo (a pound) of muscle burns 30–50 calories a day, so build 500 g of extra muscle and you'll burn 350 extra calories a week. You can increase your lean muscle mass by weight-training, also known as resistance training or strength training. Anything that puts your muscles under tension counts, so free weights and weight machines in the gym are good, as are choreographed classes which use free weights (usually called something like 'body conditioning'). You could also try a strength-training session at home with an exercise video and dumbbells. One or two sessions a week can really make a difference.

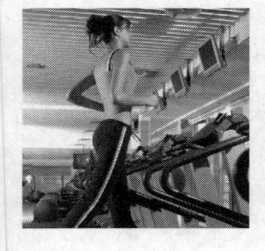
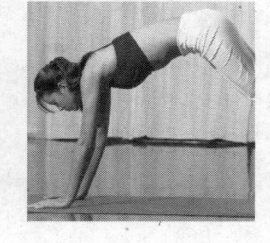

'Two thirds of people who exercise say it helps reduce stress'
DR JAMES RIPPE, Center for Clinical and Lifestyle Research, Chicago

Defining idea...

69

How did it go?

Q Aren't there drugs that raise the metabolism?

A *Yes, but they're not a good idea. Amphetamine-type drugs do speed up the metabolism, but the side effects can be serious – insomnia, depression and anxiety, for example. Herbal supplements can also be risky. Just because something is natural doesn't always means it is safe.*

Q Is it true that yo-yo dieting slows your metabolism?

A *It does in the short term, but recent research has suggested that there isn't evidence that it will have a permanent effect. It is not smart to yo-yo diet, though. Some experts still think that constantly losing and putting weight back on can result in higher overall fat levels. In any case, it does nothing for your confidence and self-esteem.*

Q I have been doing strength training exercise recently and I've put on weight! Why?

A *Have you changed shape? Muscle is three times heavier than fat and takes up less space, so it's possible to shrink in size and weigh more. Rather than keep track of your progress on the scales, try using a tape measure for your chest, waist, hips, thighs and so on. Seeing a difference in cms/inches will be a great motivator.*

17

Sweet temptation

Can you refuse the siren call of confectionery? Are you a chocoholic? Here's how to stop a sweet tooth from wrecking your weight loss plan.

Chocolate is like a really great friend. It picks you up when you're down, comforts you, is a pretty good love substitute and would never tell you that your bottom looks really big in your favourite jeans.

The feel-good factor of chocolate and other sweet foods is undeniable. Chocolate does give you a kind of chemical high when you eat it by boosting your brain's serotonin and endorphin levels, making you feel calm and happy. Other substances in it stimulate the brain's emotional arousal, giving you a lovely warm glow similar to being in love.

There's an evolutionary component to the appeal of sweet foods. Human beings have more sweet taste buds than other taste buds and we naturally prefer sweet tastes from babyhood to adulthood. Some scientists believe that humans developed

Here's an idea for you... **Try a cup of fennel herbal tea after having a little taste of something you crave. This will suppress your appetite, ensuring you don't carry on munching.**

a preference for sweet things because generally they are higher in calories and so pack lots of energy – important in hunter-gatherer times, but less so now that all you have to do is get off the sofa and go to the kitchen cupboard when you feel a bit peckish. If we were as active as we were in hunter-gatherer days and had to work hard to find our food while beating off woolly mammoths, we could stuff our faces with sweet treats and probably wouldn't put on a gram. Times have changed, but we still have our prehistoric tastebuds.

Chocolate is high in fat, often around 30% by weight, and full of calories. Other confectionery is crammed with sugars and can weigh in at 375 calories per 100 g. They will both give you a temporary rise in blood sugar and a feeling of satisfaction, but then your body will tell your brain that it didn't supply all the nutrients it wanted. Your hunger is stimulated and if you continue to munch on the sweet stuff, the process just repeats itself. The high and low swings are in response to your body asking for nutrients, not sugar.

Defining idea...

'*Research tells us that fourteen out of any ten individuals likes chocolate.*'
SANDRA BOYNTON, *Chocolate: The Consuming Passion*

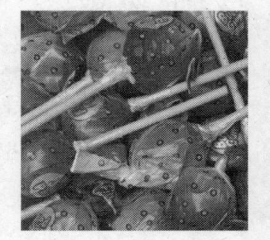

When you're trying to lose weight, it is accepted practice to stay off sweet stuff. In my experience, total denial doesn't work because the more you tell yourself you can't have

Distract your sweet tooth with a different kind of passion. See IDEA 42, *The birds and the bees*

Try another idea...

something, the more you want it. So, here's the deal. Do have a little of what you fancy, but it really does have to be a little portion. Take time to really enjoy it – sit down at the table or on a comfy chair without distractions and savour every mouthful. This way you can make giving in to temptation a positive experience while not over-eating.

You could also try having your sweet hit in a different way. For example, if you want something chocolatey and a bit creamy, make yourself a milkshake using skimmed or non-fat milk and chocolate powder, or have a hot cocoa made half with milk, half with water. A small pot of low-fat chocolate mousse might hit the spot, too. If it is crunch and chewiness you're after, try a thin scraping of chocolate spread on bread, crackers or rice cakes. A meringue with some fruit and a dollop of low fat yoghurt, fromage frais or crème fraiche on top satisfies the need for a pudding without the fat and calorie overload. Get used to reading the labels of your favourite biscuits, cakes and confectionary. By comparing and contrasting, you'll see that some sweet indulgences are much more diet-friendly than others. Life would be so much easier if you just craved broccoli, wouldn't it?

'After eating chocolate you feel god-like, as though you can conquer enemies, lead armies, entice lovers.'
EMILY LUCKETT

Defining idea...

How did it go?

Q Could I use honey or brown sugar to satisfy my sweet tooth?

A Yes, if you prefer their taste, but remember that just because something is not white and granulated, it doesn't mean it isn't sugar. Think about the number of calories you are taking in.

Q I've read that chocolate has some useful minerals in it and is good for you. Is this true?

A Yes, it contains potassium. Plain chocolate also offers iron and magnesium, but don't forget that these nutrients are coming in a fat and calorie gift-wrapped package. You can get them from other food sources at less cost to your figure.

Q Don't you think that if I give in to temptation and just have a bit of something sweet and nice, I won't be able to stop?

A You have to stop eating and start doing something else. You could: go for a walk, go to the movies, read a book, go to an evening class, have a cuddle with someone you love, have a long soak in the bath or learn to play a musical instrument. You need to distract yourself and also get absorbed in something that is more interesting (or at least as interesting) as eating.

18

Rise and dine!

If you thought skipping or skimping on breakfast would be a good way to shed weight, you need to wake up to the fact that the opposite is true. Feast on this.

Wouldn't it be great if there was a really simple trick that made us feel full of energy and sharp as a very sharp thing for hours on end? Well there is, and it is called breakfast.

Many people give breakfast a miss because they think it will help them lose weight. Research has shown that breakfast eaters tend to be slimmer than breakfast skippers. This is due in part to the fact that eating a healthy breakfast keeps you feeling full for longer. That means you'll be more able to resist a quick calorie-laden snack when you're feeling faint at 11 a.m.

Further studies have concluded that if you eat a high carbohydrate breakfast, especially breads and cereals, you'll end up consuming less fat in your daily calorie intake than if you skip breakfast. This is of significance when you're trying to lose weight. Breakfast eaters have been found to have lower cholesterol levels than non-breakfast eaters and those who choose high fat fry-ups.

Here's an idea for you...

Next time you're in the multiplex, think *Amélie* not *Slasher Vixens 2*. Heightened emotions may trigger a desire for comfort food, according to a medical study. Horror films and comedies caused a group of women to eat more, especially the women who had previously voiced concerns over their weight. Travel shows made all the women eat less. Stay calm to lose weight!

Here are a few more good reasons why having breakfast makes sense. According to one UK study, volunteers who consumed a low-fat, high-carbohydrate breakfast reported feeling less tired and muddled than those who ate nothing or chose a high fat, low carbohydrate meal. Studies on school children have shown that kids who breakfast show greater concentration in class, as well as increased problem-solving and verbal fluency abilities. This must also have some application to adults, as has been proven in tests on memory stimulation and breakfast eating. I expect you can guess that adult breakfasters showed superior skills in memory tests than those who went without!

What should you have for breakfast? Fry-ups are out, apart from a once a week treat. But you have to promise to grill your bacon rather than fry it and to choose low-fat sausages. Could you try poaching or scrambling your eggs without adding extra fat? Cereal, whether it is based on wheat, corn, rice, bran or oats, can be a good high-fibre, low fat choice – with skimmed or non-fat milk of course. Do check the label on the packet, as many cereals contain high levels of sugar. Muesli, despite its sandal-wearing, yoghurt-knitting associations, isn't always as healthy as you

might think. Many brands contain vast amounts of sugar, not to mention tasty little additions such as chocolate chips. Go for sugar-free varieties. Cooked oats have been around for centuries – the Roman historian Pliny recorded how early Germanic tribes ate porridge. As the starchy oats are digested slowly, so porridge gives a steady release of energy that lasts for hours; it is one of the most satisfying breakfasts you could choose. The soluble fibre in oats also helps to lower cholesterol levels. Prepare it with skimmed milk and it is very healthy and diet-friendly. You could try making it the traditional Scottish way with water, but personally I find that quite disgusting. Wholemeal toast with a scraping of butter and little low-fat protein is a good choice, too. Muffins, croissants and pains au chocolat are not good. Frankly, they are just cake and have no place on the dieter's plate.

Remember, a decent breakfast will make all the difference to your weight-loss plan and could make you a brighter, more cheerful person to be around.

Look at diets in a new way and watch the weight fall off. See IDEA 7, *It's never too late to change your mind.*

Try another idea…

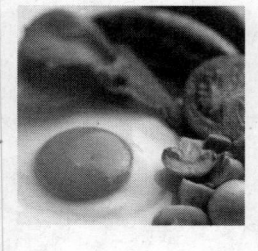
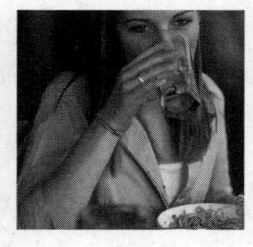

'Eat breakfast like a king, lunch like a prince and dinner like a pauper.'
ADELLE DAVIS

Defining idea…

How did
it go?

Q   **I really can't face breakfast in the morning. What can I do?**

A   *You are not alone, but it is important to try to get into the habit of breakfasting. My suggestion would be that you have something small and healthful as soon as you feel able. A banana smoothie (made with skimmed milk, low-fat yoghurt and fruit) or half a wholemeal roll with reduced-fat cheese are the kinds of foods to go for. Alternatively, just snacking on fruit throughout the morning won't do you any harm, as long as lunch and dinner are well balanced with a mix of low-fat protein and carbohydrates.*

Q   **How do I make my own muesli?**

A   *All you have to do is soak some oats overnight in some skimmed milk or fruit juice and then add some grated apple, berries or sultanas and a spoonful of low-fat yoghurt or fromage frais. You could also add a handful of nuts or sprinkling of seeds, such as sunflower or pumpkin seeds, which are rich sources of nutrients.*

Q   **Is it true that it is good to drink hot water and lemon before eating breakfast?**

A   *I don't know of any evidence, apart from anecdotal, that backs up the idea that it will cleanse your system. It won't do any harm and if it makes you feel good, do it.*

Walk yourself thinner

If you're new to exercise or just don't fancy the gym, here's a simple way to drop some weight. It's easy to start, and requires no special clothing or equipment.

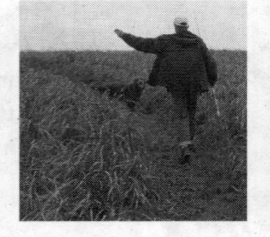

Most of us view walking as a way to get from A to B, and most of the time we'll choose to use the car or bus to get us to where we want to go.

There is a good reason to put one foot in front of the other more often: it's a great way to lose weight and stay slim. It is not expensive, it is not complicated and you can do it anywhere.

Half an hour's walking will burn up an average of about two hundred calories and help to tone up your legs and bottom. There's a catch; you won't see results with a gentle stroll to work or the shops once or twice a week. To make a difference, you'll need to walk at least three times a week, building up to five times a week, for half an hour. You'll need to do it at a reasonable pace, one that warms you up, makes

Here's an idea for you...

Make your dairy product intake low-fat. In research, obese volunteers lost 11% of their body weight over six months on a calorie-controlled diet that included three low-fat dairy portions a day.

you feel ever so slightly sweaty and leaves you feeling slightly breathless, but not so breathless that you could not hold a conversation. If you walk up some hills or on an incline on the treadmill in the gym, you'll increase the challenge and burn up more calories. It is simple. Here are a few other pointers to bear in mind:

- You don't really need specialist gear for walking, but a decent pair of trainers will support you better than ordinary shoes. If you're planning to take up hill walking or hiking, you will need shoes or boots designed for the purpose, both for comfort and safety.

- You'll work harder outdoors than inside on a treadmill as you'll have to cope with changing terrain and wind resistance. This is a good thing as you'll burn calories faster and get extra toning benefits. Regularly spending time outside has been shown to keep you emotionally fit too, boosting feelings of well-being and staving off depression.

- Wear something comfortable! It might sound obvious, but if you get wet or too hot, you'll want to give up and go back home. High-tech sports fabrics are designed to draw away sweat and protect you from wind and rain without weighing you down.

Defining idea...

'Walking is the best possible exercise.'
THOMAS JEFFERSON

- When walking, keep your tummy muscles pulled in to work your abdominal muscles and protect your back. Walk tall, avoid slumping and use your natural stride.

- If you swing your arms while you walk, you'll increase your heart rate and get more of a workout.

- For the best technique, hit the ground with your heel first, roll through your foot and then push off with your toes.

Rather than just randomly walking when you feel like it, try to schedule a daily walk, or at least every other day. That way, you are more likely to stick with it and see results in conjunction with your healthier eating habits, plus you'll be able to monitor your progress.

To reap the greatest benefits, set yourself a plan, say over six weeks, gradually increasing the length of time you walk and its frequency and the speed. For example, in week one you could walk for half an hour three times a week, slowly for 15 minutes and briskly for 15 minutes. Over the next few weeks, you would aim to add another walking session and making each one 5 or 10 minutes longer, and you would walk briskly for 20 or 25 minutes and at a slower pace for the rest of the time. By the end of six weeks, you could be walking for 45 minutes to an hour four or five times a week, and mostly at the faster pace. You'll be seeing a slimmer you in the mirror.

If you're finding you like the physical and mental effects of exercise, maybe you're ready to challenge yourself further. Go on, I know you want to. Turn to IDEA 21, *Burn fat faster!*

Try another idea...

'A sedentary life is the real sin against the Holy Spirit. Only those thoughts that come by walking have any value.'
FRIEDRICH NIETZSCHE

Defining idea...

How did it go?

Q **I love walking, but how do I stop getting lonely?**

A *Buy or borrow a dog, not just to keep you company, but also to meet other dog-walkers. Could you encourage a friend to come on walks with you, rather than meeting at the wine bar, pub or café? You could also join a walking club, or if there isn't one in your area, set up your own! Although it can be very motivating and help the time pass, for safety's sake I don't recommend listening to music through headphones, especially if you're a woman on your own.*

Q **Don't you think that walking can get a bit boring after a while?**

A *There are ways to make it more interesting, like going to picturesque places. This may not be possible every day, but you could drive to a beauty spot for your weekend walking sessions. If you are going to have dinner with friends on the other side of town, why not walk there? You could also sign up for a challenge so that you have a goal to train for. Charity walks can be fun – you meet a lot of people and have the satisfaction of really achieving something, both for yourself and others. There are plenty of organised charity walks at home and abroad, from an easy 5 km walk around your local park to serious trekking in Nepal. Fancy hiking up the Himalayas? Now that's a real challenge!*

20

Detox diets – con or cure?

If you've heard that detoxification diets can help you slim down, you've probably been tempted to try one. But what do they involve and are they safe?

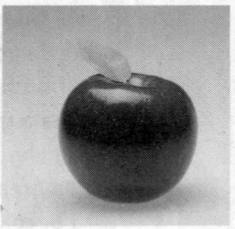

The urge to purge is not a new idea.
The ancient Aztecs were keen on enemas,
while in 19th-century Europe some doctors
argued that removing the colon made sense
because it is where the body stores its toxins.

Fasting has long been a feature of some religions. Mostly, however, we're drawn to detoxing as a way to cleanse the body rather than the soul and hope to lose weight in the process. This is what countless magazines, books, celebrities and health gurus sell us.

Detox fans see it as something to be done a couple of times a year to improve digestion, energy levels, skin and to kick-start weight loss. Usually they'll take the pattern of eating only fruit and raw vegetables and drinking juices and water for a few days. Then over the next few days they reintroduce other foods, such as

Here's an idea for you...

Yoga-inspired detox breathing is great for de-stressing and will take your mind off food. Inhale very slowly and deeply, but without straining. Then exhale quickly, as you would if you were sneezing. Continue this breathing pattern and try to become aware of your abdomen tightening and releasing and how calm, heavy and relaxed your body feels.

steamed vegetables, soups, fish and poultry, wholegrains, nuts and seeds. Red meat, alcohol, coffee and dairy are usually banned. There is nothing wrong with cutting out red meat, alcohol or even coffee, though I have never seen any hard evidence that a cup or two of coffee a day is anything other than delicious.

I don't like the idea of cutting out an entire food group, such as dairy, unless you actually have an allergy. These kinds of detox diets tend to only be for a week or two, and won't do you any harm, but will they do any good? Most doctors agree that your body is perfectly capable of eliminating toxins without the help of a special diet. In fact, the only form of detoxification that many of them recognise is the one for alcoholics when they stop drinking. Believers will counter that the medical establishment is simply behind the times and that because our modern bodies are subjected to pollution and antibiotics and additives in food, they need all the help they can get. Many detox aficionados also claim that the process is cathartic, helping you get in touch with your deepest emotions, which could lead to far-reaching changes in your life. But navel gazing is all you can do when you're light-headed and too weak to get off the sofa. Ouch! That was mean, wasn't it? I do have friends who swear by their January detox and look and feel fantastic. Personally, I find detoxes hard work. I'm for everything in moderation: eating low fat and healthily, with plenty of variety. If you want to avoid pesticides and additives, buy organic food.

FASTING

**Beware of disordered eating.
See IDEA 36, *Dieting danger*.**

Try another idea...

This is a step beyond detox diets, but is also recommended as a way to cleanse and boost weight loss. The problem with fasting is that it makes you feel weak and dizzy, and any weight you lose will find its way back as soon as you eat normally. The bottom line is that the occasional one-day fast won't hurt you, but please don't try it for longer than a day unless you're under professional supervision. Psychologists have commented that fasting attracts individuals who want to punish their bodies. It's hard not to be down on yourself when you're overweight, but don't punish yourself. Self-loathing and guilt are common feelings experienced by dieters, but they sabotage your good intentions and progress. A healthy attitude to food and your body is the secret of success.

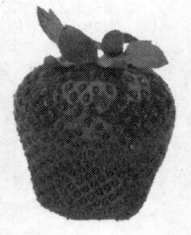
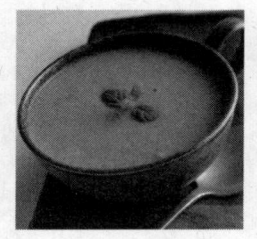

'I believe this idea of the build-up of toxins is absolute rubbish and I won't change my mind until the detoxing lobby can prove what they claim with properly controlled trials'
PROFESSOR JOHN GARROW, quoted in *Zest* magazine

Defining idea...

85

How did
it go?

Q I think I'd find a full-on detox too difficult. Is there a sort of detox-lite I could follow?

A   *You could try cutting out processed foods, alcohol and sugary products such as cakes, ice-cream and confectionery for a week and see how you get on. You are bound to lose a few kilos. It's really just healthy eating, so it should get you thinking more about the food choices you normally make. It may also stimulate your palate and you could find you prefer the taste of real food to refined foods.*

Q What about herbal detox drinks?

A   *Readily available in health food stores and chemists, these drinks make the same sorts of cleansing and weight management claims as many other diets. I can honestly say, having tried a few, that I haven't experienced any great effects. One or two have made me feel more energetic than usual but I lost no weight. Try them yourself if you don't mind spending the money. Just don't expect miracles.*

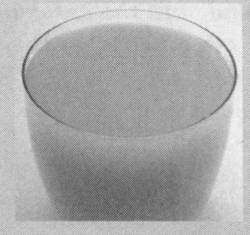
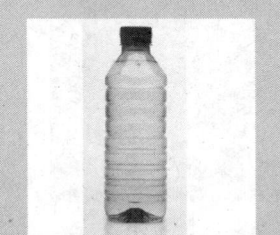

Burn fat faster!

Eating less and moving more will result in weight loss. If you rev up the exercise part of the equation, you'll lose kilos quicker.

Taking a bath burns calories. And, given the choice, who wouldn't prefer a nice long soak to a nice long session on the rowing machine in the gym?

Most daily activities, such as watching TV, doing housework and sleeping use energy, but they are unlikely to exceed your energy intake from food. The secret to burning fat faster is to maximise the fat-burning potential of everything you do, from your daily chores and activities to proper workouts. Here are some tips for you to mix and match as you like.

Try working out for longer
If the prospect of an intense workout at the gym or a 15 km hike around your local park horrifies you, try working out less fast, but for longer. For example, walking briskly for an hour burns the same amount of calories as running for half an hour.

Here's an idea for you...

Following a good workout, after an hour, go for a healthy protein and carbohydrate snack, such as a tuna and salad sandwich. This will help your body through its 'after-burn', when it replaces short-term energy loss with energy from your fat stores.

Have a more energetic day

You can burn up to 300 calories more simply by being more active in the way you do everyday things. Instead of ambling along to work, stride briskly. Do those dull old household chores you've been putting off for ever, such as cleaning the windows, scrubbing the kitchen floor, tidying the garden and redecorating the bedroom. Put some good old-fashioned elbow grease into it and you've got yourself a workout. Why not start your day in an upbeat mood and dance to a few songs on the radio or on your CD player? And when you next go to the shops, walk instead of driving or taking the bus.

Defining idea...

'Consider joining a group or exercising with a friend. Commitments made as part of a group tend to be stronger than those made independently.'
AMERICAN COLLEGE OF SPORTS MEDICINE fitness book

Build some muscle

Use weights, either on gym machines, in a workout class or as part of a home fitness routine. This will help you burn fat and not just because simply lifting weights uses energy. Pumping iron (I know, it's such a male term, but women, please take note) builds muscle tissue, which is metabolically more active that fat tissue. Muscle uses more energy than fat

just to exist, so the more muscle you have, the more calories get used, even when you're resting. You really don't need to look like Arnold Schwarzenegger for this to be true.

Learn to love intervals

I don't mean going off mid-performance to have an ice-cream or a glass of wine, I mean interval training. The idea is that you can increase the amount of calories you burn during any exercise by increasing your speed, the intensity or the duration, even for brief intervals. If you are walking, swimming or cycling, you could go steady for about 15–20 minutes, then go faster for a couple of minutes, then slow down again and speed up in random bursts. To earn extra good marks, increase the duration and frequency of the intervals of harder work. It's tough, but really effective.

Remember, the fitter you are, the better your body becomes at using its fuel, which translates into a leaner, more toned you. The more exercise you do, the quicker you'll see results. This makes it worth learning to love exercise.

Weight loss is about calories in versus calories out. But where do they hide and how many do you need anyway? Turn to IDEA 2, *Food accountancy made simple.*

Try another idea...

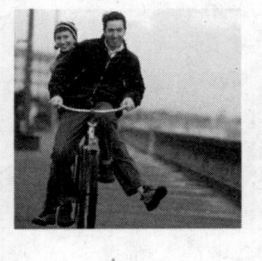
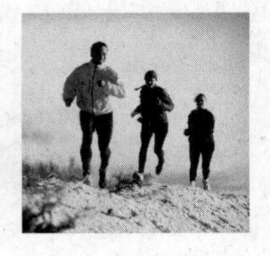

'My idea of exercise is a good brisk sit.'
PHYLLIS DILLER

Defining idea...

How did it go?

Q **I don't really want to pump iron and get lots of muscles. What kind of exercise should I do in the gym that avoids muscle development?**

A *To bulk up you need to use specific training techniques and work very, very hard – much harder than a normal, regular exerciser could ever dream of. Don't give it a second thought, since you won't suddenly become the Incredible Hulk without trying. Instead, think about this: kilo for kilo, muscle takes up less room than fat. This is why many women who take up weight training find they drop a dress size.*

Q **When I lift weights, my muscles go all shaky. What's that about? Is it a sign that I'm ill?**

A *It sounds like it's a normal reaction, and that you are doing good things in the gym. For the best results when weight training, you need to repeat the exercise until you experience muscle exhaustion – that's when you think you really can't squeeze out another repetition and, you guessed it, your muscle starts to shake. If you give up before you reach this point, you're not working hard enough and won't see the results you want. If you've only just started exercising, you might well reach this point after four to five repetitions. As you continue, it will take longer and longer to get there.*

22

I want it and I want it now

Run, hide or play dead and a few other bright ideas to control the food cravings that well up in most of us when we diet.

If your appetite for a certain food is really strong, or you'll go to any lengths to have what you desire, that's a craving.

In the past, it has been thought that cravings represent a nutritional need. Some experts, especially those with an alternative medicine background, still maintain that is the case. I think it's rather curious that we invariably crave sweet, fatty things as opposed to a nice big serving of spinach. There is no doubt that at certain times your cravings can be related to what is going on in your body. This seems to be particularly true for women and may be hormone-related. Many women experience strong cravings just before menstruation, for example. It is also common to have cravings when you're pregnant. I couldn't eat enough baked beans when I was pregnant, which was not very glamorous. Men don't get so many cravings. It seems we all grow out of cravings in the end; the over-65s have fewer cravings than younger people. It is thought this is because our appetites reduce with age, together with a weakening of the senses of smell and taste.

Here's an idea for you... **Green tea can raise the metabolic rate. If you drink four or five cups a day, you could burn up around 70 calories – for doing very little! Drinking green tea could lose you nearly half a stone over a year. Put the kettle on!**

The bad news is that people who are trying to lose weight experience the most cravings. Much of this can be put down to psychological factors. Remember when, as a child, you were told not to do something and it made you want to do it even more? It's the same with dieting. Self-denial in itself just makes you want to have whatever you have told yourself you are not allowed to have.

Diets that are very restrictive become incredibly dull and foods that are banned become disproportionately attractive. In contrast, a healthy long-term approach to losing weight, using a balance of nutrients and portion control, won't encourage cravings because there's no real deprivation. You also won't become desperately hungry if you're eating sensibly, which will curb cravings and mean that the double cheeseburger and fries you are fantasising about will remain in the burger shop where they belong.

If a craving sneaks up on you like an uninvited guest who won't take the hint that you don't want their company right now, you could try one of these three tricks:

■ Bring on a substitute.

If it's chocolate you're craving, would a glass of chocolate milk made with skimmed milk do? You could try grating a couple of squares of chocolate on top. If the subject of your lust is ice-cream, go for a lower fat version or try sorbet.

■ Pay attention to portion size

Buy a smaller version of your favourite food craving, such as a kid's size, a travel size, just not a family size! This way you can't overindulge. Or, measure out a small portion of what you fancy, sit down and really concentrate on enjoying it. When you've finished, get involved in a non-food related activity.

■ Give in and don't beat yourself up

Denying yourself a craving could lead to a full-scale binge.

It's also worth seeing if you can identify a pattern in your cravings – for instance, check if they occur at certain times of the day. Work out if how you usually feel at that time of the day. The more you understand your eating habits, the easier it is to tackle them and not allow them to interfere with your goal to lose weight.

Exercise helps to control your appetite. If you're not a gym fan, read IDEA 35, *Shape up from home*, which suggests another approach,

Try another idea...

'Food is like sex. When you abstain, even the worst stuff begins to look good.'
BETH McCOLLISTER

Defining idea...

How did it go?

Q **Why is my craving for sweet foods intensified when I'm premenstrual?**

A *Lots of women say that they experience this. Our bodies do require extra calories just before menstruation. The trick is to improve the overall balance of your diet. You could also try taking a multivitamin supplement with zinc and evening primrose oil. Don't deny yourself, but be careful not to binge. As well as employing distractions, this is also a time of the month when you could probably use some pampering. A massage, for example, will make you feel good, and lessen the bloated, cranky feelings of PMS. It will also stop you thinking about food for a while.*

Q **Are there any ways I could 'train' myself out of a craving, like you train a puppy not to do certain things?**

A *You could try 'de-temptation' training. List six or seven foods that you regularly crave and put them in order of importance. Take the food craving you care least about from your selection and carry some of it around with you all day in your bag, briefcase or pocket. At the end of the day throw it away or give it to someone else. Work through your whole list to prove to yourself that you can resist giving in to your cravings. Some people swear by this method, and even if it doesn't completely remove the cravings, you'll probably learn quite a lot about the whys, whens and hows of these unwelcome urges.*

Make your kitchen more diet-friendly

Decent equipment and a little low fat cooking know-how can transform the way you eat. It's fun to learn, too.

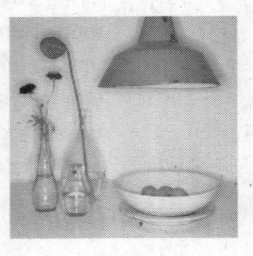

I have heard it said that you should never trust a skinny chef; I never trust them with the double cream, because they just don't care about calories.

The proliferation of celebrity chefs with their TV shows and books is undoubtedly a good thing in as it has definitely reawakened our collective interest in food and cooking. However, these people, pleasant as I'm sure they are, do not care about your diet. What you do in your own kitchen is of paramount importance in the battle of the bulge. The good news is that it's easy to serve up food that is calorie-conscious, yet still delicious. Here, in no particular order, are a few of my top tips for slimmingly wonderful food preparation methods and techniques:

1. Get used to grilling as a less fattening way to cook meat and fish than frying. You can do it without using any extra fat at all. If you find that your grilling is getting a bit dry, simply brush on a small amount of an unsaturated fat, such as olive or sunflower oil. Note the word brush; it's quite different to drench.

Here's an idea for you...

Slouching and eating don't mix! Lying down makes you eat more than when you're sitting up straight at a table. When you're lying down, food passes through your gut more slowly and it takes you longer to realise that you are full.

2. Invest in a steamer to cook your vegetables. Boiling boils most of the nutrients away and makes them all school-dinner soggy. You can even be adventurous and steam fish.

3. When serving vegetables, don't dollop a knob of butter on top. A few chopped herbs, such as parsley or mint, add oodles of flavour without the calories.

4. Buy good quality, non-stick cookware so you can reduce or cut out the need for cooking with fat. Nothing lasts forever, though, and non-stick coating can wear off over the years. Check your pans to see if they need replacing.

5. Use proper measures. While it's fun and terribly TV chef to measure using your eye and just throw everything together, in real life this means it is easy to add unnecessary calories and produce overly large portion sizes.

6. Braising and poaching are a couple of failsafe healthy cooking methods that you can use for fish and meat. Just use stock, milk, water or juice and chuck in the relevant herbs and spices.

7. If you're making a casserole or meaty sauce such as Bolognese, you could try dry frying the meat first and draining away the excess fat before you add in your other ingredients.

8. Always look to see if there is a reduced fat version of your ingredients. For example, coconut milk is a staple of many cuisines, but is very high in saturated fat. You can find brands with half the fat, which is worth it if you use it a lot. Double-check that you can use reduced and low fat butter/margarine products for cooking, as some are only suitable for spreading.

What's a healthy balance of foods on your plate? See IDEA 4, Pyramid selling.

Try another idea...

Just because you're losing weight, it doesn't mean it's all bland deprivation in the kitchen department. And if what you are producing tastes like cardboard, add a new cookbook to your shopping list.

'The kitchen is the great laboratory of the household and much of the weal and woe as regards bodily health depends on the nature of the preparations concocted within its walls.'
MRS BEETON, *The Book of Household Management*

Defining idea...

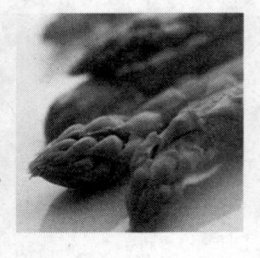

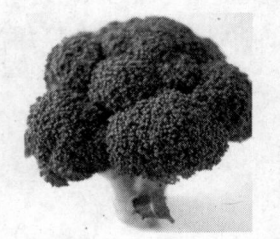

Q   How can a dish have a creamy texture without cream?

A   Just add a little reduced-fat crème fraiche or yoghurt. Although it's not the lowest fat option, a light Greek yoghurt has a creamier taste than regular low-fat yoghurt.

Q   I love bacon and want to cut it out completely, but what substitutions could I make?

A   In cooking, you could try swapping bacon for sun-dried tomatoes. Rinse the oil off them or reconstitute dry ones in water. They will produce a flavour that is as rich as bacon. You could also try turkey rashers, which look like bacon. They are perfectly tasty and a lot less fatty.

Q   What about microwaving?

A   Some people are mistrustful of microwave ovens, but I think they're great because you rarely need to add fat to whatever you're cooking in them. They're also brilliant when you're late, tired or lazy because you can whip up something healthy and tasty in half the time that it would take to go to the take-away on the corner. Make the microwave your friend, and use it to make a wholesome, hot meal instead of giving in to the attractions of commercially prepared take-aways that are full of fat, salt and sugar.

24

Trip ups

They say travel broadens your mind, but it can also thicken your waistline. Here's how to holiday without piling on the pounds.

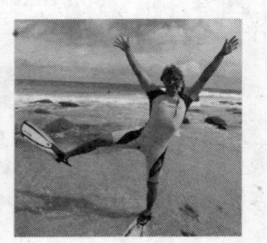

Looking at your holiday snaps can be a turning point in deciding to lose weight. Seeing how plump you look in them can be quite a shock.

I remember eagerly shuffling through my photographs after returning from a sojourn in Portugal. I was looking for the ones in which I might look as though I was related to Cindy Crawford, but no, I looked hideously out of shape from every angle in every picture. There were a lot of me at tables, laden with the remnants of blow-out meals and several empty wine bottles. Cruelly confronted with my personal excess baggage, I vowed that I was going to get a grip and be slim and toned by my next break.

The aftermath of a holiday can be scary, but often it's the prospect of going on holiday that fills us with fear. Away from our normal routines, we worry about how we're going to eat in a calorie-conscious way to avoid returning with an extra three kilos as a souvenir. If you go to somewhere really remote and exotic, you might

Here's an
idea for
you...

Eat fiddly food. It could save you calories. Things like fresh artichoke, crabs, lobster, shrimps with their shells on, and mussels require some effort to consume, so you eat more slowly. This stops you eating too much too fast.

come home a stone lighter thanks to some nasty tummy bug, but otherwise, travelling and staying abroad is likely to trip up your diet plans.

This doesn't mean that you shouldn't go on holiday! You can't put life, fun and new experiences on hold while you try to get to your target weight. The key is knowing your way around foreign menus, choosing dishes wisely, watching the portion sizes and going easy on the local beers, cocktails, vino, sangria and port or whatever other alcoholic temptations are on offer.

Here's a whistlestop tour of popular holiday destinations and the pros and cons of local cuisine:

SPAIN

Go for: gazpacho, stuffed peppers, grilled fish, salads, paella, mussels, grilled chicken and rice, tortilla.

Skip: fried dishes, whitebait (they're cooked in batter, so it's a snack with more than 300 calories), fish served with oily sauces, albondigas (fatty meatballs) and chorizo (a high fat sausage).

GREECE

Go for: pitta bread, salads, baked fish, stuffed tomatoes, grilled fish, fresh fruit, seafood kebabs, lamb and pepper kebabs, tzatziki and hummus dips. When you order salad, ask for the dressing on the side.

Skip: baklava sweets, moussaka (a high-fat dish), meatballs, taramasalata (just a tablespoon is 50% fat and contains 200 calories), and spicy sausages.

ITALY

Go for: fish dishes, thin-base pizzas with vegetable toppings, pasta with tomato, vegetable or seafood sauces, parma ham with melon, seafood salad, bread sticks, tuna and bean salad, and grilled chicken (ask for sauce on the side).

Skip: pasta with creamy or buttery sauces, pizza with salami, extra Parmesan, chargrilled vegetables (drenched in oil), pesto sauce. Avoid creamy sauces such as carbonara.

FRANCE

Go for: consommé soup, grilled trout, ratatouille, salads, bouillabaisse, salad-filled baguettes, lower fat cheeses such as brie, camembert and goat's cheese, and French onion soup (but don't eat the floating cheese).

Did you know that sleep plays a part in weight loss? Flip to **IDEA 29**, *Snooze and lose*, to find out more.

Try another idea...

'**The trouble with Italian food is that five to six days later you're hungry again.**'
GEORGE MILLER, British writer

Defining idea...

101

Defining idea...

'**The quality of food is in inverse proportion to a dining room's altitude, especially atop bank and hotel buildings – airplanes are an extreme example.**'
BRYAN MILLER, *New York Times* restaurant critic

Skip: Creamy and buttery sauces such as Béarnaise or à la Normandie, buttered vegetables, patisserie, croissants, and pain au chocolat.

USA

Go for: Tex mex – bean burritos, chicken fajitas, vegetable chilli tostadas, low-fat or fat-free muffins, yoghurts and ice-cream. In the USA you can get any variation on a menu, but you need to ask. The downside is the enormous portions they give you.

Skip: burgers, fries, cheesecake, brownies, potato skins, tortilla chips, fried steaks and Caesar salad, which seems healthy, but has a dressing that whacks up the fat and calories.

THAILAND

Go for: fish cakes, prawn or green papaya salad, stir-fried vegetable dishes, soups (avoid those with coconut, a rich source of saturated fat), meat or seafood pad ka pau (stir-fried with garlic, basil and chilli), whole baked fish.

Skip: Curries (often swimming in coconut milk) and satay sauce (delicious, but a calorie colossus).

Q **I enjoy exercise and want to keep it up while I'm away. Any suggestions?**

How did it go?

A *Ring in advance to check if your hotel has a gym or an arrangement with a local health club. Perhaps they could also assist you in hiring a bike during your stay. You could check if your room has a video so you could take along a couple of exercise tapes. A skipping rope is a fun way to do some cardiovascular work, while a resistance band can take the place of weights. Don't underestimate the benefits of swimming or walking on beaches and around the sights either.*

Q **Although I can control what I eat when I get there, I find the actual travelling tricky. How do I stop eating something that I don't really want because I am too hungry to resist.**

A *The simplest thing to do is to pack your own little food bag for your journey with plenty of fruit and low-fat snacks. That way you won't be caught out and have to eat a burger because there was no choice on the train/at the airport. Don't forget that most airlines can provide for a special diet, as long as they have enough notice. Some are better than others, but it's always worth asking for a low-fat meal or a vegetarian option, which should at least guarantee some fresh fruit and vegetables.*

103

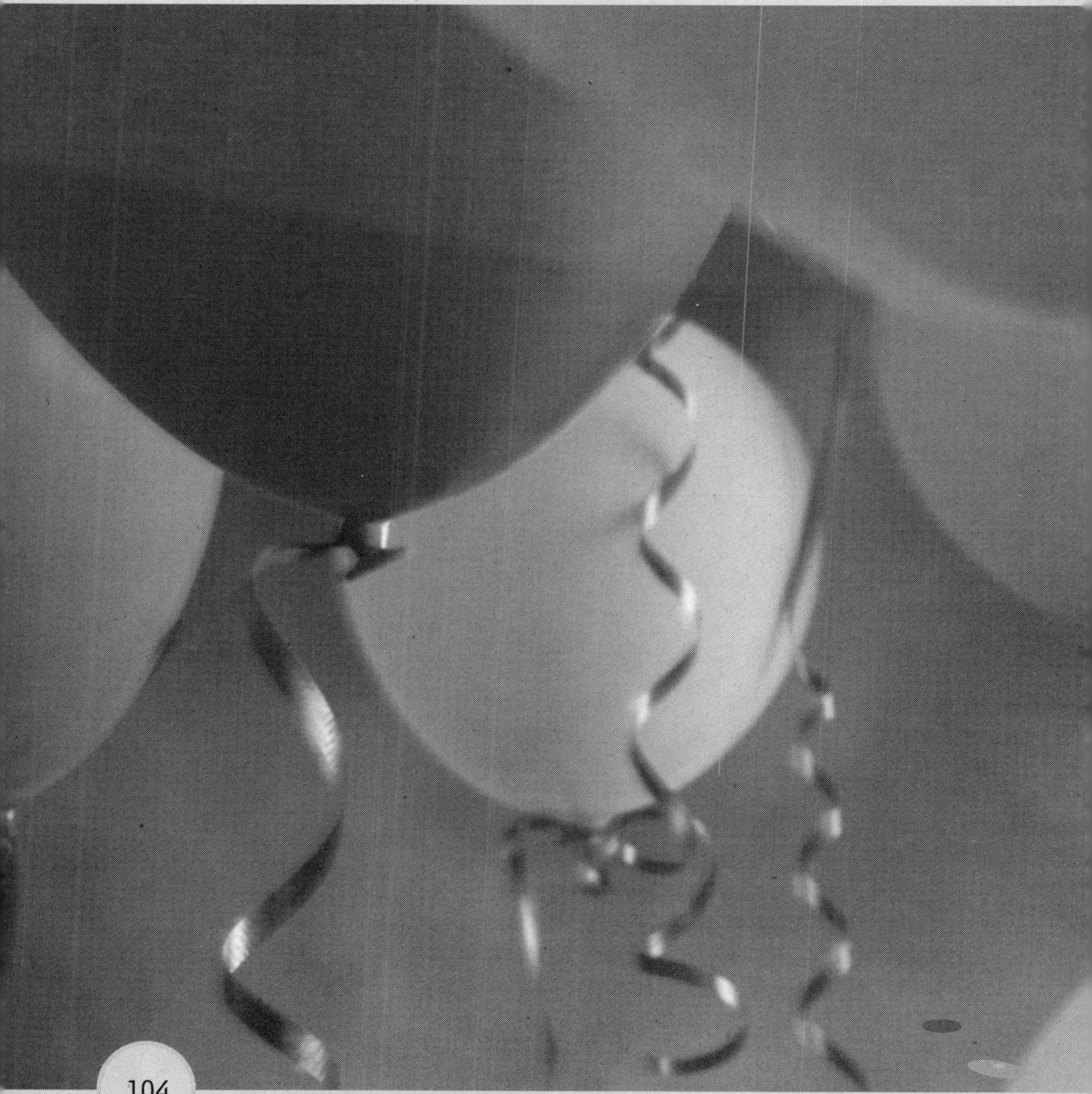

The morning after the night before

Special events always seem to be popping up to put your eating plans under severe strain. Here are some tricks to help you stop falling off the diet wagon.

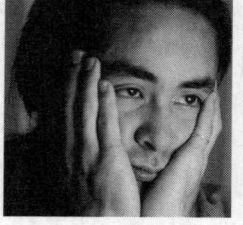

Weddings, birthdays, anniversaries, new job, new home — they are all great excuses for a party and could lead you into temptation. Don't let your good diet intentions fall by the wayside.

It's hard to resist free-flowing alcohol and high-calorie snacks and treats in a happy, loud atmosphere. How easily those handfuls of peanuts can slip down. More wine? How about a cocktail? Have a slice of cake. Taste this cheese. The next thing you know, you've completely overdone it.

Come the morning, you wake up feeling bloated, perhaps a little hungover, cross and disappointed in yourself. Your reaction could be to give up your diet. Or obsess about the precise amount of calories and fat consumed. It's important not to let these negative feelings take over. Firstly, it's unlikely that your one-off excesses will

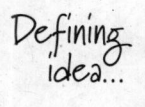

Here's an idea for you...

Play with plate size. If you eat from an enormous plate, chances are you'll fill it with an enormous portion or feel short-changed because there doesn't appear to be much on it! Choosing a smaller plate and piling it up is a sneaky way to trick yourself that you're having a big meal.

lead to weight gain. You need to overeat by around 3500 calories to put on half a kilo (a pound) of fat. Any bloated, fat feeling you may be experiencing is more likely to be water retention after eating lots of salty foods, such as crisps, nuts, pies, pizza and so on. Take some time to think about how you feel and then reframe your thoughts in a positive way. So for example, instead of dwelling on the idea that as a result of your over indulgence you've totally blown your diet and may as well give up, say to yourself 'I've been losing weight steadily and after my break yesterday, I'm confident and eager to get back to my healthy habits today'. And rather than thinking you can never go to another party because you'll pig out, try to get some learning from the experience. Which foods in particular couldn't you get enough of? Was it the alcohol that was your downfall, both in terms of the empty calories and the fact that alcohol relaxes the willpower? Did you continue to eat when you felt full? Identifying the pitfalls should mean that come the next party, you'll have some tactics to cope. For instance, if you have a soup or salad or piece of fruit before you go out, you'll feel a little fuller and therefore more able to avoid picking at calorie laden-snacks. You could also try having a large glass of water in between every alcoholic drink. Maybe you could mingle with fellow guests in an area away from the food, to avoid snacking without really thinking about what you're doing. Conversation could be another diversionary tactic. After all, it's rude to speak with your mouth full!

Defining idea...

'One more drink and I'd have been under the host.'
DOROTHY PARKER

As for feeling tired the morning after the night before, you need some damage-limitation tricks. Chances are you'll be craving carbohydrates to boost your energy levels and, if you're hungover, fatty foods too. A healthy eating plan will get you back on track though.

For many of us, losing weight gets harder as you get older. For some good reasons why, immerse yourself in IDEA 33, Stop the middle-age spread!

Try another idea...

Start the day with a large glass of water to combat dehydration, then have a slow-energy release breakfast to ensure you don't get snacking urges mid-morning. Try something like porridge, a slice of wholemeal toast, with a thin scraping of butter or low fat spread and jam or reduced sugar baked beans or a smoothie (just blend half a pint of skimmed milk with a pot of low fat yoghurt and some fruit of your choice). Drink another couple of glasses of water during the morning and if you need to snack, eat fruit, crackers and jam, a fruit scone or a rice cake, spread thinly with peanut butter. A huge salad with some low fat protein for lunch should fill you up healthily. If you include watercress in your salad, you could help combat the bloat as it's a natural diuretic. Have an early evening meal of simple grilled fish or meat with plenty of vegetables. If you cut out starchy foods, such as pasta, rice and potatoes with this meal, you'll save on calories, helping to balance out yesterday's splurge. An early night will ensure you look and fabulous the following day!

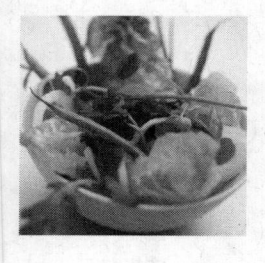

'When I read about the evils of drinking, I gave up reading.'
HENNY YOUNGMAN

Defining idea...

How did it go?

Q   **I can't help but mooch around the day after a pig-out. How can I start the day more positively?**

A   *Go for a walk, swinging your arms and breathing deeply. You'll feel energised and have burned a few calories. On your walk think about how you'd like to feel today. Keep that feeling in mind and plan how else you could fuel it. Once you get home, rather than slobbing around in an old tracksuit, get dressed up to give yourself a lift. If you need more encouragement, phone a friend or a member your family who you know will make you feel good and who you can have a laugh with.*

Q   **It's the buffets that I find the killer at parties. How can I negotiate my way round one in the most calorie-conscious way possible?**

A   *Buffets are difficult, especially as it's easy to go back and forth without anyone noticing. Rather than having a little portion, so you feel it's OK to keep going back for more, promise yourself you will make only one visit and put your whole meal on the plate so you can see exactly how much you're eating. Foods to load up with are vegetables and salads. You should also try to stick with lean meats and grilled foods (but check they're not swimming in a pool of oil). Avoid pastry, creamy dips and too many salty snacks.*

26

Fancy a calorie-free dip?

It's easy to turn a dip into a workout. What's more, splashing around is so much fun that it won't even feel like exercise.

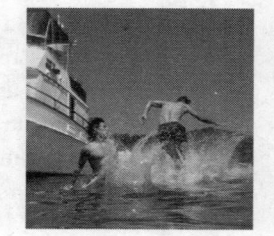

Like it or not, we all know that a sedentary lifestyle does us no favours in terms of health and fitness, not to mention the slimming stakes.

Many people shy away from 'formal' exercise such as sports and the gym because they find it dull, hard to do or hard to fit into their lives. That's why I'm suggesting swimming, which most of us view as an enjoyable thing to do rather than a chore. In my experience, there seem to be very few people who really hate it. I am one of those people, but that's because I nearly drowned as a kid and wouldn't go back into to the water for years – so I choose the gym over the pool every time.

Swimming is great exercise, easy on your joints and lots of fun. You can even take your kids along. Just make sure that someone keeps an eye on them whilst you do a little more than splash about, using the following ideas.

Here's an idea for you... **Saddle up! Horse riding is a great alternative exercise routine. Just sitting in the saddle strengthens your stomach and back muscles, and tones your thighs, bottom and legs. It provides an aerobic workout too.**

- **Use different strokes to maximise the benefits** – If you vary the strokes you use, you won't get bored with endless laps of front crawl. Breaststroke works on the chest muscles, shoulders, upper back, arms and thighs, while backstroke focuses on the upper back as well as the arms and stomach muscles. Crawl works the shoulders and upper back, the buttock muscles and the quads at the front of the thighs.

- **Try floats for extra resistance** – Use a float for extra muscle toning. For the lower body, simply hold your float out in front of you and kick your legs to work your legs and bottom. If you hold the float between your legs so you can't kick them, you can concentrate on working on your arms.

- **Maximise fat burning potential** – Rather than swimming along at a gentle pace without getting your face wet, you'll have to get your heart rate up to burn lots of calories. One way to do this is with interval training, which means swimming fast for a length or two, then swimming more slowly. Just as you feel you're starting to recover, pick the pace up again and so on until the end of your session.

Defining idea... **'The cure for anything is salt water – sweat, tears or the sea.'**
ISAK DINESEN

- **Keep it up!** – As with any exercise you have to do it consistently to see results. Swim three times a week for twenty minutes as a starting point and you'll feel fitter and more toned in a month. If you're very overweight, you'll see a difference much sooner. In order to keep seeing results, you should increase the length of time you spend in the pool, and aim for five sessions a week.

You've improved your swimming technique, now polish up your shopping skills with IDEA 37, *How to be a smart (slim) shopper.*

Try another idea...

- **Breathe right** – Breathing correctly stops you becoming exhausted too quickly or getting frustrated at taking in mouthfuls of water. Think of breathing for swimming in the same way as breathing when you're walking down the street. You should neither hold your breath or take in enormous gulps of air. With the crawl, for example, when you need to take a breath just turn your mouth to your right or left shoulder. When you put your head back into the water, look forward rather than down. This will help with exhalation as your windpipe is more open. Breathe out by letting the air trickle out slowly instead of blowing it out. Develop a rhythm and you'll be able to keep going for longer.

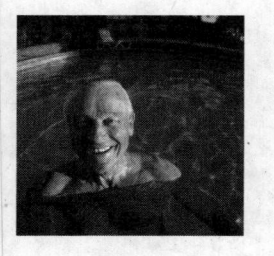

Efficient swimmers seem to "knife" through the water with little effort. Like human torpedoes, they streamline themselves to become as small as possible in the direction they intend to move.
WES HOBSON, CLARK CAMPBELL and MIKE VICKERS, *Swim, Bike, Run*

Defining idea...

Q My swimming technique is not really that good – it's limited to back and breast stroke. Am I really exercising properly?

A *Swimming lessons aren't just for kids. Most pools offer the services of an instructor, so go for it. You'll feel a difference in just a few sessions.*

Q I want to swim at lunchtime, but by then I'm starving. You can't swim on a full stomach, so what should I do?

A *Try a quick snack, such as a piece of fruit and a large glass of water, half an hour before swimming. It should take the edge off your hunger.*

Q I like water, but I get bored with swimming. What can I do to make it more fun?

A *Try aqua aerobics, which is fun for just about everyone. Some exercises are done holding on to the side and others use floats. Most sessions include some sort of routine in the middle but you're never out of your depth. Try a few different classes, as instructors have different styles, and you'll like some more than others.*

Can beauty products help you slim?

Lotions, potions and treatments promise all kinds of miracles, including inch loss and wobble firming. But are they worth the money?

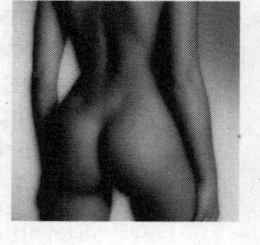

It's an appealing idea. Rub in this cream twice a day for six weeks and your flab will melt away.

A friend of mine once remarked that these creams should come with a symbol on them, featuring a slice of cake with a cross through it meaning that to lose weight, you have to watch what you eat as well as, or even rather than, spend money on some gimmicky product. But he's a cynic and a man – and men generally don't believe in the powers of applying creams to themselves. They prefer it if you do it for them, coupled with a back rub, after eating a fabulous meal you've cooked for them, and that you've also shopped for and cleaned up after – not to mention put the kids to bed, fed the cat and done a little recreational vacuuming. But enough man-bashing. This idea is as much for them as it is for women.

Here's an idea for you... **Get a fake tan. It can make you look slimmer and leaner by sculpting, shadowing and highlighting muscles and curves. For the best results, have it applied in a salon. It will usually last for about five days.**

Depending on your background, beauty treatments can be very useful for getting in shape or a waste of time, money and effort. The cosmetics industry is always able to wheel out a boffin from their laboratories to produce clinical studies proving that X cream really does help you lose inches, refine your silhouette or firm your curves. Meanwhile, most other doctors and scientists will say that what you apply from the outside doesn't make a blind bit of difference. Advertising claims are strictly regulated and can only go so far, so it can be hard to know how effective these products really are. The better magazines and newspapers do some investigatory work and produce information and recommendations of their own.

I believe that some of these treatments do have an effect, though it might be short-lived. I also think that the psychological element can't be underestimated. There's no doubt that looking after yourself does make you feel good. When you feel good, you're motivated, positive and confident, which is how you need to feel to spur you on to losing weight.

Here are my opinions of what's on offer:

SALON TREATMENTS

These usually involve being wrapped, massaged or painlessly zapped with some sort of electrical current. Massage is undoubtedly soothing and is claimed to stimulate your lymphatic system, which drains waste fluid from your tissues. You'll feel good afterwards, but not thinner. Wraps can shrink inches, but it's just fluid loss – they

are fab for feeling a bit thinner for a special occasion. You can't beat them for a short-term boost. Electrical impulses stimulate your muscles by working them while you lie back and read a magazine. You would see better results with regular exercise.

For more on looking good while you're going down in size, see IDEA 38, *Alternatives to kaftans.*

Try another idea...

FAT-BUSTING CREAMS

Despite the claims, I really don't believe you get results unless you eat less and move more too. Still, they do make your skin feel very smooth and soft and strokable.

COLONIC IRRIGATION

This is very controversial. It is based on the principle that toxic deposits are stored in your large intestine. When these are flushed out, it kickstarts the metabolism and helps elimination. If having a speculum inserted in your anus and having gallons of water sloshing around your insides is your idea of a good time, go right ahead! While many alternative practitioners say it's perfectly safe and even emotionally rewarding, conventional doctors reject the idea, even saying it's downright dangerous.

'After forty a woman has to choose between losing her figure or her face. My advice is to keep your face and stay sitting down.'
BARBARA CARTLAND

Defining idea...

How did it go?

Q **A friend recommended skin brushing as a way to combat cellulite. Will it work?**

A *I am a fan of skin brushing. This is where you stroke a dry bristle brush in sweeping movements over your limbs and torso, always working towards the heart. It definitely makes your skin feel great and gets the circulation going. I don't think it will get rid of cellulite, though used in combination with massage, diet and exercise, it will help to hold it at bay.*

Q **I read about some slimming tights recently. Can you tell me more?**

A *Coffee tights look like normal tights but are impregnated with caffeine which slowly gets absorbed through the skin. The idea is that this speeds up the metabolism, leading to inch loss. One test had all the volunteers losing inches from their waists and hips. Usually I'd be cynical, but I think I might just give these a go myself. You can find out more at www.palmers-shop.com.*

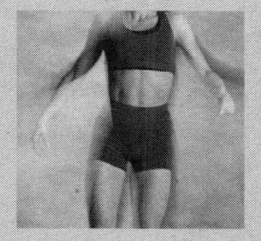
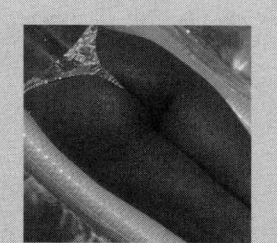

Members only

Slimming clubs promise results, but who are they for and will they make more of a dent in your pocket than your fat reserves?

Our reasons for finding it easy to gain weight and hard to lose it are as individual as our musical preferences. If yours include a lack of motivation and encouragement, try a slimming club.

Millions of people the world over belong to slimming organisations. Although the majority of clubbers are female, men are signing up too. Experts agree that the big established clubs do a good job, by providing support, which is incredibly important when you're trying to lose weight. They also offer plenty of information, advice and tips on long-term weight loss. Of course, not all clubs are created equal; for example, some are more expensive than others. Some include an exercise session, while others barely mention exercise at all. Before joining up, it's a good idea to prepare a list of questions that you can ask the trainer or group leader. This way you should be able to work out if the club will be right for you. Try these for starters:

Get everyone in your office or household to write down their favourite comfort foods. Notice any gender bias here? Men and women eat different kinds of comfort food. Men prefer things like mashed potato and pasta, while women prefer instant snacks such as chocolate and biscuits. Is this because men don't expect to have to cook them for themselves?

1. Is there any evidence that this club's methods work? As well as testimonials and member success stories, do they have any press clippings from magazines and newspapers? Are these publications independent, or do they only have clippings from their own in-house publications?

2. What are the costs and payment structure? Will you have to pay extra for special sessions, special foods or supplements recommended by the club?

3. How convenient will the meetings be for you, both in terms of time and geography. Are there options to follow the programme on–line or by post?

4. What are the club rules? Does it focus solely on diet, and if so, what are the basic guidelines you will follow? Is exercise included in sessions or recommended? Do they have vegetarian options? Ask about things like motivational talks and image consultants – these are extras that will really give you value for money.

'I have a mind to join a club and beat you over the head with it.'
GROUCHO MARX

5. What would a typical day's menu look like? Better to find out now!

6. What about aftercare? When you reach your target weight, do they offer a maintenance plan? Is that included in the price, or does it cost extra?

7. Can you sit in on a session to see what it's like? Getting a feel for the format, what's expected and what the other members are like, is so important – make sure you feel happy with the support network on offer.

Have you discovered the wonders of water yet? It's great for your energy levels, for your skin and, of course, your waistline. Go to IDEA 15, *Water works*.

Try another idea...

As well as the big name diet clubs, your local doctor or hospital may well run a weight-loss programme, and your local gym may offer one too. Do not respond to flyers, posters and funny little ads in newspapers saying something like 'Wanted! Overweight people to lose 30 lb in 30 days. No hunger! No Exercise!' These sorts of operations usually have a product they are pushing hard, such as a slimming pill or a meal-replacement shake. You may well be invited along to a meeting where various 'before and after' case studies will be trotted out in front of you and a few salespeople will speak with evangelical fervour about the product. Then, *bam!* 'Here's your month's supply.' And have you guessed? It costs nearly as much as your monthly salary. Seductive as it might seem, losing a vast amount of weight quickly is not sustainable. It will be water and lean muscle mass that disappears, only to reappear when you start to live normally again. If you try to do it with some unproven diet pill you could be putting yourself in all kinds of other health dangers, too. Go for the tried and tested methods.

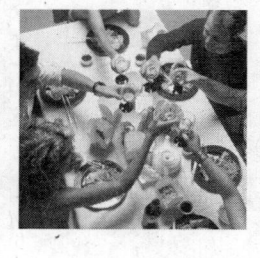

'Women are more likely to lose weight and keep it off in a group than on their own.'
BBC Diet Trials 2003 findings

Defining idea...

119

How did it go?

Q **Is there a specific club you could recommend?**

A *I find Weightwatchers impressive and know a lot of people who have lost weight with them and kept it off. Sarah Ferguson, the Duchess of York, is a famous fan, although admittedly they pay her. Weightwatchers offers a well-balanced diet which uses a points system and no foods are forbidden. You can earn extra points for exercising, and you can hold them over until the following day, which is useful if you have a dinner date, for example. They have their own branded food which members are encouraged to use. This makes life easy, but I still prefer home cooking. Plenty of tips are given out during the meetings. Do check out who else operates near you. Most of the large organisations have online services too, but I think that personal contact works best.*

Q **Aren't all the people who go horribly competitive? Will I be the sad fat one at the back?**

A *Sometimes a little competition isn't a bad thing. As long as it doesn't get out of control – like spiking your rival's scales – it's good for motivation. Maybe you should take some support along with you. Would a friend or your partner come, for instance? Keep going and soon you'll be the slim one in the front.*

Snooze and lose

What has sleep got to do with weight loss? A lot more than you probably think. So get your pyjamas on. I'll tuck you in and explain.

One famous Hollywood actress allegedly owes her beauty and slender frame to very large amounts of sleep. Apparently it is not unusual for her to spend an entire 24 hours in bed, snoring away.

I'm sure that her personal chefs, trainers, makeup artists, hairdressers, acupuncturists, aromatherapists and all the other flunkies also play a part in maintaining her in peak physical condition, but the notion of sleep as a powerful aid to beauty and wellbeing makes perfect sense. As well as giving your body the time to recharge and repair itself, a good sleep makes you feel on top of the world. Just think how awful you feel without it: tired, lacking in concentration and energy, bad tempered and hungry. Research in the US has revealed that people who don't get enough sleep are more likely to go for high-sugar, high-fat foods and drink. The idea is that if you're not getting energy from rest, your body will encourage you to turn to quick-energy food.

Here's an idea for you...

Be careful with that coffee. Did you know a large full-fat latte packs in a hefty 260 calories? A cappuccino with skimmed milk has only 100 calories while black coffee is virtually calorie-free. Which one do you usually choose?

If you're not getting enough sleep on a prolonged basis, it could interfere with your body's ability to metabolise carbohydrates by up to 40%, according to another US study.

While we're asleep, our brains go through various stages, from stage one, which is light, drowsy sleep through to deep or slow-wave sleep and then on to Rapid Eye Movement (REM) sleep, in which our eyes move rapidly under our closed lids and our brain waves are active, although the body is paralysed. Experts generally agree that bodily repair happens in deep sleep and brain repair happens during REM sleep. You need both to be at your physical and mental best. Disruption of REM sleep has been found to lead to an increase in appetite.

HOW MUCH SLEEP DO YOU NEED?

This varies from person to person. Most of us sleep for between six and ten hours a night, with the average around eight hours. Whatever leaves you refreshed and full of energy to face the day is the right amount for you. As well as quantity, the quality of your sleep counts too and there are things you can do to maximise it. So if you've been feeling tired, sluggish and rather peckish all day, check your 'sleep hygiene' as the sleep scientists like to call it.

SIX SUGGESTIONS FOR BETTER SLEEP

- Keep your bedroom for sleeping. Try not to take work to bed, eat in bed or even watch TV in bed. TV encourages snacking and also doesn't create a restful atmosphere. Your bedroom should be a comfortable temperature, dark and quiet.

- Stimulants such as alcohol and caffeine are best avoided before bedtime as they can cause twitching and tossing and turning. This might not wake you up, but it will affect the quality of your sleep and leave you hungry for high calorie snacks the next day.

- Keep to a regular bedtime and waking up time whenever possible. If you're sleeping badly, it might be worth forgetting the weekend lie-ins, since they will interfere with your body's natural rhythm.

- If your partner snores or next door's cats like to serenade you at night, try earplugs.

- When your mind races or you feel stressed out and anxious, visualise yourself putting your worries in a drawer and locking it, telling yourself you'll deal with it in the morning. Or read a few chapters of a non-demanding book. Don't read anything that will make you think too deeply or get agitated!

- Make yourself a warm drink of milk (skimmed, of course). Although there's no real proof this helps you feel sleepy, there's something very comforting about it.

Omitting carbohydrates from your diet can lead to sleep problems. What are the other pros and cons of high-protein, low-carbohydrate diets? See IDEA 40 *Trust me, I'm a doctor.*

Try another idea...

'Early to bed and early to rise makes a man healthy, wealthy and wise.'
BENJAMIN FRANKLIN

Defining idea...

How did it go?

Q I often get cramps in bed at night. Is it due to dieting? Am I lacking some nutrient?

A *This is unlikely; actually cramps are usually thought to be a result of waste products collecting in the muscles because of poor circulation. Regular exercise can combat this, as well as burning up extra calories and so helping weight loss. You could also try this stretch: stand about a metre away from the wall and lean towards it, keeping your heels on the floor. Hold for 10–15 seconds and repeat.*

Q What should I eat when I need an energy boost that won't wreck my diet?

A *You could just try a brisk walk to revive yourself. Sometimes a change of scene is all that's needed. Or eat something that will provide a long-lasting boost, such as fruit, a wholemeal fruit scone, some low-fat cheese or a slice of chicken on a cracker or crispbread, or a bowl of low or no sugar cereal with skimmed milk. And remember, if you are getting sufficient and regular sleep and plenty of exercise, you may not need so many energy boosts anyway.*

What does it say on the label?

It has a little healthy eating logo on it, so it must be good for you, right? Reduced fat means I can eat a bigger portion too, doesn't it? No and no! Learn to read labels and help yourself lose weight.

I'm something of a label freak and it's not just because I like a little bit of Gucci and Prada. If you read food labels, you can transform your body because you know much more about what you are eating.

It's not some nerdy hobby of mine. I had to start reading labels when my daughter was diagnosed as having a peanut allergy, as nuts can be hidden in all kinds of food and a reaction can be potentially fatal. Once you start reading labels, you discover interesting things – juice drinks with vegetable oils in them, for instance, or

Here's an idea for you... **Check the labels of various loaves of bread next time you're at the shops. Bread is a healthy food to eat, especially if it's wholemeal, but the fat content of a slice can vary quite dramatically between the brands, from around 60 calories a slice with 0.9 g of fat, to 115 calories a slice with 2.7 g of fat and even more!**

something you thought looked like a delicious fruity yoghurt that is just fruit-flavoured, not full of fruit. That 100 g (3.5 ounces) of your favourite cheddar cheese might turn out to add up to 410 calories and 34 g of fat.

As a starting point, you should know that food labels have to tell us things like the sell-by date and also state the country of origin. There has to be a list of ingredients too, with whatever the food or product contains most of named first and the rest listed in descending order. This is interesting when something looks full of meat, for example, and then you see that meat is actually the third thing listed rather than the first! Labels also give a nutritional breakdown, usually expressed per 100 g, but sometimes as a percentage of the RDA, which is the recommended daily amount suggested by the government and calculated to prevent nutritional deficiency in at least 95% of people. You can check the RDA against calories, fat, protein and so on. All of this is useful when you compare similar-seeming foods in the supermarket. It all becomes slightly more complicated when you start seeing extra little logos and words such 'lite' or 'reduced fat'. When you're trying to lose weight you're more conscious of these extra labels, but don't just take them at face value. Here's what they really mean:

- **Lite/light** – Although manufacturers are encouraged to say what they mean by this, there are no real rules to say how much fat and how many calories should be in something that describes itself this way. The only way to work out whether it is as diet-friendly as it appears is to check the nutritional label yourself against a standard, i.e. non light, version. Check it against the per 100 g breakdown and you'll be able to judge for yourself what the difference is. Light in fat can still contain as many calories as a standard product because sugar has been added to compensate for example.

Think you might have a food allergy? Turn to IDEA 39, *I can't eat that because my allergy means it'll pile on pounds.*

Try another idea...

- **Low fat/fat free** – By law you can't be misled on this one, but it's still not straightforward. The UK Food Standards Agency suggests to manufacturers that 'low fat' should only be claimed when the fat content is less than 3 g per 100 g. 'Fat-free' should be for foods that only have a trace of fat – under 0.15 mg per 100 g. Claims of '90% fat-free' used to be used quite freely and implied that it was perhaps a better bet than low fat. However, it basically meant that a food was still 10% fat – so it was actually not as good as low fat. Confused? Luckily, voluntary guidelines for labelling mean that this particular description is being used far less, but if you do see it, you have been warned!

- **Reduced fat** – It sounds good, but the recommendation is that it can only appear on foods that have less than three quarters of the amount of fat of the standard product. Again, to really understand what you're getting, you'd have to

Defining
idea...

'*It helps to know your labelling law here: a strawberry yoghurt must contain some strawberry. A strawberry-flavoured yoghurt has had a brief encounter with the fruit, while a strawberry flavour yoghurt has not even been within sight of a strawberry.*'
FELICITY LAWRENCE, author of *Not on the Label*

check against the original product. Reduced fat taramasalata dip, for example, still contains 25 g fat per 100 g. So it's better than regular taramasalata, but not necessarily the best choice of dip (tomato-based salsa is an alternative).

Finally, beware 'healthy eating' style logos and labels. Quite often when fat is reduced in these types of products, fillers are used to bulk them up, and the sugar and salt contents may be high too. Maybe the calories are reduced because it's a tiny portion! As ever, do a comparative label check.

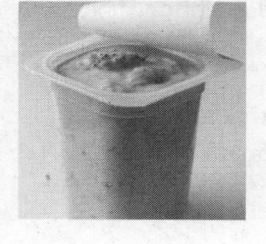
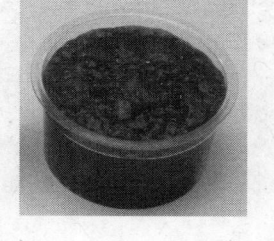
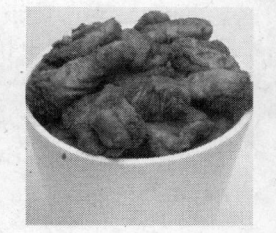

Q   **If 3g per 100g is low fat, what is a lot of fat?**

A   *As a rule of thumb, 20g of fat or more per 100g is a lot of fat.*

Q   **What about organic foods? Aren't they healthier?**

A   *Well, they certainly don't include as many additives which has to be healthier. Hydrogenated fats and artificial sweeteners are usually banned too, but they're not necessarily lower in fat or sugars (sugars can be 'natural'). Again, you really need to study the label closely to see what you're getting from a weight-loss perspective.*

Q   **I've heard the term 'hidden sugars'. What are they and how can I spot them?**

A   *These are simply sugars that are a little less obvious, i.e. you can't see them, or don't recognise the names they hide behind! They turn up in all sorts of things from burgers to baked beans. So as well as natural, raw and cane sugars, which are probably reasonably easy to spot, look for things ending in 'ose' – sucrose, lactose, dextrose and also malt extract, corn syrup, honey and molasses.*

How did
it go?

129

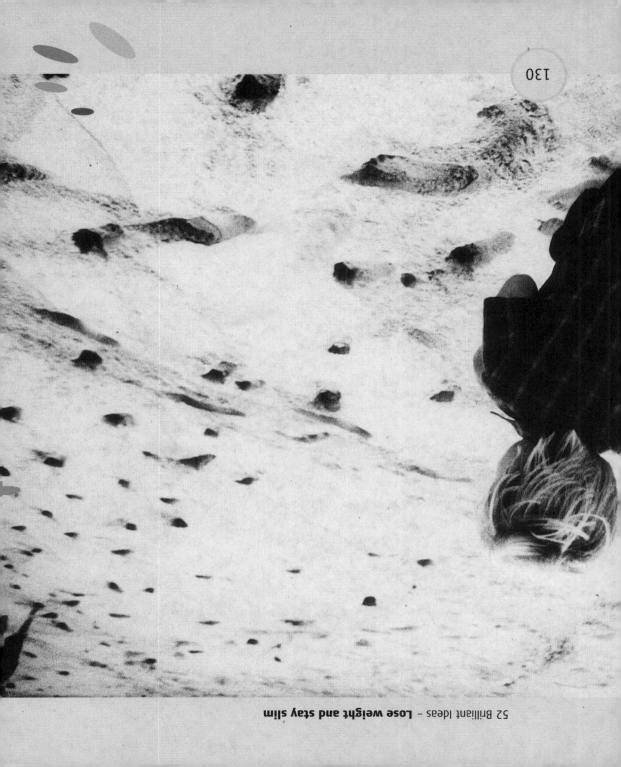

Easy ways to lose a pound a week without trying too hard

**Simple food swaps, cutting back on high calorie treats and
pushing yourself to be a little more active can help you
achieve realistic, long-term weight loss. Mix and match these tips
and you will look and feel slimmer with minimum effort.**

There is always a less fattening choice of snack
to be made, or a calorie-minimising way to cook.
Take one of my favourite meals, the Caesar
salad. It's a salad, so it must be good for you,
right? Wrong!

Unfortunately, the Caesar salad has one of the most fattening dressings known to
the hips, plus enough cheese and croutons to demand its own place setting at
dinner. What can you do, apart from gaze at it longingly from across a crowded

Here's an idea for you... Chew sugar-free gum or clean your teeth after a meal or a snack. As well as cleaning your teeth and giving you sweet breath, it sends you a psychological message that you have finished eating and that it is time to do something else. Make a clean break when your meal ends so that you really know that it is over.

room? You can make a lighter version, that's what. Just replace the fried croutons with baked ones, reduce the cheese drastically and go very light on the oil. There's always a solution, you see.

One of the best solutions to losing a little bit of weight every week is to make changes that are so simple, you'll barely notice them. It's safe and possible to lose half a kilo (a pound) a week if you shave 500 calories per day from your food intake (or expend it through activity). The maths behind this is that 3,500 calories equals half a kilo (a pound) of fat. So, divide 7 days into 3,500 and you get that magic 500 number. Do some more maths and you'll see that 500 g a week is 2 kg a month and 12 kg in six months. Get started with the following clever little ideas:

Say no to crisps

This is one of the most popular snacks, but a regular 40 g bag has around 200 calories and 10 g of fat. Even lighter versions come in at slightly over half of that amount. So if you stopped having a bag each day at work, you'd save at least 500 calories a week.

Avoid large portions

A large burger, fries and fizzy drink will easily stack up to 1000 calories, if not slightly more. If you can't cut them out, at least opt for the regular or small sizes which will cut the calories in half.

Watch what you drink

On a night out, three 175 ml glasses of white wine will cost you nearly 400 calories. Three spritzers will be half that. A half pint of strong lager clocks up around 160 calories, while a half of ordinary strength is about 80 calories. Steer clear of cocktails too – a pina colada is easily 225 calories, while a vodka and slimline tonic is just 60.

On your bike

Eco-friendly, fun and jolly good exercise, an hour's cycling should take care of nearly 500 calories.

Sandwich swap

If you have a little low fat salad cream in your lunchtime sandwich instead of lashings of butter, you could save up to 500 calories during your working week.

Rethink your Saturday night take-away

Choose chicken chow mein and boiled rice over sweet and sour chicken and fried rice, you'll save around 500 calories.

Walk more

If you walk to work, the shops or just for fun (but at a reasonably brisk pace) you'll burn up around 250 calories an hour.

Got a sweet tooth? Try IDEA 17 *Sweet temptation.*

Try another idea...

'Another good reducing exercise consists of placing both hands against the table edge and pushing back.'
ROBERT QUILLEN

Defining idea...

Wash the car

Save money and burn energy by valeting your car. Wash it, polish it and vacuum it inside and you'll use up a few hundred calories,

Have a skinnier coffee

You could save yourself 170 calories if you opted for a regular white coffee, made with skimmed milk, rather than a cappuccino made with full fat milk.

Party snacks

Think such small little nibbles don't count? If you had two tablespoons of tzatziki dip that would add up to around 40 calories. Two tablespoons of taramasalata, however, is 130 calories. Thick meat pate on French bread can cost you about 250 calories, whereas a small helping of smoked salmon on rye bread is a mere 130 calories. A cocktail sausage is around 70 calories. Wrap it in pastry and serve it as a sausage roll and you're looking at 200 calories.

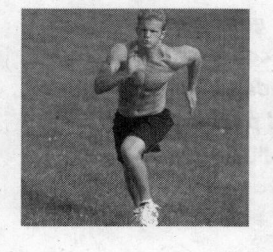
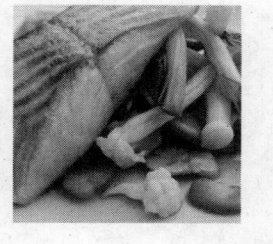
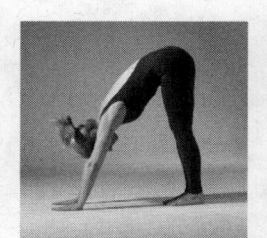

Q My weakness is cheese. How can I lose weight and still indulge?

How did it go?

A *Keep your portion sizes matchbox small and enjoy a delicious ripe piece of fruit with it. Some cheeses are also more heavyweight than others. Cheddar, for example, is around 124 calories per 30 g with around 10 g of fat. The same weight of camembert is about 90 calories with 7 g of fat, while feta is 75 calories and 6 g of fat. Check labels to make comparisons and the best choices. You could also try grating cheese to have on toast or a cracker rather than slicing it, so you still get the taste, only fewer calories.*

Q I'm too busy to walk or cycle, so I can't really burn up extra energy that way, can I?

A *Ultimately you're going to have to find a way to schedule some exercise into your life. You could start by breaking it down into smaller chunks. For example, if you took half an hour's walking a day as your target, you could break it down into three ten minute sessions, say a walk before breakfast, one at lunchtime and one in the evening. I don't think that's impossible for anyone.*

Q Does it help you lose weight if you don't eat after 6 p.m.?

A *There isn't a proven link between eating in the evening and gaining weight. You might eat more over dinner, especially if you eat out, but your metabolism isn't slowing down as dusk falls. It does when you're asleep though!*

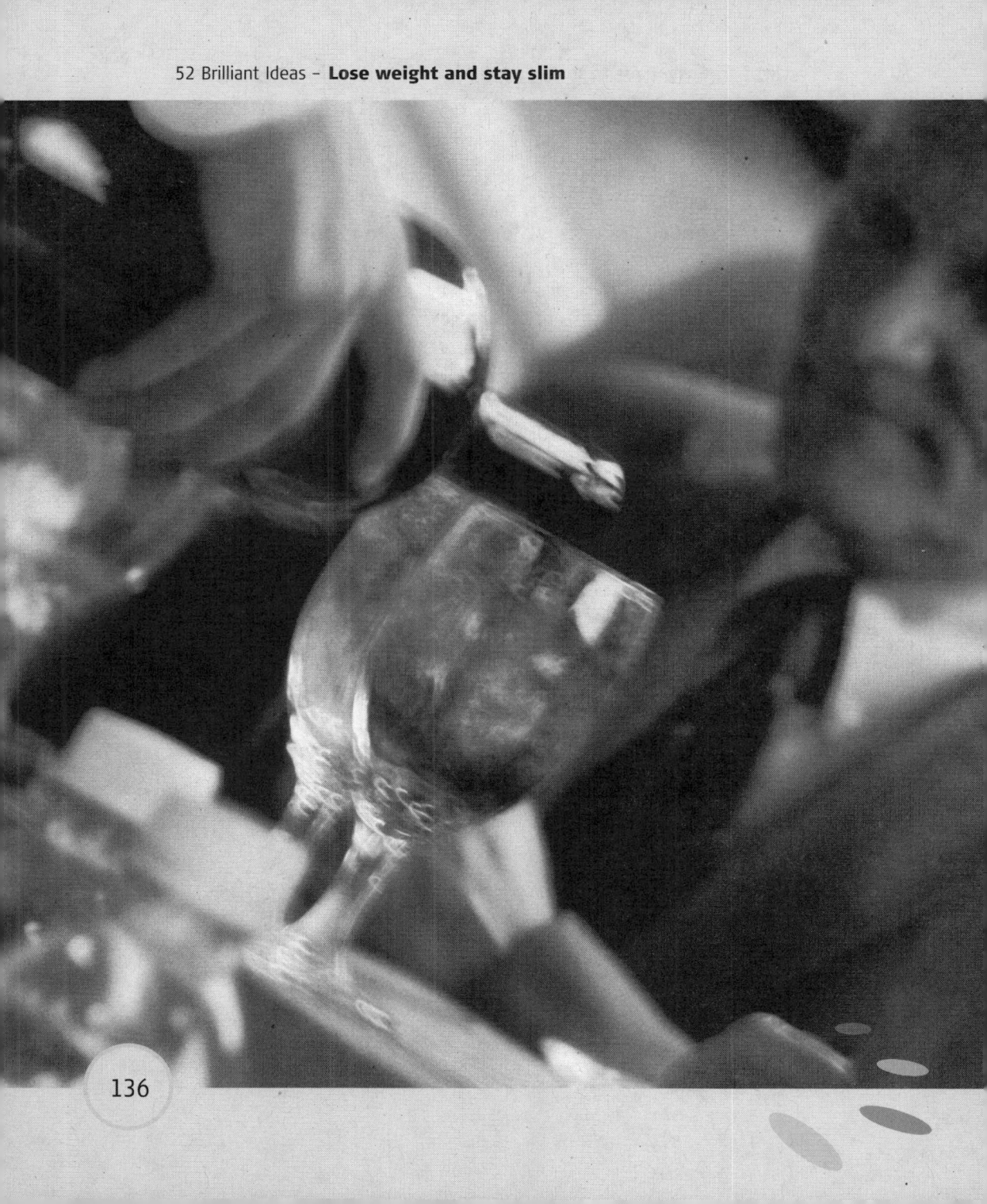

High spirits

Sociable, mood-enhancing, delicious … but alcohol can also be ruinous to your diet. When should you call time on your drinking?

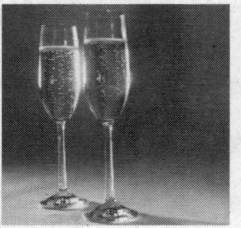

Some diets expressly ban alcohol. Others allow you a few measures a week. Personally I follow the 'everything in moderation' school. The point is that if you deprive yourself of too much, you won't keep up with your programme.

The trouble with alcohol is that one glass so easily leads to another. Or four. And that's where the problems can lie.

The UK recommended guidelines for alcohol consumption are 21 units for men and 14 for women. These are quite conservative recommendations, so a few extra units every now and then won't pose any serious health risk. You do need to be unit-aware. A unit is always disappointingly small, I think – a half pint of beer, a small (125 ml) glass of wine and a single measure (25 ml) of spirits. Often, it's hard to keep track of how many units you've had, especially if you are drinking at home or

If you're eating out, save the alcohol for during the meal rather than tucking in to the aperitifs too. As well as cutting back a few calories, this will leave you with a clear head when you come to order. Alcohol can have a strange way of making deep fried camembert or kalamari look like the perfect choice for dieters!

ordering say a 'large' glass of wine in a restaurant. Some restaurants appear to be serving up half a bottle of wine in a glass these days, which might seem good value for money but can stack up to four units and a few hundred calories. Interestingly, doctors reckon that people underestimate their alcohol consumption by 50%, which is why it's a good idea to record your intake over a period of a few weeks to assess if you need to make some changes. The health dangers of excess alcohol include liver damage, mood swings and malnutrition. Of course, regularly drinking to excess requires professional help. It's estimated that a regular daily intake of eight units by men and six by women can lead to long-term damage, with 20% of heavy drinkers going on to develop cirrhosis of the liver. Spreading your alcohol consumption over a week, rather than binge drinking is thought to be healthier for the liver, not to mention your head. Try to keep a few days alcohol-free too.

ALCOHOL AND DIET

Alcohol is full of calories, which gives the body an instant energy hit, but not much else, as alcohol has few nutrients to boast about. If you calculate that in order to lose a pound a week, you need to cut 500 calories a day – 3500 calories make half a kilo (a pound), which, divided by the seven days of the week, equals 500. A strong

lager can clock up 350 calories, so it's not hard to understand why cutting down on alcohol makes sense. Then there's the fact that alcohol seems to make you snack. How quickly handfuls of peanuts and crisps slip down when you're enjoying a few cocktails! How much easier is it to have a burger or huge ham, cheese and mayonnaise sandwich after a few drinks than start cooking yourself something healthy?! And while there are a few people who can't face food the morning after the night before, the majority of us just can't help feeding a hangover. There's no doubt that alcohol weakens the resolve, so resolve to keep it under control.

There are less fattening choices of drinks of course. If you have a white wine spritzer instead of a large (175 ml) glass of wine, i.e. use half the amount of wine and top up with soda or carbonated water you will save half the calories. Strong lagers are usually twice as high in calories as ordinary strength lagers. Slimline or diet mixers will also help to reduce the calorific impact of tipples such as vodka and tonic. So you can save calories and still have a good time!

Try another idea...

It's hard to resist free-flowing drinks and canapés when you're in the party mood. But how do you deal with falling off the diet bandwagon? See IDEA 25 *The morning after the night before.*

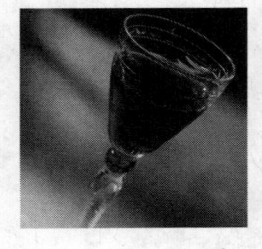

Defining idea...

'Only Irish coffee provides in a single glass all four essential food groups: alcohol, caffeine, sugar and fat.'
ALEX LEVINE

How did it go?

Q   I'm always reading that wine is really good for you. Is this true?

A   *Research has suggested that wine, and red wine in particular, can help protect against heart disease and stroke. More recently, it was discovered that an antioxidant in red wine, reservatrol, also protects against lung diseases. Most of the evidence is slightly skewed to favour middle-aged and elderly men, more than younger men and women though. The best advice is to stick within the recommended safe units and enjoy, rather than thinking you're doing yourself any great health favours!*

Q   I find it difficult to stop at just one glass of wine. Just as with biscuits, I open a packet and eat the lot. I can easily sink a bottle by myself.

A   *Me too. Addictive personality or just plain greedy, who knows? There is of course a health issue here. If you're doing that often, you could develop quite a serious alcohol problem. But on a lighter note, one way to deal with this is to buy expensive wine and create a bit of a ritual around it. Decant it or put it in an ice bucket. Promise yourself you will really enjoy two glasses only. Wait until an appointed hour and the drink it slowly and savour it. Have some food with it too. If you're out, designate yourself the driver, so you can't drink more than a glass or two.*

33

Stop the middle-age spread!

As you get older, gaining weight is easier and losing weight is harder. Here are a couple of common reasons why, and what you can do about them.

Previous generations accepted that a few bulges in all the wrong places was just what happened as you aged. But in our far more lookist, sizeist, ageist society, that just won't do.

There's no doubt that after the age of about thirty it gets much harder to shake off excess weight. This is particularly annoying if you don't think you're overeating. There could be some very good reasons why this is happening, as well as some good excuses. The key is to identify the potential physiological changes that apply to you personally and act on them.

Here's an idea for you...

Set the table, draw the curtains, light some candles and enjoy a leisurely supper. Your environment can have a huge impact on how much you eat. The noisy, colourful atmosphere in fast food restaurants and cafes stimulates the appetite. Try to relax over your food in a more subdued atmosphere.

COULD YOU HAVE A THYROID PROBLEM?

An underactive thyroid (hypothyroidism) is a common condition, especially in women, with two in every hundred experiencing problems. Its classic symptom is weight gain.

The thyroid gland controls the body's metabolic processes, how quickly calories are burned up and how energy is used. When you have an underactive thyroid, your metabolism will be sluggish, you'll probably feel tired and low and you may have poor concentration. Other symptoms include high blood pressure and muscle and joint pain. A blood test will reveal the condition, which is treated with thyroxine (one of the thyroid hormones). If you suspect you have a thyroid problem, see your doctor.

IS STRESS MAKING YOU FAT?

Some people barely eat anything when they're under pressure, so the weight falls off them. For most of us, though, the opposite is true. This is not simply to do with the comfort eating and extra snacking that we indulge in when we're wound up. It seems there is hormonal connection to stress which causes a certain kind of weight gain.

Our bodies react with the 'fight or flight' response when we're under pressure. In Stone Age this was helpful when, say, we were being attacked by a wild animal, but today we can just as easily feel like this when we're late for an important meeting and stuck in a traffic jam. The body responds to a stressful scenario by saying, 'OK we need extra fuel here to cope', and releases the hormone cortisol, which helps us

to use glucose stores for fuel. The cortisol stays in the bloodstream after the stress levels have calmed down, continuing to stimulate the appetite to replenish the glucose stores. So, stress makes your body want food, even though it hasn't actually burned off any extra calories. The result? Weight gain. Some experts also say that cortisol-related weight is stored around the abdomen, rather than thighs and buttocks, which is not a good place to store fat because of its association with heart disease.

A glass of wine after work or biscuits with a cup of tea will mount up to extra calories! Keeping track of what you're eating (and where you're sabotaging your dieting efforts) is easy with a food diary as explained in IDEA 6 *Get the write habit.*

Try another idea…

If it sounds as if it could be happening to you, try two things. First, make sure that you have a good supply of healthy snacks in anticipation of stressful moments. If you've got chocolate, crisps and pies around, that's what you'll eat. If you have crudités, wholemeal rolls with a healthy filling, fruit and so on, they will satisfy your stressed-out urges just as well. In the longer term you need to find ways of dealing with that stress through exercise, massage, therapy or maybe even a serious life change.

We can always make plenty of excuses for why we have put weight on and why we can't shift it. Think about the real reasons you are in this situation. Is your life very sedentary? Do you eat enormous portions? Do you snack on confectionery without even noticing? If you're making excuses to yourself all the time, you'll never reach your goals.

'Several excuses are always less convincing than one.'
ALDOUS HUXLEY

Defining idea…

How did it go?

Q **My lifestyle is sedentary and I know it's not helping my efforts to slim down. How can I start getting more active?**

A *Why not try the 'three minutes an hour' rule? Once an hour, get up and walk, skip, dance, run up and down the stairs or whatever else you can think of for at least three minutes. Over the course of a day, it should add up to a minimum of thirty minutes, which is getting towards the amount you need to do to start seeing and feeling some of the benefits of exercise.*

Q **I'm always eating on the run, so end up grabbing high calorie snacks. How do I stop?**

A *Try to make healthier choices. Could you prepare your food at home and take it with you? Make it a rule to always sit at a table, chew slowly and taste what you're eating. That way, you can get back in touch with your body and its relationship with food.*

Q **I work in a high pressure job which I enjoy, but I realise it could be affecting my weight. Are there any instant de-stressing ideas?**

A *If you can get outside for just five minutes and be in some green space, or even just look at a window box, you'll reduce stress levels, lower your blood pressure and feel clear and focused, according to US research.*

34

Suck it out: the surgical route to fat loss

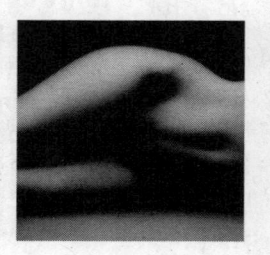

An alternative to dieting or the icing on the cake when you've lost weight and need a boost? It's not without risks, so here's what you need to know about cosmetic surgery.

If you don't like your long toes, you can get them shortened. You can swap an 'outie' belly button for an 'innie'. You can even buy J Lo's bottom for yourself.

Cosmetic surgery has come a long way. It is now possible to sculpt away that excess fat. The downside is that it's expensive, it isn't always successful and it might not make you any happier. Surgery is not a good alternative to eating less and being active, which is the safe and sensible approach to weight control. Personally, I do feel that surgery is a last resort, but if you have lost lots of weight and the fat loss has left you with loose rolls of skin, a tummy tuck might give you a confidence boost. The most important thing is to do lots of research, ask questions and find the best possible surgeon.

Here's an idea for you... **Try an instant image change with a haircut. Layers can make your face look slimmer as can highlights. For men, a short, sharp haircut can make you look more George Clooney than Billy Bunter. Great hair works wonders.**

Any surgery carries risks, such as infections, bleeding and reactions to anaesthetic. It's also important to see several surgeons before committing yourself to a procedure and ask them plenty of questions, including the following:

- How often have you performed the procedure?

- What kind of anaesthetic is used and who will administer it?

- How long will the procedure take and how long will the results last?

- Where will the incisions be and what level of scarring might I be left with?

- What's the recovery time?

- Can I see 'before and after' pictures and testimonials from other patients?

WHAT SURGERY IS ON OFFER?

One option for fat removal is liposuction, where a narrow metal tube is inserted into the fatty area via an incision in your skin. The surgeon moves the tube back and forth and sucks out the fat with a vacuum pump, leaving the nerves and blood vessels intact. There are variations in techniques, but that's the general idea. There

is a maximum amount of fat that can be removed from an area, so you might not be able to sculpt off as much as you like. It also doesn't affect cellulite (the lumpy, dimply bane of many women's lives) and can leave skin loose. Following the procedure, your skin usually retracts and is bruised and uncomfortable. Healing can take a long time, with lumpiness and swelling taking up to six months to disappear. It's definitely not for the faint-hearted. Neither is a tummy tuck (abdominoplasty). With this procedure, excess skin and fat can be removed and muscles tightened. There are mini, standard and extended versions. All leave a scar, from a low one at the level of the pubic hair to one that extends around to the back. Are you feeling faint at this point? Me too, but let me tell you about a couple of new developments. The latest high-tech techniques include LipoSelection by Vaser, which uses advanced ultrasound technology to separate out the fatty tissue from the rest before it is removed. This is claimed to be more precise, gentler and less painful, with a quicker recovery time. There is also the lower body lift, which pulls up all your slack skin around the hips, thighs and stomach. It is claimed to smooth out cellulite, flattening lumpy 'orange-peel' skin. You can also get arm and breast lifts, and just in case your hands don't match your newly slim and lifted body, there is now plenty that can be done, from getting rid of bulging veins to plumping up saggy hand skin with your very own recycled bottom fat! Excuse me, I must go and lie down as I'm feeling rather queasy.

Enough of fat in our bodies (and having it sucked out). What you really need to know about is fat in food. Learn more in IDEA 9, *Fats: the good, the bad and the downright ugly.*

Try another idea...

'I was going to have cosmetic surgery until I noticed that the doctor's office was full of portraits by Picasso.'
RITA RUDNER

Defining idea...

147

How did it go?

Q **How much do these sorts of operations cost?**

A *Prices depend on individual surgeons and hospitals, and the specific techniques used. However, the cost of a tummy tuck and liposuction would probably pay for gym membership, a personal trainer, a nutritionist and goodness knows what else for at least a year.*

Q **How do I find a surgeon?**

A *As well as seeking out personal recommendations, check that they are members of a professional body such as The British Association of Aesthetic Plastic Surgeons (BAAPS). New BAAPS members, for example, have to be recommended by two others who are aware of their ability, skills and knowledge.*

Q **Is there such a thing as a toe job?**

A *Yes. It involves making little incisions, cutting a bit of bone out, then reattaching the tendon. Result? Prettier toes.*

35

Shape up from home

While cash undoubtedly helps, you don't have to join an expensive gym to lose weight and get fit. If you're motivated, there's plenty you can do from home.

There are lots of little things you can do around the house to be more active. Everything counts, even hiding the TV remote control so you have to get up to change channels and the volume.

To really burn calories and see a difference in your body, the level of activity has to be revved up a few notches. For many people, exercising from home is the ideal solution, as it fits in with almost any lifestyle and can work for every budget. Here are some ideas to get you started:

FITNESS VIDEOS

These are very cost effective, provided you use them regularly and don't simply file them beside your complete collection of Bond movies. Go for a variety so that you don't get bored too quickly, and choose whatever you think looks like fun, whether

Here's an idea for you... **If you've been running for a while and enjoy it, why not join a running club to keep your motivation high? Or you could sign up for a charity fun run, such as the Race for Life series. Or dare you think about training for a marathon? Check out www.coolrunning.com.**

it's dance-inspired or a celebrity fat-burner. Make sure that at least one of them has a body sculpting or resistance training section so that you get all-round benefits. For the resistance training you'll need to use stretchy bands or dumbbells, which are available at sports shops and some department stores. In an emergency you can use a can of beans or bag of sugar in each hand instead!

Do the resistance training section of a fitness video two or three times a week and the faster, more aerobic section three to five times a week. After just a few weeks you should notice that it's getting easier and that you're starting to firm up. If not, have you just been sitting on the sofa watching it? As your new eating habits and the exercise work together, your body fat will gradually decrease.

A HOME CIRCUIT

With just a few pieces of equipment, you can set up your own version of a fitness circuit. All you need are a skipping rope, a mat or a couple of thick towels to protect your joints from cold, hard surfaces, some stairs and a resistance band such as a Dyna-Band, which comes with an illustrated sheet of exercises, .

Start with a warm up by walking up and down the stairs or around the block. Next, skip or stair-step for one minute, followed by twenty repetitions of a toning exercise from the resistance band sheet such as an upper body exercise. Then, do your minute's aerobic exercise again, followed by another toning session. This time, do a

lower body move or some stomach exercises. Continue the circuit for about fifteen minutes and aim to do it twice a week. To progress, all you need to do are more repetitions or different toning exercises and longer aerobics sections. Add a purely cardiovascular activity to the two sessions of circuit training and you'll be slimmer and more toned in just a few weeks.

For another exercise idea that's easy to fit in to any lifestyle, look at IDEA 19, *Walk yourself thinner.*

Try another idea...

RUNNING

This is a fantastic way to burn fat, tone your legs and boost your fitness. Running requires a good pair of running shoes and comfy clothing; do go to a specialist sports shop to get them. An easy way to start is to walk for a few minutes, then run for a few minutes, then walk again and so on. As you progress, you'll be running more and walking less! You could also invest in a heart monitor which transmits your heart rate to a wrist display, to check you're working at the right level. To burn fat you need to work at about 70% of your maximum heart rate – make that a goal for later if you're just starting out, rather than trying to do it straight away. To work out your maximum heart rate, subtract your age from 220 and multiply that figure by 0.7. Another way to check if you're running too hard is if you're unable to speak! It's better to run, jog or even walk more slowly for longer, than it is to go hell for leather and collapse in a heap after ten minutes.

'The best thing about running is that it can give you whatever you need – whether that's a better body, quiet time to think, or something more radical like the confidence to make life-changing decisions or tackle an "I didn't think I had it in me" challenge.'
SUSIE WHALLEY and LISA JACKSON, *Running Made Easy*

Defining idea...

How did it go?

Q **I've got a couple of fitness videos, but how can I find the time to do them?**

A *Schedule time for exercise, just as you note down an appointment in your diary. It might sound pedantic, but it should ensure you take your efforts seriously! Remember you don't have to do the whole video in one go. You could do one section in the morning and one in the evening, or one today and one tomorrow. The key is to keep doing something and build on your success.*

Q **I think I've reached a fitness plateau. How do I know if what I'm doing is worth it?**

A *Why not try a personal training session? A trainer can gear workouts to your needs and goals and help with motivation. Just a few sessions can put you on the right track again.*

Q **I was thinking of buying a mini trampoline to work out on at home. What do you think?**

A *These are great for injury rehabilitation because they reduce the stress on the joints. However, if you're uninjured, it is hard to work vigorously enough to improve your cardiovascular fitness on a trampoline. Impact activities like jogging, aerobics and so on are good for improving bone density, which is something you wouldn't get bouncing on your trampoline. If you think it will be fun and it will get you to do something, then go ahead. If you're already exercising regularly, though, save the money for a new pair of trainers or personal training session instead.*

36

Dieting danger

Disordered eating is frightening, confusing and poses severe health risks. While the causes are complex and not fully understood, everyone should be aware of the danger signs of eating habits that are getting out of control.

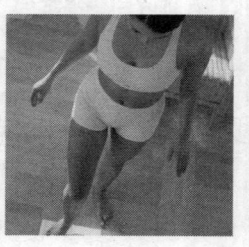

Contrary to popular belief, eating disorders are not a modern illness — they have been going on for centuries. What is true, is that they now seem to be on the increase.

Much disordered eating is kept secret until it becomes patently obvious that there's a problem, so it is hard to put any real figures on how many sufferers there really are. More and more people are coming forward for help and treatment for themselves or their friends and family members.

Eating disorders are difficult to understand, whether you're a sufferer or watching someone else suffer, but I think it is especially hard on the latter group. Why does someone who has starved themselves still insist they're fat? What is going on in the mind of someone who looks perfectly gorgeous yet steals away to the bathroom a few times a week to vomit? How can they be ashamed of what they've eaten and afraid to gain weight when they are obviously thin?

Here's an
idea for
you...

Get yourself along to a self help group. Talking to others who have experienced the same issues and problems and can offer support and understanding without blaming you or making you feel guilty, can be a real help.

Some experts think there is a link between dieting and developing eating disorders, especially bulimia. The theory goes that dieting makes you hungry, which makes you binge, which then makes you feel guilty. In susceptible people, a purge (vomiting or using laxatives), helps to deal with the guilt and 'remove' the calories.

There are millions of us who diet without developing these kinds of illnesses. What has been discovered is that people who have eating disorders also share certain personality traits – they are perfectionists, who are eager to please, yet who have low self-esteem. When these factors are combined with family troubles (divorce, bereavement) or indeed certain family attitudes to weight and food, the spiral into illness can be quick. Ultimately, eating disorders are usually about control.

Treatment is available, but success is dependent on the individual accepting help. Even then, there are a proportion of people who will continue to obsess about weight and food for the rest of their lives. Anorexics will usually be referred to a specialist psychiatrist who is experienced in eating disorders, which may be enough to get attitudes to food and eating back to somewhere approaching healthy. However, some anorexics will be hospitalised because of the lack of fluids and nutrients in their bodies, which is even more distressing, not only for the carers, but for the sufferer themselves as they feel themselves losing what little control they have in their lives. For bulimics, anti-depressants have been found to help reduce bingeing, but psychological treatment is essential too.

Check whether your own eating habits and attitudes, or those of a friend or family member, could indicate signs of disordered eating. If you're concerned, see your doctor, contact a self-help group or check The Eating Disorders Association at www.edauk.com.

The following is not an exhaustive list, but some common indications that issues exist or are beginning to develop include:

- Not eating in front of others, claiming to have just eaten or having prepared a meal for others.

- Being secretive around food

- A strong fear of gaining weight, although you have an acceptable weight or are even underweight.

- Distorted body image – believing you're fat when you're at an acceptable weight or underweight

- Recurrent bingeing – eating too much in a short space of time, i.e. within a few hours.

Focus on developing a healthy body image. Turn to IDEA 11, With friends like you, who needs enemies?

Try another idea...

'It's important to remember that eating disorders are very complex conditions and are not about dieting going too far. The vast majority of people who diet don't have eating disorders.'
LYNDEL COSTAIN, *Diet Trials: How to Succeed at Dieting*

Defining idea...

155

■ Shame and guilt after eating leading to using laxatives, or making yourself vomit

■ Obsession with exercise – working out several times a day for a couple of hours at a time

■ Judging yourself solely on looks

■ Ritualistic eating habits such as cutting food into tiny pieces

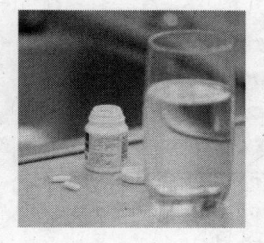 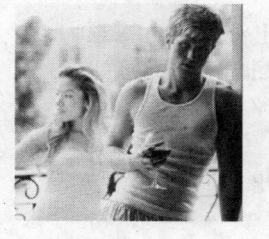 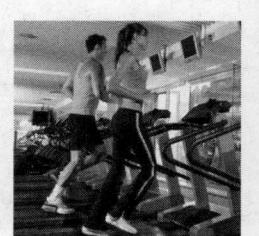

Q **I think about food all the time, especially about what I've just eaten and what I'll eat next. I don't have a problem, do I?**

How did it go?

A *Maybe not, but it doesn't sound as though your relationship with food is all that healthy either. Sorry to sound nannyish, but you could probably use some professional support, via a nutritionist or friendly doctor.*

Q: **I have a friend who has dieted as long as I've known her. I'm sure she's anorexic but she gets really angry if I try to talk to her about it. What can I do?**

A *Of course you want to help, but often this will be perceived as criticism or pressure which will only make things worse. All you can do is be there, listen, love and support. Once your friend has recognised she has a problem, you can lend practical support in finding help, going along to medical appointments and so on.*

Q **I binge, but don't vomit or use laxatives. So I'm ok, aren't I?**

A *Many binge eaters eat to escape their emotions, but then feel that food makes them out of control. If you binge but don't purge, you may well also be very overweight. Medical help is essential to get you out of this behaviour. Pluck up the courage to ask for it. You won't regret it.*

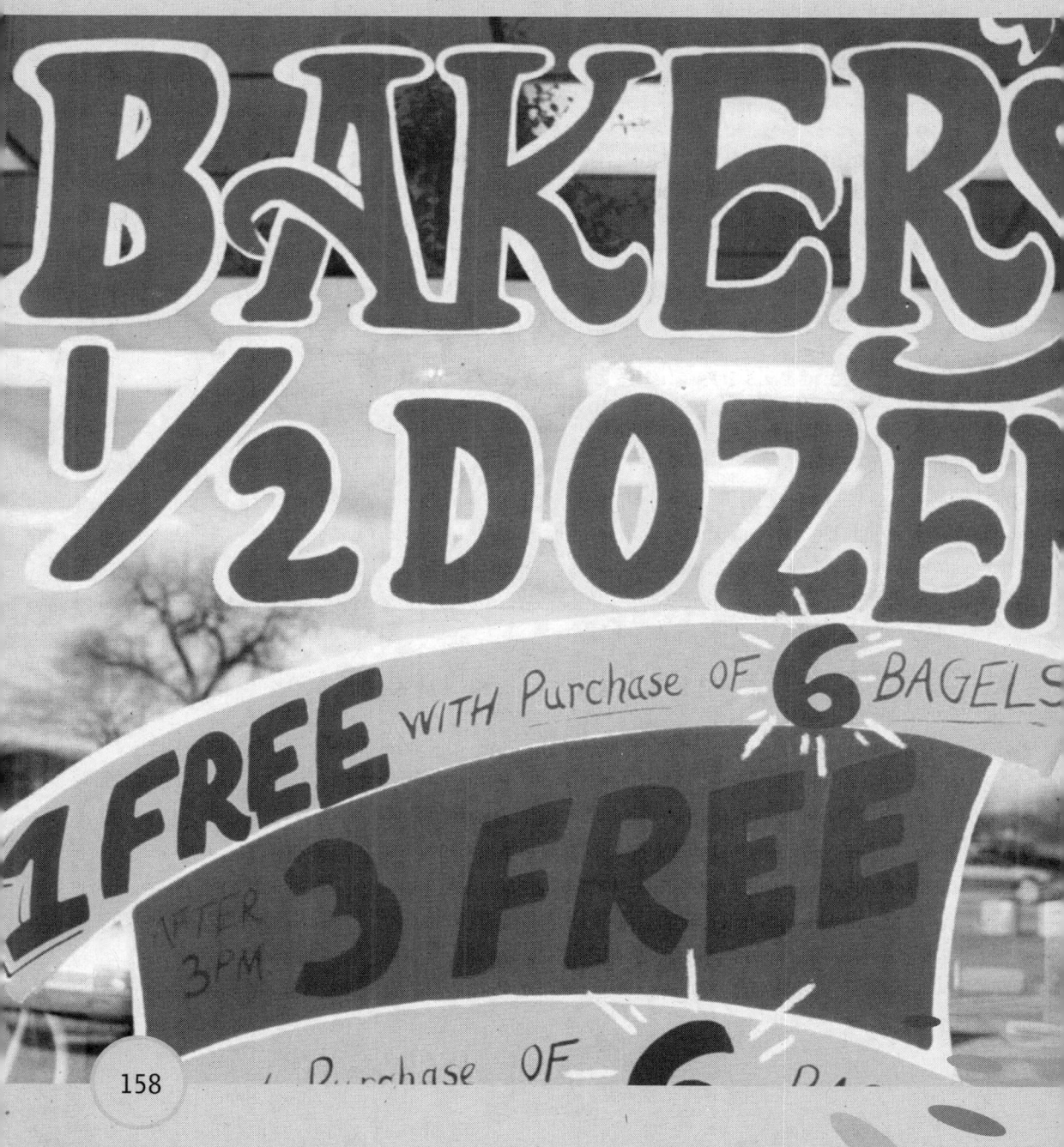

How to be smart (slim) shopper

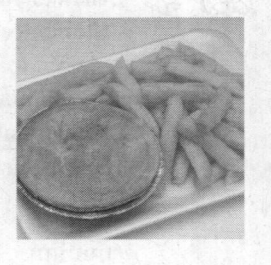

You can save yourself pounds (£s and lbs!) by shopping wisely. Here are a few tricks to help you make the leanest deals and find the best buys for your thighs.

Good intentions are a commendable thing, but soon lose their rose-tinted glow if that's all they remain. Translate them into action, and keep going.

Losing weight means getting on and doing it, not just thinking about it. It means being prepared, which is where being a savvy shopper comes in. What's the point of deciding you'll prepare a delicious low-fat meal if all you have in the house is some ready-made pastry, a string of sausages and some out-of-date double cream? How can you protect yourself from a snack attack when all your larder contains is a family-sized bag of crisps? Shopping for food might well be a chore, but haphazard shopping will cost you dear in the weight-loss stakes. Here are some things to think about:

Here's an idea for you... **Chop bananas into bite-sized chunks and freeze them. They then become healthy, delicious, almost ice-creamy treats to snack on. You can freeze grapes too or make your own ice lollies by freezing fruit juice.**

Do not go shopping when you're hungry. Your eyes will be seduced by all the high-fat, calorie-rich possibilities on offer, while your body says "feed me, I'm hungry, feed me now". This will get you thinking about an impromptu picnic in the supermarket car park, so have a meal or snack before you go. Take a list too. That way, you'll buy everything you really need and minimise the threat of impulse buys . Let's be honest, no one buys extra cabbage on impulse – you know the sort of temptations I'm really referring to.

If you can, plan some easy, healthy meals you can cook yourself and shop for the fresh ingredients. Get away from an over-reliance on convenience foods and slash fat and calories from your diet. Even if they have a healthy eating or reduced fat logo, check the labels to see what you're really getting. Low fat only counts if it is 3 g or less per 100 g. Avoid special offers, super-sizes and multi-buys unless they're healthy and low fat. Short of wearing a mask over your eyes and nose, it's difficult not to notice the lovely aromas and free samples all around you so you just have to accept that supermarkets are run by clever people who want to sell you lots of things. Even the way they lay out their stores is a cunning ploy to ensure you see everything they offer. As well as the tips above, you have to be strong and say "No thanks, not today". A trip around the aisles should end up looking something like this:

IN THE TROLLEY

Fill it up with:

- Wholegrains – they're not less calorific than white, refined produce, but they have more fibre and will keep you feeling full for longer

- Lots of colourful fruit and vegetables

- Low-fat dairy produce

- Lean cuts of meat, chicken and turkey (the white meat is lower in fat than dark)

- Fish, including a portion or two of oily fish, such as salmon, tuna, mackerel and herring

- Dried fruit to snack on – it's calorific, but OK if you keep servings small; low-fat/reduced-calorie cereal

- Low-fat and cereal snack bars – but still check the label for the better buys

Done the shopping and missed your opportunity to do an exercise class? You need help with your support network. See **IDEA 51**, *Support act.*

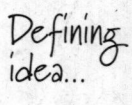

Try another idea...

'I can spend hours in a grocery store. I get so excited when I see food, I go crazy.'
CAMERON DIAZ

Defining idea...

THINGS TO LEAVE ON THE SHELF

- Cereals with added sugar (pick out the sugar free ones and choose oats if you like porridge or making your own muesli)

- Biscuits and cakes, crisps

- Sausages, meat pies and pasties

- Anything with pastry

- Battered and bread-crumbed meat and seafood (all that extra fat and calories)

- Sugary jams and spreads (choose sugar-free versions)

- Full fat ice-cream – why not try frozen yoghurt instead?

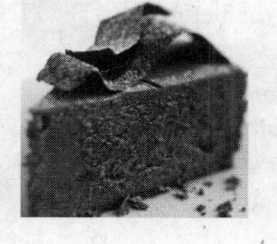
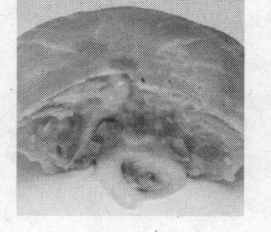
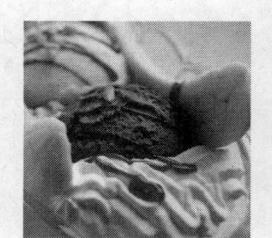

Q **I need another snack idea. Do you have any?**

A *Try making your own popcorn. Buy your corn kernels and add 50 g to a saucepan in which you've heated one tablespoon of oil. Put the lid on, and they'll pop in a few minutes. You can experiment with flavours. If you have a sweet tooth, try adding some cinnamon or grated orange rind. For a savoury snack, add curry powder, black pepper or garlic powder. It's tasty, low fat, high fibre and has a few B vitamins.*

Q **Any other tips for distraction? I'm not sure I can make it past the cake counter in one piece.**

A *Perhaps you could start viewing your shopping trip as part of your daily exercise plan. Buy a pedometer, which measures how many steps you're taking and how many calories you're burning. 10,000 steps a day, which is not as hard to achieve as it sounds, will go a long way to keeping you fit and healthy.*

Q **I shall get bored with grilled chicken breasts for the rest of my life, won't I?**

A *I think you're being over-dramatic. There are lots of easy, healthy, low fat cook books out there to inspire you. Besides, you could get creative with store cupboard condiments alongside your grills. Have you ever heard of salsa, mustard, balsamic vinegar, horseradish and chutney? Have some fun and surprise yourself!*

How did it go?

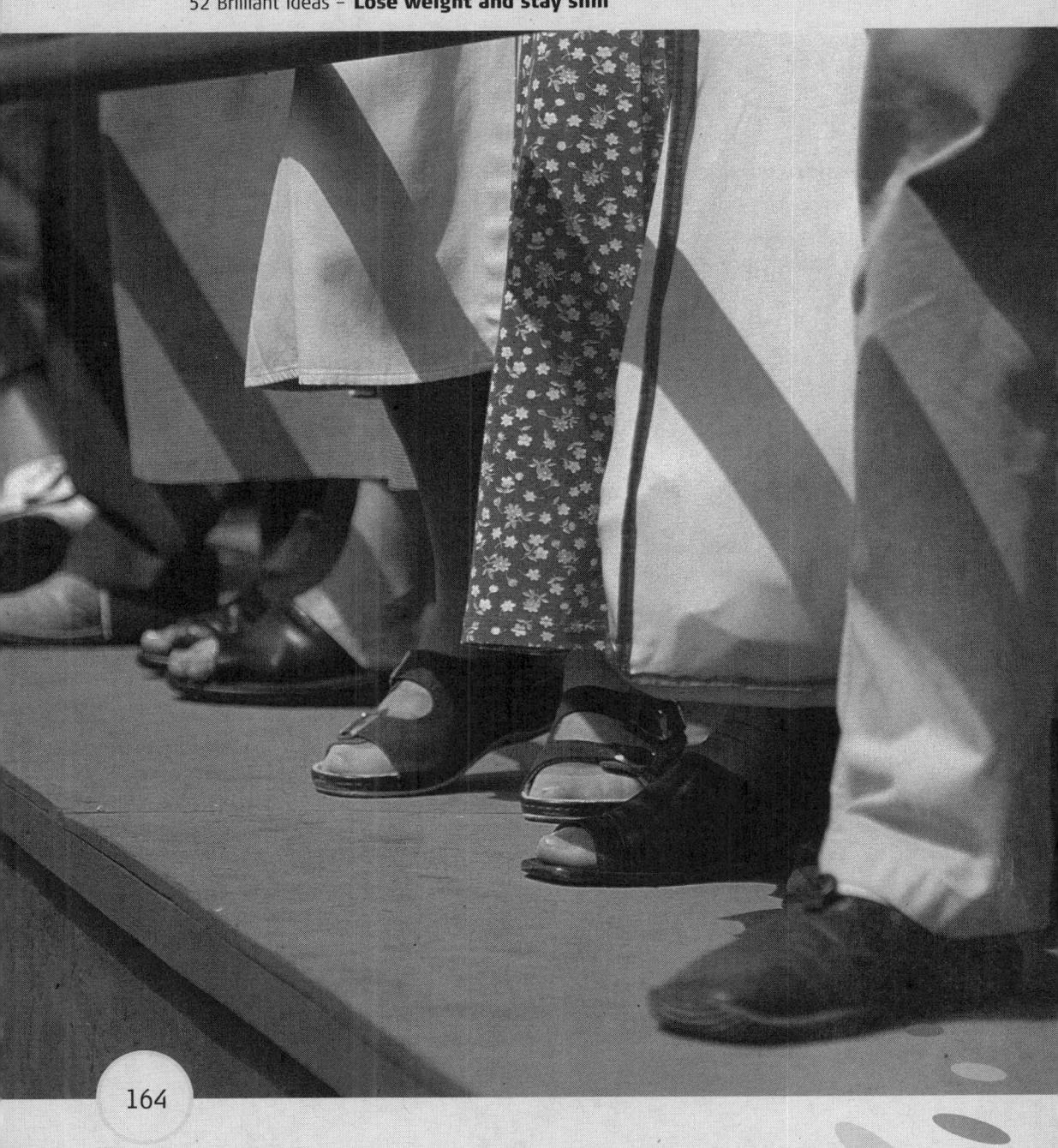

38

Alternatives to kaftans

Being groomed and stylish is confidence-boosting whether you're just starting out on your weight loss plan or already beginning to change shape.

As well as looking good, it will make you feel good about yourself. A few sartorial tricks will go a long way to making you appear thinner than you are.

Stylish, streamlined dressing isn't a question of size or money, despite the famous remark of Wallis Simpson, the Duchess of Windsor, that 'one can never be too thin or too rich'. The extraordinary amount of choice on the high street now means that whatever your budget or measurements, you'll be able to find clothes that suit you. It wasn't ever thus. Not so long ago, unless you were a 'size tiny', all that was on offer was a tent, a kaftan or baggy tracksuit. Manufacturers and retailers have woken up at last to the fact that people come in all shapes and sizes and want to look good. Of course, it's not just what you wear, it's the way that you wear it too. Here are some super-useful tips for dressing well and dressing to look slimmer:

Here's an idea for you...

Go through your wardrobe and throw away anything that is baggy and shapeless or too tight. Try on doubtful items and take a long hard look at yourself in the mirror. Does it flatter you? Any doubts, chuck it out.

FOR WOMEN

- To disguise a big belly, don't wear your tops tucked in. Try a chunky low slung belt worn over a loose top.

- An A-line skirt is great for hiding big thighs and bottoms.

- Combat trousers and narrow tight-fitting trousers will maximise every curve. Try a boot leg cut or flares to take the emphasis away from a large top half.

- Keep detail simple. Lots of pockets, buttons, bows, prints and zips look over-fussy and can make you appear wider.

- If you have a large bust and arms, say no to thin spaghetti straps and ruffle necks. Keep it simple with tailored shirts and jackets and v necks.

- A long jacket hides a fuller figure. Boxy jackets just make you look square-shaped.

- Beware anything that is too small – and this includes your underwear – as you will just bulge out.

- Go for fabrics that drape, such as cotton, lightweight knits and jerseys as opposed to fabrics that cling, such as satin and Lycra.

- Skirts that end just below the knee tend to make your legs look longer.

- Beware of shoes with ankle straps, which have the effect of cutting off your legs and shortening them. Heels are great for extra height and leg lengthening, as are boots. If you have big calves, go for boots in a stretchy material. They go with practically anything.

- Wearing one colour, or complementary tones of a colour streamlines your body. As a general rule, darker colours are more slimming.

- Leggings and other Lycra trousers and shorts should be kept for the gym.

- Wide-legged trousers flatter pear-shapes. Trousers that do up on the side will also minimise a belly and bottom.

FOR MEN

- Avoid jackets and tops with extra padding as they'll just make you look bulkier.

- Steer clear of shapeless, bulky jumpers for the same reason.

- If you've got a big belly, go for trousers and a jacket in the same colour to streamline. Single-breasted jackets are more slimming than double-breasted.

- Buy the right size! Anything clinging over a large belly looks slobby.

For more on body shapes, go to IDEA 47, *Spot reduction: the facts and the fiction.*

Try another idea...

167

Defining idea...

'*Looking stylish is not about following fashion, losing weight, being rich or succumbing to the knife. It's about dressing to show off what you love and hiding what you loathe about your body.*'
TRINNY WOODALL and SUSANNAH CONSTANTINE, *What Not To Wear*

- Dark coloured jeans are more flattering than light denim ones.

- Beware of heels for men. Cowboy boots or shoes with a built-in heel won't make you long taller and leaner, they'll just make you look silly and sad.

- Shirts with a vertical stripe will make you look slimmer, as will a tie that is simple and predominantly one colour. Cartoon ties and mad prints are best worn by the very young.

- Go for looser fits and ensure that you can do your trousers up somewhere near your waist.

- Choose fine knits that skim the body. A v neck lengthens, and is especially good if you have a large neck. A polo neck can make you look square-shaped.

Q   **Are there any rules about handbags?**

A   *Little fussy bags may be cute, but can look silly on a larger frame. If you need to take a small one out in the evening, keep it chic, simple and one colour. An oversized bag doesn't do much for creating a longer, leaner silhouette, especially if the weight of it has you leaning to one side just to walk along the street. If you're large-busted, it will just add to the top-heavy look. A medium-sized bag that is colour-coordinated with what you're wearing is the way to go.*

Q   **What about all the shaping underwear you can buy. Is it worth spending the money?**

A   *Yes it is and there's a lot to choose from, from bras that minimise the bust to pants and tights that trim the tummy, bottom and thighs. Just make sure you buy them in the right size to start with, otherwise they'll create rolls of flab outside the garment!*

Q   **What about jewellery?**

A   *Keep it small and neat to distract the eye. A big choker necklace, for example, will emphasise a chubby neck, just as a chunky bracelet will cover, rather than show off, a slim wrist. For men, a nice chunky watch works better on big hands and wrists than on small ones.*

How did it go?

169

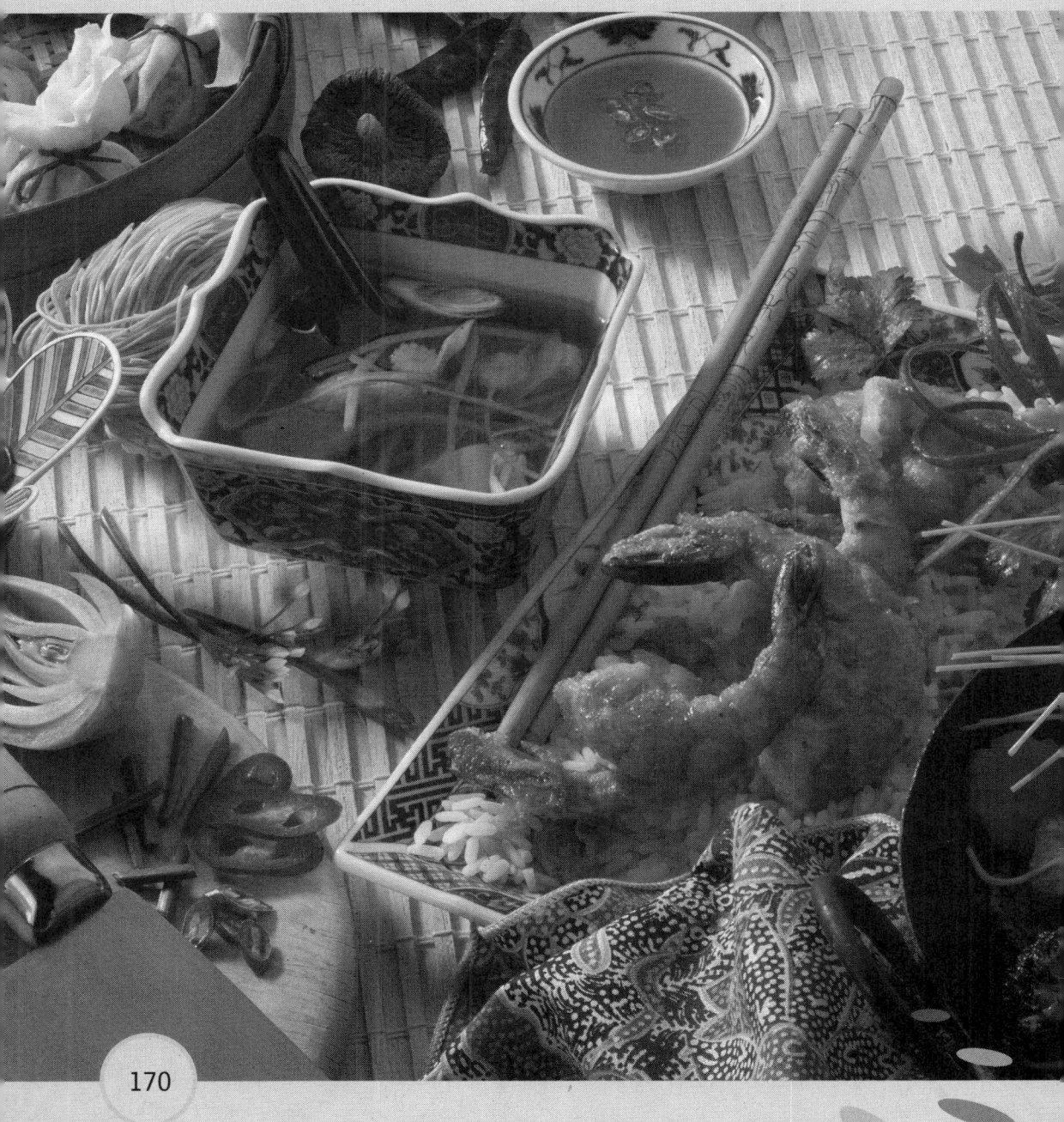

I can't eat that because my allergy means it'll pile on pounds

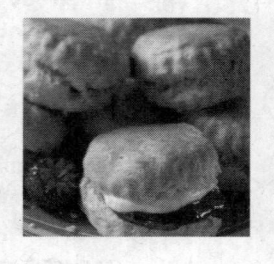

Food allergies and intolerances are very real. They can be fatal. But can they make you fat or is it just a fashionable excuse?

Lots of people latch on to the latest fad in allergies to justify their poor eating habits, which does not do them, or the genuine sufferers, any favours.

Years ago I had a raft of food allergy tests because it was the late 80s and it was 'in' to blame weight gain on certain foods. Apparently if I gave up courgettes I would lose that extra half stone I wanted to shift. Give them up? We were barely on first name terms! It was a waste of time and money. Years later, via my daughter, I came to understand real food allergies. She's allergic to peanuts, as are increasing numbers of people these days, and that's not fun. In fact, it can be fatal. So what are allergies and intolerances all about and how do they affect us?

Here's an idea for you...

In a study on laughter, one group sat quietly in a room while another group watched a stand-up comic. Blood samples taken later showed that the group who had been laughing had a significant increase in their immune system boosters, such as T-lymphocytes, and reduced cortisol, the stress hormone.

A proper food allergy occurs when your body responds to a substance with an immunological reaction. That is, it releases histamine and other chemicals into your blood stream to fight the invader. It may make your skin itch, cause hives or an asthma attack. It can also lead to changes in the blood vessels and swelling of the tongue and throat. The most severe reaction is anaphylactic shock, in which you're struggling for breath and could die. Avoidance of the allergen is the best course of action. Sufferers also get used to carrying an adrenaline injection pen with them.

Food intolerances don't involve an immunological reaction, but can still be unpleasant. They include enzyme defects. For example, a lactose deficiency makes you unable to digest lactose, the milk sugar, and can cause various bowel problems and migraines. You can also suffer pharmacological reactions in response to various components of food, such as amines in coffee and chocolate. Other foods can have an irritant effect, causing quite alarming symptoms such as palpitations and chest pains. A reaction to monosodium glutamate used in Chinese restaurant food can do this – and make you think you're having a heart attack! Food intolerances can be difficult to pin down, too. Your symptoms can be anything from migraines to anxiety, to aching muscles or water retention. You know there's something wrong, but nine times out of ten your doctor will say you just have to live with it.

Defining idea...

'I'm allergic to food. Every time I eat it, I break out in fat.'
JENNIFER GREENE DUNCAN

With all of these, it's essential to be properly diagnosed by a doctor or nutritionist who can do various sensitivity tests and help you with a food elimination diet where you cut out what you think you could be sensitive to and gradually reintroduce it, watching for a reaction.

All of these issues are very real, but various diet gurus and alternative health practitioners jump on the food intolerance bandwagon and say if you only give up X and Y, you'll not only feel fantastic, but drop loads of excess weight into the bargain. Not true! It is hard to lose weight. It takes time, discipline and lifestyle changes. The desire to lose weight also makes you vulnerable to quackery; how reassuring it is to be told that your weight problem has nothing to do with anything except your intolerance to, say, wheat or dairy products.

These unscrupulous types often base their spurious claims on wheat and dairy products, because intolerance to these foods is relatively common. Dairy products can be a problem if you're lactose-intolerant, for example. Wheat can also be an issue, but you would probably be diagnosed by a conventional doctor as having coeliac disease, which is when your body reacts to gluten, a constituent of wheat. Symptoms include extreme tiredness, abdominal pains, aching joints, moodiness, migraine, asthma and a stuffy nose. Coeliac disease prevents you from absorbing nutrients properly, resulting in

Try another idea...

Stuck on that last half a stone? Check out the ten-point plan in IDEA 49, *Stuck on those last 7 lb.*

Defining idea...

'**Given that the most common sources of food intolerance are wheat and milk, such therapists can achieve a reasonable success rate by diagnosing sensitivity to these two foods in all their patients.**'
JONATHAN BROSTOFF, *The Complete Guide to Food Allergy and Intolerance*

various deficiencies and weight loss, and you have to follow a wheat-free diet more or less permanently.

The upshot is that while you could have an intolerance to foods, diagnosis is difficult because of the wide variety of symptoms. Don't let anyone hoodwink you into thinking you have an intolerance which means you can't lose or stop gaining weight. You'll just end up spending a lot of money without getting the results you deserve, like me and my courgettes. See an allergy specialist or nutritionist to rule out anything serious and then concentrate on tried and tested methods of weight loss.

How did it go?

Q   Crikey, what can you eat if you can't eat wheat?

A   *If you're told you have to go on a gluten-free or wheat-free diet, it can be terrifying at first. You have to read food labels very carefully; even stock cubes can contain wheat flour, for example. You'll find that plenty of shops now stock special gluten free ranges however, and it is fine to eat rice, buckwheat (despite the name, it's not wheat), millet, corn, potato flour, and many more flours and grains. Arm yourself with a good wheat-free cookbook.*

Q   Aren't there pills you can take if you are lactose intolerant?

A   *You can eat a more varied diet if you use lactose replacers that help digest the lactose if taken at the same time as milky food. They are quite widely available. It is worth trying different brands to see which works best for you.*

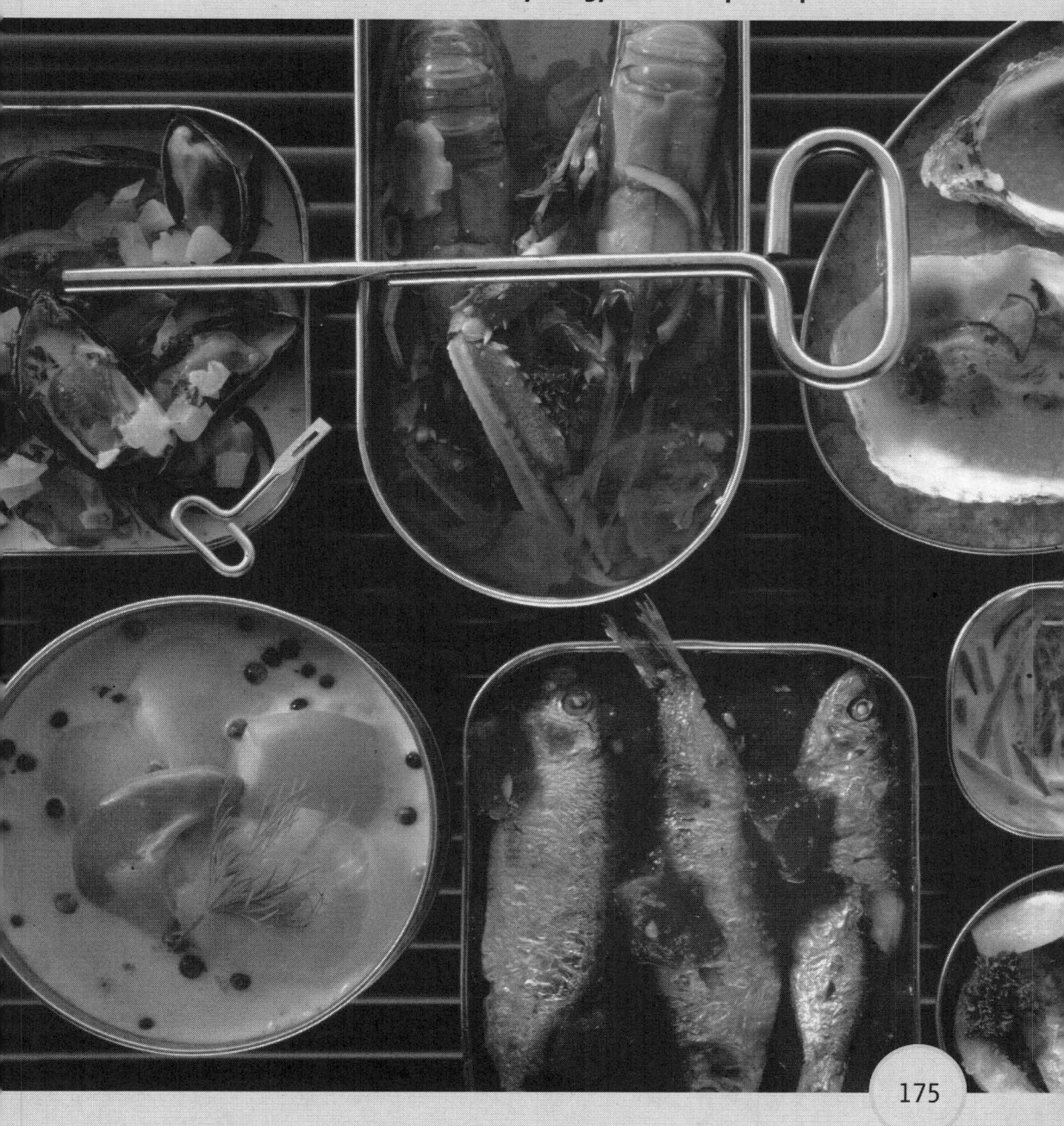

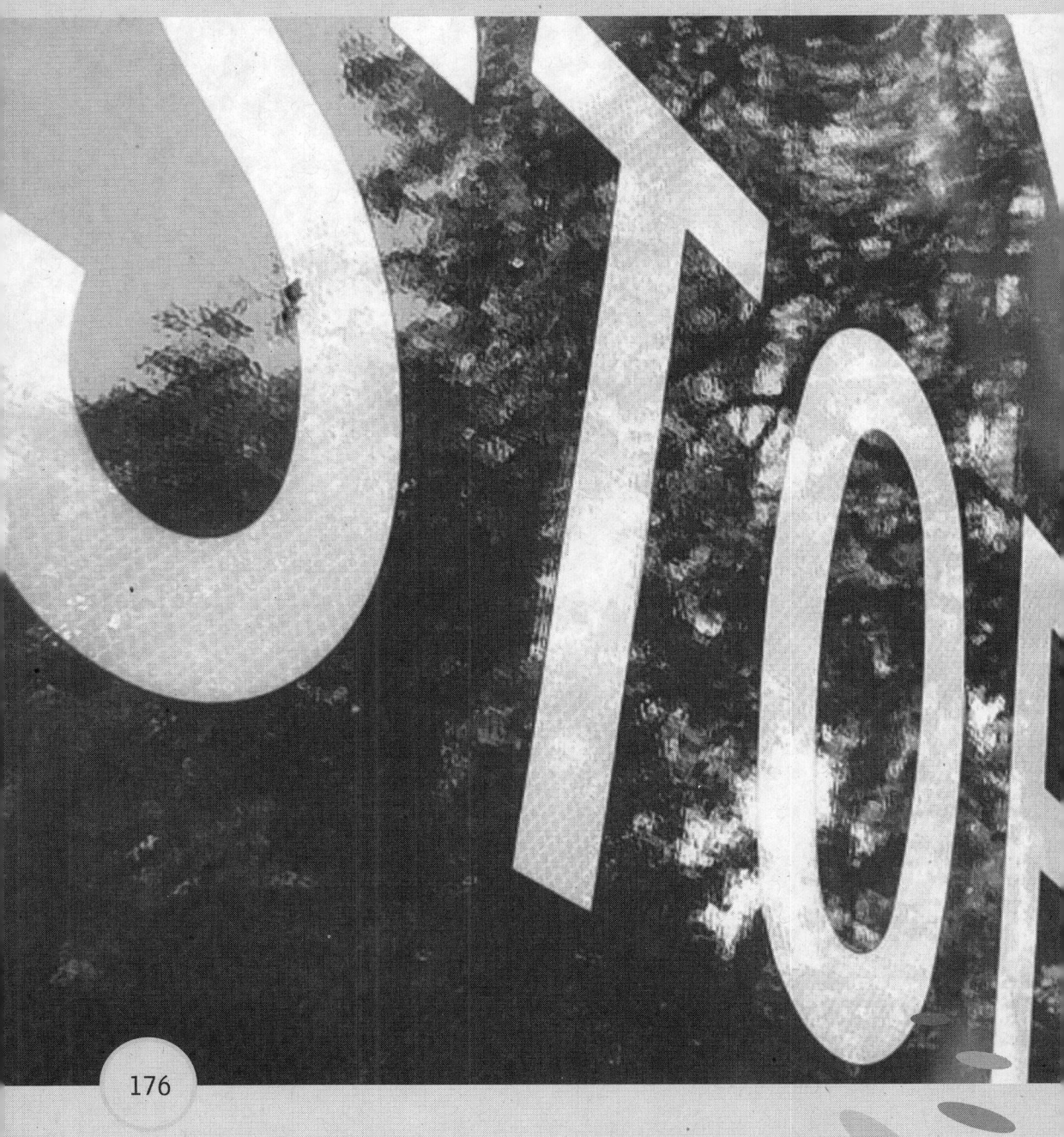

40

Trust me, I'm a doctor

The Atkins diet and other low carbohydrate/high protein diets are in fashion, but they are as controversial as they are popular. Would eating this way work for you, and is it safe?

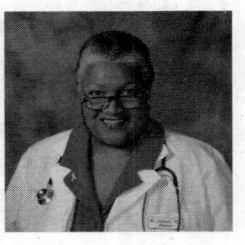

You can't open a magazine or a newspaper these days without seeing some reference to the late Dr Atkins and his amazing diet. His ideas have reached millions through his books.

I know lots of people who swear by his methods and say their lives have been changed, but there are many doctors, nutritionists and other health professionals who have rubbished his views. Others have taken his ideas and refined them. Atkins maintains that traditional low-fat diet recommendations have led to diets high in carbohydrate instead, which are all wrong for our metabolisms. He also says that fat isn't the baddie it is made out to be – at least, not all fats. Is this a case of the mainstream being slow to catch on? After all, Atkins pointed out that it took us centuries to accept that the world was not flat!

Try a carb curfew. Pioneered by British health and fitness expert Joanna Hall, the rule is to eat no carbs after five o'clock. It's a neat way to avoid excess carbohydrates, cuts some calories, and you don't go to bed feeling bloated.

It is beyond the scope of this chapter to go into all his ideas in detail, but let's look at some of the main premises:

THE ATKINS THEORY

We should be concentrating our efforts on our insulin levels, which control sugar levels in the body and how the body stores fat. If you eat a lot of carbohydrates, insulin is released which encourages the body to store the energy from food as fat. You can be 'insulin resistant', which means your body releases very high levels of insulin just to maintain normal blood sugar levels, encouraging more fat to be stored.

Switching to low levels of carbohydrate intake leads your body to burn fat as its energy source, rather than glucose from carbohydrates. Eating fat doesn't affect your blood sugar and, contrary to popular opinion, can be good for your health. Fat also helps you to feel satisfied after eating.

'The perfect diet for those who love food.'
NIGELLA LAWSON

IN PRACTICE

The Atkins diet requires you to start on an induction plan that lasts a minimum of fourteen days. It's pretty strict, including rules such as eating no more than 20 g of carbohydrates a day, which should come from salad greens and certain other 'acceptable' vegetables; no fruit, bread, grains or dairy foods other than cheese, cream and butter; plenty of poultry, fish and meat; no caffeine, processed foods and refined sugars. As you progress, you move through another three phases,

culminating in your lifetime maintenance plan. Each phase changes what you can and can't eat; for instance, later on you eat less fat than in the beginning.

Read up on another eating formula that gets the thumbs up from many experts. Turn to IDEA 43, *What's the next big thing?*

Try another idea...

You have to follow the diet to the letter or it won't work, and it's not for the short term – it's a way of eating for life.

WHAT'S THE VERDICT?

Critics have raised concerns about high fat intakes because of the risk of heart disease, but there are studies that show that the diet can have a beneficial effect on cholesterol levels and fats in the blood in the longer term. Kidney damage is another charge levelled at the diet, but there's no real proof. Atkins makes it clear that the diet is not for those who have kidney disease, or for pregnant women and nursing mothers. If you're diabetic, speak to your doctor about the diet. Diabetics can follow the Atkins diet, but only under very careful medical supervision.

Would I recommend it? Despite the fact that it flies in the face of most mainstream thinking, if you're fit and healthy, give it a try. It's down to personal experience in the end, and whether you can stick to it. I couldn't, although I still try to keep my carbohydrate intake controlled. I have also noticed that men seem to get on better with it than women. It must be the lure of all that meat!

'Atkins has never been about no carbs. It's about choosing the right carbs in the right amount.'
Dr STUART TRAGER, Medical Director of Atkins Nutritionals Inc.

Defining idea...

How did it go?

Q Is it true that you get constipation and smelly breath doing the Atkins diet?

A *Yes, some people do get constipated, particularly in the early stages. You should drink plenty of water, which should help. Atkins suggests taking a tablespoon of psyllium husks, coarse wheat bran or flaxseed meal each day. The breath thing is to do with ketones, which are fat breakdown chemicals and most common in the induction phase. Some perceive it as odd, sweetish smelling breath, others as horrid. Water, chewing parsley and frequent teeth-cleaning should sort it out.*

Q What about all the health benefits of fruit and vegetables? We're always being told to eat more, but here you're not allowed them.

A *Dr Atkins isn't against fruit and veg at all. There are restrictions during the first phase, but plenty of fruit and vegetables are allowed thereafter. He's not too keen on starchy ones, such as sweet potatoes, peas and corn. He thoroughly approves of berries.*

Q What happens if I have a massive carb binge?

A *You will get sent straight to the head teacher's office for punishment! If you do have a binge, you just have to go back to the strict induction regime for a few days. And sit in detention by yourself, writing lists of the carbohydrate contents of various foods...*

Does being overweight really matter?

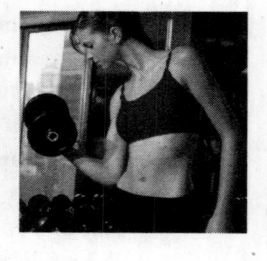

Perhaps you never got back into shape after having kids or maybe you've always been a little plumper than you would like. How do you know if it's really a problem?

A very attractive, curvaceous woman in her early sixties once said to me, 'Eve, darling, don't ever get too thin, it's so ageing.' And she was right!

I have friends who are in their early thirties and are incredibly proud of their skinny little size 8 or 10 frames, but look at least ten years older with their dried-up faces and flat little bottoms. I think a few curves and a couple of extra kilos are flattering and sensual – and that goes for men too.

When does a little plumpness become unacceptable? It depends on your viewpoint. If carrying a *few* extra kilos doesn't bother you, then it is not an issue. If it annoys you because you want to be in better shape, or it diminishes your confidence or stops you wearing the clothes you want to wear, then you should do something about it. If you have more than a few extra kilos, it does start to matter and when you're properly overweight it starts to matter very much indeed.

Here's an idea for you... **Get out your tape measure and calculator. Divide your waist measurement by your hip measurement (in centimetres). If the result is more than 0.95 for a man or 0.87 for a woman, you are apple-shaped. If you are apple-shaped, with more fat around your middle, your risk of heart disease is greater than if you're pear-shaped, with more fat on your bottom.**

Fatness is a worldwide epidemic. In the UK alone, it is estimated that two-thirds of men and half of women are overweight, with one in five being obese, that is at least 12.5 kg (28 lb) overweight. Experts are predicting that one in four adults will be obese by 2010.

Obesity makes everyday life uncomfortable is so many ways, such as being unable to run for a bus, a lack of choice in clothes, rude stares and comments from other, thinner, people, and sleep and fertility problems. It is also the commonest cause of ill health and potentially fatal diseases. Obesity contributes to heart disease, diabetes, gallstones and some cancers. Just being overweight – and that's more than say a kilo or so – can raise your blood pressure and give you problems with cholesterol. Even dental decay is more common in overweight people.

In case you're in any doubt as to why being overweight does matter, here are some fat facts to consider:

According to the British Heart Foundation, heart and circulatory disease is the UK's biggest killer. Although the numbers are in fact slightly lower than twenty years ago, this is because of medical advances, not because we are getting healthier! There are other risk factors too, such as smoking, poor psychological health and inherited infirmities, but the truth is that 30% of deaths from coronary heart disease are

directly linked to an unhealthy diet. The World Health Organisation estimates that somewhere between 1 and 24% of coronary heart disease is due to doing less than two and a half hours of moderate activity a week.

For another good health reason to get yourself in shape, see IDEA 45, *Could you have diabetes?*

Try another idea...

The fatter you are, the greater your risk. A weight gain of just 10 kg doubles your risk of heart disease. Reducing your weight even by 5 or 10% can have a beneficial effect on cholesterol levels.

Excess weight plays a part in high blood pressure, which can lead to blood clots, stroke and heart attacks. You can reduce these risks through diet: less salt, lower fat consumption and a huge increase in fruit and vegetable consumption.

Although the exact relationships are not fully understood, diet and cancer have an association too. A recent report suggested that as many as 40% of cancers have a dietary link. Breast cancer risk rises with a high fat diet or being overweight.

Clearly there's still a lot of research to be done, but it is certain that being overweight isn't fun and it isn't clever – and it can be about a lot more than the way you look.

'Imprisoned in every fat man a thin one is wildly signalling to be let out.'
CYRIL CONNOLLY

Defining idea...

183

How did it go?

Q **I smoke and know I should give up, but I'm already overweight. I don't want to put on even more weight, which always happens when you quit. What shall I do?**

A *Lots of people find that they put on up to 5 kg (10 lb) when they give up smoking. It's thought that nicotine somehow increases the metabolic rate. When you stop it lowers, which means if you eat the same amount, you will gain weight. Also when you first stop, you can't help snacking more (often out of boredom). This does tend to even out over a period of months. One way to keep weight gain down is to up your activity levels – as much as for distraction as burning up energy! Ultimately the benefits of not smoking have to be worth it. You could also try talking to your doctor about drugs, such as Zyban, that could help you quit without piling on the pounds.*

Q **How does diet affect your cholesterol levels?**

A *Firstly cholesterol isn't all bad, in fact it's needed by the body, but it's about the levels of the two kinds of cholesterol. HDL cholesterol is the good stuff, but LDL is the one you want less of. Trans fats (when liquid oils are hardened by hydrogenation in the manufacturing process) and saturated fats (found in meat, cream, butter, full fat milk and so on) cause LDL to rise, while fibre, vegetables and poly- and monounsaturated fats (think olive oil, sunflower oil and fish oils) not only lower LDL, but also boost levels of HDL cholesterol.*

42

The birds and the bees

There's a lot to be said for putting some loving into slimming. Oh come on, don't be shy, everyone does it, you know. Let's talk about sexercise.

Not all the good things in life are bad for you, although it often seems that way when you're trying to lose weight. Sex is definitely slimming.

Although you might be thinking you'd prefer a family-sized bar of fruit and nut chocolate to sex, or just a nice cup of tea, as Boy George once said, it's time to start thinking of love and sex as powerful weapons in your weight-loss armoury. How so? Being in love inspires you like nothing else. You look and feel great, feel happy and full of confidence. It's a great base to start your weight loss plan from because you feel so motivated. And sex? It burns calories, should make you feel good, oh and so much more. So, let's slip into something more comfortable, put some romantic music on the stereo and have a grown up chat.

Here's an idea for you...

Try a sensual aromatherapy massage to get you both in a loving mood. Just add five drops of your chosen essential oil to 20 ml of a carrier oil, such as almond or sunflower. Lavender, rose and camomile are all good relaxers. If you throw in a few drops of juniper or cypress that's supposed to be good for cellulite too!

LOVE AND SEX LESSON 1

Sex is a great booster for your self-esteem. Despite the fact that if you're trying to lose weight you might feel self-conscious about the way you look, learning to let yourself go is important for intimacy. Besides, virtually all research shows that men have no idea what cellulite is and that women go for personality, not looks (well, maybe they go for looks second). The key is to try to stop dwelling on what you don't like about your body. And when your partner compliments you, even if it is only about your ears, accept it, believe it and enjoy it. If you feel more comfortable with the lights out, turn those lights out or light a few candles, which makes everyone look like Richard Burton and Elizabeth Taylor, Brad and Jen, or Shrek and Princess Fiona. Oh, you know what I mean. It makes everyone look good. And if you feel the need for some covering, a sexy negligee, corset or nurses outfit won't fail to impress. Chaps, there's nothing sexier than you just out of the shower wearing a clean white towel wrapped around your middle, your hair slightly wet, your body lightly oiled, a faint hint of Eau Sauvage...gosh, I'm getting quite carried away.

Defining idea...

'I'd like to meet the man who invented sex and see what he's working on now.'
ANONYMOUS

LOVE AND SEX LESSON 2

Sex helps you win the battle of the bulge. According to a study in the US, if you make love three times week, you'll burn approximately 7,500 calories a year, which is

the same as jogging 120 km (75 miles). Not bad, eh? Of course you do have to actively participate, as opposed to lying there wondering what you're going to eat tomorrow, but still, even kissing burns a few calories a minute. Sex also releases endorphins, those feel-good chemicals that you get after exercising, plus it relaxes you, which is useful as there's a definite link between stress and heart disease as well as weight gain.

If that's got you going, rev yourself up even more with IDEA 16, *Metabolism masterclass*.

Try another idea...

LOVE AND SEX LESSON 3

Sex helps you to sleep, which is a good thing as long as it's not in the middle of a love session. Lack of sleep has been shown to increase snacking and the urge for high-calorie quick energy foods.

LOVE AND SEX LESSON 4

Sex makes you look younger and helps you stay healthy. All that stress reduction and the increased blood supply that you get with regular love-making makes you look more youthful. It boosts your immune system and could help to reduce cholesterol levels. The younger you feel, the more you'll feel like having sex. And of course, sex is a way of strengthening your relationship, of feeling cared for, cherished and respected, which boosts your self-esteem, which means that anything is possible, including losing weight. See, it's all connected.

'Being deeply loved by someone gives you strength, while loving someone deeply gives you courage.'
LAO TZU

Defining idea...

187

Q We're so busy, we don't have time for romance. What can we do?

A   *Try something out of the ordinary to get away from ordinary everyday life. Book into a B&B for a night, have a sexy finger food picnic by candlelight in the garden or in front of the fire, take a day off work and go to the countryside or the beach and walk, or chat about anything as long as it's not domestic stuff or work-related. Take the time to really listen to your partner too, even if you think you have heard the jokes and moans a million times before.*

Q What aphrodisiac foods are there that won't blow my diet?

A   *The aroma of almonds is said to induce passion in women. It's OK to eat a few as well. Chickpeas were fed to stallions by the Romans for mating purposes and they were thought to work well on men too. A sprinkle of nutmeg on your food might be worth a try – it's been prized as an aphrodisiac by Chinese women for centuries. Ginger, chillis, cinnamon and cloves are also said to boost blood flow and make you sweat slightly, two things that could heighten feelings of arousal – or just make you want to step outside for a breath of cool air. Lean steak is rich in B vitamins, zinc and iron, which can all affect sex hormones and the libido. And then there are always oysters, which are full of zinc. Even the act of swallowing them can be very erotic.*

What's the next big thing?

Heard about the glycaemic index? If you've been left feeling confused, not to mention hungry and still overweight by other diets, perhaps the GI diet or one of its relatives could be the one for you.

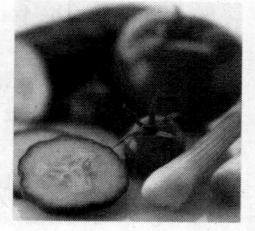

Celebrity fans of the glycaemic index (GI) way of eating are rumoured to include Kylie Minogue. If it could give you a bottom like hers, you'd be mad to not give it a whirl, wouldn't you?

I've got lots of time for this kind of diet because it's easy to follow and live with. It works for vegetarians, too. The GI diet is basically pretty healthy and I've seen people achieve great results with it. So what's it about?

Originally developed during research for diabetes, the glycaemic index is a measure of how quickly you digest various foods and convert them into your body's energy source: glucose. Glucose, or sugar is rated at 100 and everything else gets scored against that. So cornflakes come in at 84, for example, while oatmeal is 42.

Here's an idea for you...

Next time you are shopping, see if you can find GI information on the food label. As well as the full GI listings and information that is available in specialist books, some forward-thinking supermarkets are starting to label products with a low GI and medium GI rating.

Eating low GI foods means you're satisfied for longer, while those with high ratings on the index not only make you feel hungry again quicker (cue snacking), but also trigger off various processes that lead to fat formation and fat storage. However, that's not the whole picture. The GI diet, to take one of my favourites (by Rick Gallop) also promotes eating a combination of low GI foods that are low in sugar and fat, therefore calories too.

Foods are rated red light – avoid, amber – eat occasionally and green – as much as you want. Is this starting to make sense?

The GI diet also recommends playing with balance of your plate, which is not a circus trick, but still a clever kind of juggling. It means creating a mix on your plate that is a little different to mainstream healthy eating guidelines, of 50% vegetables, with another 25 per cent of meat or fish and the remaining 25% rice, pasta or potatoes. As far as serving sizes go, moderation and common sense are encouraged, but suggestions such as 100 g (4 ounces) of meat and 40 g (1.5 ounces) of dry weight pasta are given. Fruit and vegetables tend to be unlimited, though they have to be the green-lighted ones. For instance, boiled new potatoes are 56 on the index, while a baked potato is 84.

What might your breakfast look like on the GI diet? Here's a taster:

- You could have fresh fruit, although not all fruits are green-lighted. Melon for example is out as it's quickly digested. As juice is processed and therefore digested more quickly, whole fruits are better.

- Porridge and sugar-free bran cereals are allowed, as is wholemeal bread that is labelled stoneground – this means less of the fibre is separated, i.e. it'll take longer to digest. A bread serving is one slice and to be eaten sparingly.

- You can have skimmed milk and low or no-fat yoghurts, with artificial sweeteners to keep the calories down.

- No butter is allowed, so you have to shop for non-hydrogenated soft margarine.

- Spreads such as reduced sugar or sugar-free jams are fine.

Try another idea...

What are the secrets of successfully maintaining your weight loss? As well as a healthful diet, there are other tricks you need to know to IDEA 52, *Zen and the art of weight loss maintenance.*

Defining
idea...

'I decided to try this diet. To my amazement and delight I lost the twenty pounds that had been plaguing me for so long.'
RICK GALLOP, author of the *GI Diet*

What you can't have are sausages and regular bacon (a bit of leaner back bacon or lean ham is fine), full fat dairy products, white refined produce, such as baguettes, muffins and croissants and dried fruit or fruits that are canned in syrup. My only real gripe as far as the breakfast goes is that coffee isn't allowed – well, only the decaffeinated sort. This is due to caffeine increasing insulin production and reducing blood sugar levels, which makes you hungry.

Overall, the diet is supposed to be a way of eating for life, rather than using as a short-term diet. As it's healthy and easy to follow, that doesn't present a problem. Yes, there are things you have to cut out, some temporarily and some long term, but in truth, they're things that ultimately don't do you health or weight any good anyway. The diet also endorses exercise – an essential in my book! So, yes, this one gets the green light from me.

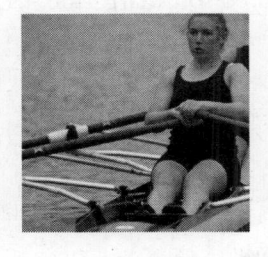
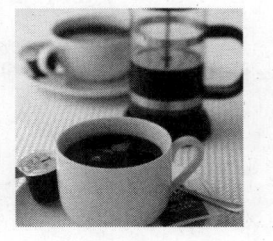
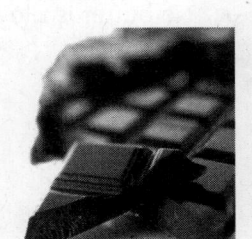

Q How long will it take me to lose weight on the GI diet?

A The first phase is supposed to take between three and six months based on a 10% reduction in your weight. Although this might sound quite a long time, it does mean that you're losing weight at a safe rate, as opposed to losing lots at once and then plateauing. Besides, it's not really that long in terms of the rest of your life. If we can really establish a life-long habit of healthy eating and exercise, we may never have to diet again. Wouldn't that be wonderful?

Q Are there variants of the GI eating plan, just like there are variants of the high protein/low carbohydrate diets?

A Yes there are and they all have subtle differences, though using the index as the basis for their recommendations. There is also a plethora of GI cookbooks – a worthwhile investment if you like the sound of eating this way.

Q What does the GI diet say about chocolate and alcohol?

A They are strictly forbidden! No, just kidding. You are allowed the occasional bit of chocolate, as long it's one of those with a high cocoa content, which usually have less fat and sugar than regular chocolate. Alcohol is allowed after you've done the first phase of the diet, but always only in moderation.

How did
it go?

193

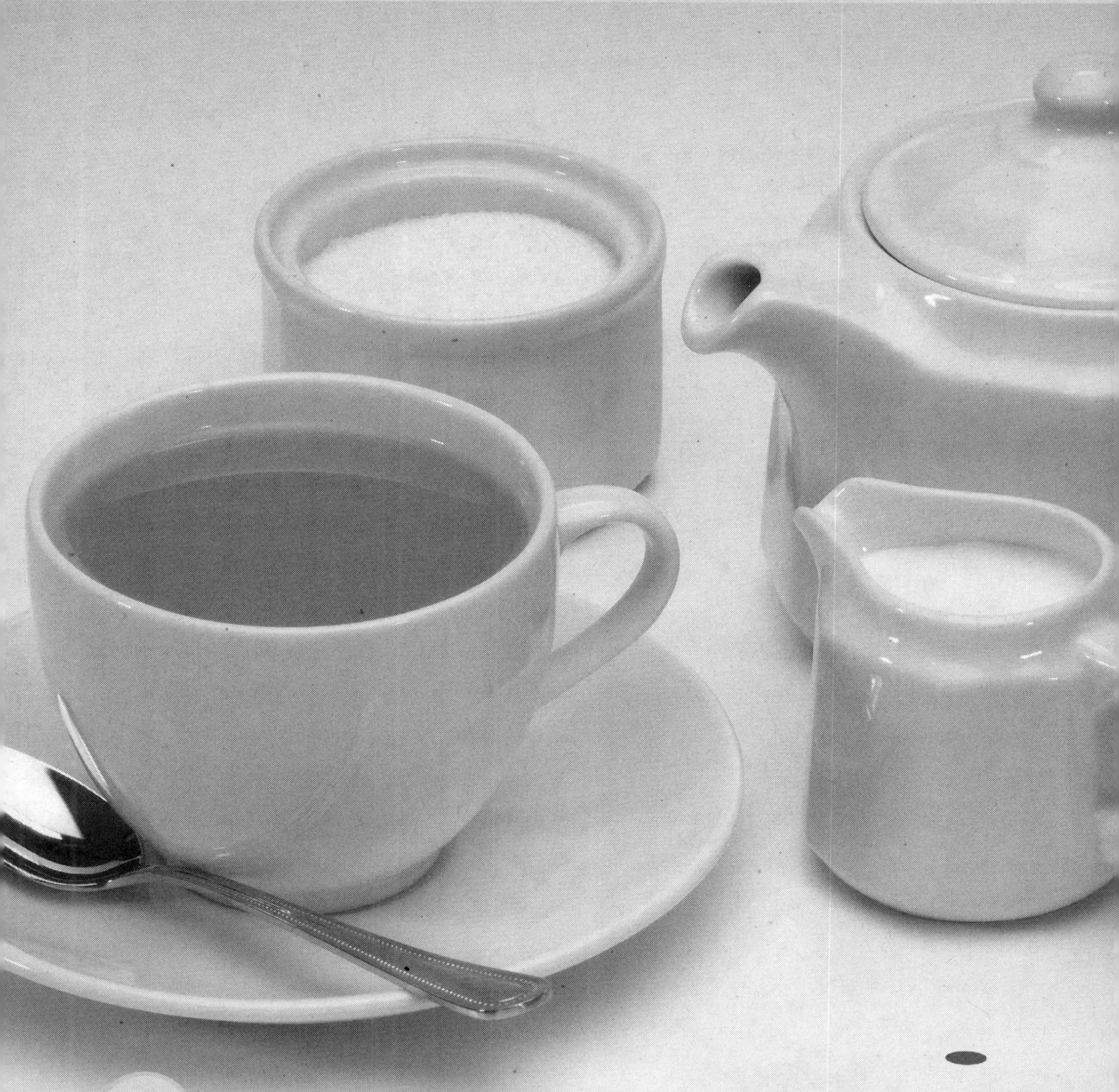

44

Time for tea (would you like black, green, herbal or slimming?)

It's a seductive idea: sip tea and watch the weight melt away. But can a tea ever really be more than a refreshing drink?

Let me read your tea leaves. I see a large shape saying this cup of diet tea was a waste of time. Stick to sensible eating and more exercise instead of lying around drinking your brew of 'Bye Bye Fat'.

We all like an easy option, and what could be easier than sipping yourself slim with a fat-busting tea? Health food stores offer some of these super-charged brews, but it's on the internet that you're really spoiled for choice. And it's also on the internet that you can say or sell just about anything you want and get away with it. As with many things in life, not all everything is what it seems, and tea is no exception.

Here's an idea for you... **Make your own herbal tea or infusion. Use a teaspoon of dried herbs or two of fresh to a cup of boiling water. Pour the water over the herbs and leave it covered for five to ten minutes. Before you drink it, strain it.**

Let's take black tea, which is the regular tea you find everywhere, and green tea first of all. Both contain flavonoids with myriad health benefits including protection against heart disease. This is proven, so drink up and you'll do yourself some good. Just use skimmed milk and limit the sugar. Green tea has been in the spotlight recently, following various research projects. It has been linked with having a preventative effect on all kinds of diseases, including certain cancers, as well as having the ability to lower cholesterol and, to speed up fat oxidation, i.e. to burn calories quicker. Further research is needed in all these areas, but it's safe to say that if you like the taste of green tea, you've got nothing to lose apart from just possibly a few kilos.

TRIED AND TRUSTED?

Herbal teas go back a long way and are used in both traditional Chinese and Indian medicine. They're popular everywhere as an alternative to regular tea and coffee and in some countries are used as "cures" for common complaints, including for example, fennel as an aid to digestion and camomile to ease anxiety and promote sleep. Of course quite how healing they are is a matter for debate, primarily because they may not in fact contain enough of the herb to have any effect. But still, a herbal tea whose ingredient you recognise won't do you any harm at all. It's the blends that are given compelling weight-loss promising names that you need to be cautious about.

In fact, many people think diet teas, which contain ingredients such as licorice root, senna and buckthorn, should really be called laxative teas because that's what they do to you! In small amounts they can just be a little, well, inconvenient, as you have to run to the loo rather a lot. If you consume them in large amounts, you're asking for trouble. Others act as diuretics, especially if they have dandelion, parsley or juniper as ingredients, so you lose water weight. Then there are the diet teas that contain stimulants such as yerba mate, kola nut and guarana. They're OK in small doses, but if you're sensitive to the ingredients or have just a little too much, you'll get palpitations, the jitters and have difficulty sleeping. It's rare, but there's a risk of heart attack. Since the only reason you'll be drinking the teas that are marketed as slimming aids is to lose weight (most of them don't actually taste that great) and as there's absolutely no proof that they can help, I'd leave them well alone. Stick to a nice cup of real tea, or traditional herbal tea that doesn't make any other claim than it tastes good!

But aren't there useful supplements and medical diet pills that could work for me? Yes, there are, but they are aids to weight-loss, not substitutes for exercise and a good diet. Turn to IDEA 46, *Couldn't I just pop a pill?*

Try another idea...

'Drinking a daily cup of tea will surely starve the apothecary.'
CHINESE PROVERB

Defining idea...

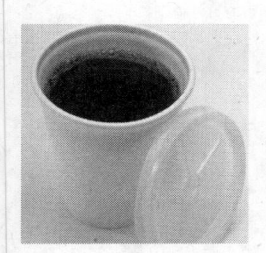

197

How did it go?

Q Doesn't normal tea have caffeine in it, so can't it give you the jitters too?

A *Yes, tea does contain caffeine, but at far lower levels than coffee, regular cola drinks and chocolate bars. You'd have to drink an awful lot to get twitchy side effects, unless of course you were particularly sensitive.*

Q It's a diuretic too, isn't it?

A *According to recent research, no. You'd have to drink five or six cups at one sitting to clock up the 250–300 mg of caffeine needed to create a diuretic effect. In fact, it is now acknowledged that tea can contribute to your daily fluid intake, which is recommended to be 1.5–2 litres a day. In the UK, most people drink on average three to four cups of tea. That might sound like a nice bit of trivia, but it shows that some seemingly old-fashioned habits really aren't so bad after all.*

Q How should you drink it?

A *You can drink it hot with milk or lemon or cold with ice. It's up to you. It won't affect the health-giving properties of green or black tea, so drink it the way you like it. Ideally, though, don't drink it with meals, as it decreases the absorption of iron from foods.*

45

Could you have diabetes?

Diabetes is increasing on a global scale. Even more concerning is the fact that you could be a sufferer without knowing it. Here's what is has to do with diet and activity levels

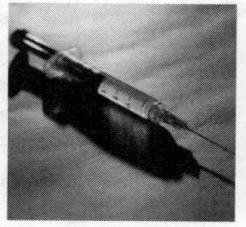

Diabetes is a chronic and incurable disease with nasty complications, such as blindness, kidney failure, stroke and nerve damage.

Diabetes is not new – in the 17th century it was called the 'pissing evil' – but it is on the increase. There are two types of diabetes. Type 1 is more commonly found in children and young adults and is treated with a strict diet and insulin injections. It's Type 2 that is on the increase and is strongly linked to obesity and a lack of activity. There are other risk factors over which we have no control, such as genetic inheritance, simply getting older and your ethnic origin – Asians and Afro-Caribbeans do seem to be at a higher risk. Eating lots of sweet things, contrary to popular belief, doesn't cause diabetes, but it leads to weight gain, which does increase your risk. It's a fact that 80% of people with Type 2 diabetes are overweight. The fatter and less fit you are, the greater your risk.

Here's an idea for you...

How can you get five fruit and vegetables into your daily diet? Try having one piece of fruit at breakfast, plus a piece of fruit after lunch or as an afternoon snack; have a salad with lunch or dinner and two vegetables (not potatoes) with your other meal.

Type 2 diabetes used to be more common in middle age, but increasingly it's affecting younger people too. Those with the condition either don't produce enough insulin or what is produced doesn't work effectively, which means that the body can't use glucose properly and levels remain high in the blood. Some of the symptoms of undiagnosed diabetes include increased thirst, a need to go to the toilet often, especially at night, lethargy and tiredness, blurred vision, regular thrush and genital itching, plus weight loss when nothing else has changed regarding your lifestyle. Doctors say many people have these symptoms on and off for years before eventually being diagnosed as diabetic, which is easily done with a simple blood test.

In the past, if you were diagnosed as having diabetes, physical activity was discouraged and, a high fat/low carbohydrate diet prescribed. How times change! Now exercise is encouraged, just as it is for everyone to improve their health and control weight. As a role model, look to Sir Steve Redgrave, five times Olympic Gold medal winner and a diabetes sufferer! Diet-wise, the reason a high fat diet was recommended was to make up for the lack of calories that resulted from following a low carbohydrate diet to keep sugar levels stable (fat doesn't boost sugar levels in itself). Diabetics are more at risk of heart disease as a result of the condition, but of course, the high fat diet increased this risk! Luckily, nutrition has moved on, with eating guidelines for diabetics pretty much in line with general healthy eating recommendations. As well as using medication and being under strict medical supervision, most diabetics can control their condition and also lose weight by

eating in the most healthful way. The eating guidelines also work as a preventative and can be used by everyone. In brief, they are:

- Eat regular meals featuring starchy carbohydrates of the whole grain variety, i.e. wholemeal bread and cereals, rather than refined carbohydrates.

- Cut down on fat, especially saturated fats found in animal products. Choose low fat and monounsaturated fats such as olive oil.

- Eat more fruit and vegetables!

- Cut down on sugar and sugary foods, especially sugary drinks which cause blood glucose levels to rise quickly.

- Cut down on salt to keep blood pressure in check and drink in moderation. Diabetics in particular should be careful of drinking on an empty stomach, as it can precipitate hypoglycaemia – dangerously low blood sugar levels.

Try another idea…

IDEA 48, *The incredible bulk*, tells you more about the benefits of unrefined foods, fruits and vegetables.

Defining idea…

'**According to one recent study on diabetes care conducted in the US, on average for every 1 kg (2 lb) in weight a person puts on over the normal range, their risk of developing diabetes increases by about 9 per cent.**'
JUDITH MILLS, *The Diet Bible*

How did it go?

Q   **What about special diabetic foods?**

A   *Most experts say they are unnecessary and a waste of money.*

Q   **Isn't Type 2 diabetes just a mild form of the illness?**

A   *No, it needs to be taken seriously. Four out of five people with the condition die prematurely from heart disease. There's also an increased risk of stroke, diabetic vetinopathy which can lead to blindness, and nerve damage in the hands and feet. Action is essential, both if you've already been diagnosed and also as a preventative measure with weight control being an important strategy. Recent research has shown that complications are prevented if blood glucose levels are normalised with Type I diabetes. Most experts believe the same for Type II diabetes too.*

Q   **Surely it's not that big an issue? What about all the plagues and epidemics?**

A   *The World Health Organisation thinks it is a big issue. It is predicting a global epidemic of diabetes, which means that it already is an issue for you and it will definitely be an issue for your children and the ones you might have in the future. Do ask your doctor for a test if any of the risk factors apply to you and also if you have any of the symptoms described above.*

46

Couldn't I just pop a pill?

You would think there would be safe, effective, fat-reducing pill that you could buy at the pharmacy. Some would say it's already here in the form of supplements and certain prescription drugs. So what's the truth?

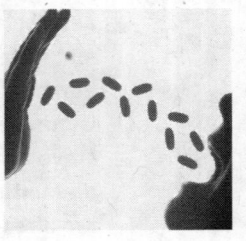

Some years ago when I was editing a health and fitness magazine, we all got very excited about a new fat-busting product that built lean muscle mass. It was a powder that you mixed with water and drank daily — sadly it didn't seem to work.

Eight of us decided to give it go. After a week, seven had given up due to stomach cramps and diarrhoea. The eighth (it was me) carried on. My stomach was fine and I decided I must be quite tough, but at the end of the two month long course I didn't look, weigh or measure any different.

Here's an idea for you...

If you want a herbal appetite suppressant, scientists have now isolated the active molecules in the *Hoodia gordonii* plant, used by tribesmen in the Kalahari to stave off hunger pangs whilst on hunting trips. Some products are already available, being sold as appetite suppressants and anecdotally are getting good reviews. However, more research is needed.

There are many supplements that promise appetite suppression, weight loss and increases in lean muscle mass. These products are widely available through pharmacies, health food stores and of course the good old internet. Often you might find a trainer at your local gym recommending them too. But do any of them actually work? Let's look at a few of the most popular:

Chromium picolinate

Chromium is needed to help insulin transfer glucose and nutrients from the bloodstream to the cells and plays a role in energy production. It's found in foods such as mushrooms and broccoli. The lure of supplements that combine chromium and picolinate is the potential of losing fat and gaining muscle tone – this is based on the results of a number of studies. However, further research hasn't been able to duplicate the original claims and indeed some research has subsequently made links between high levels of supplementation, DNA damage and a host of other nasties. In fact, at time of writing, this substance is facing a ban in the UK.

Chitosan

This is made from crushed crab and lobster shells! The theory is that the fibre from the shells binds with and absorbs the fat from your food before it is metabolised. Some studies have shown it can help weight loss, but there are no large scale convincing trials, so who really knows? The downside is that chitosan will also

decrease the absorption of fat-soluble vitamins, plus you'll experience a laxative effect. It is not recommended – especially if you're allergic to shellfish!

Is there any merit in diet teas? Probably not, and they are certainly not a miracle cure. See IDEA 44, *Time for tea*.

Try another idea...

Creatine

Creatine is used by athletes and perhaps a few chaps in your local gym to increase muscular performance. Most studies have been short term. It's not one for average dieters.

Amino acids

These are readily available as pills and powders, but despite the hype there's no proof that they will increase muscle mass or burn fat as a supplement. The only approved use of amino acids is for the intravenous feeding of people with specific health conditions such as kidney disease. You are better off with protein foods such as meat and eggs and plenty of exercise.

DOCTOR'S ORDERS

Producing a weight-control pill is truly one of the Holy Grails of pharmaceutical companies, because anything that even half works is a veritable goldmine. There are already products available. You may have heard of sibutramine, marketed as Reductil, and Orlistat (or Xenical) to name a couple. Trials of a drug called

'People usually spend more time researching their next car or computer purchase than selecting their supplements.'
FELICIA BUSCH, *The New Nutrition*

Defining idea...

Rimonabant have also been successful in both weight loss and helping smokers to quit without piling on pounds. At the moment the drugs that are licensed can only be given to you on prescription from your doctor. So what would happen if you went along and asked for your doctor for one of them? As non-pharmacological means of losing weight are still the first line of treatment, you'd probably be sent away with a diet sheet, an appointment with a dietician and advice on getting more physically active. However, if you have a BMI of 30 or more or have been trying without success to lose weight through lifestyle changes, your doctor may well prescribe one of the drugs.

In conclusion, beware of supplements that promise weight loss and muscle tone with no effort. At best they just won't work and will be a waste of money. At worst, they could be dangerous, especially if randomly combined with other supplements and medicines. And if you're not obese, you probably won't be advised to pop a prescription pill. So, it's back to good old fashioned sensible eating and exercise, truly tried and tested and suitable for everyone.

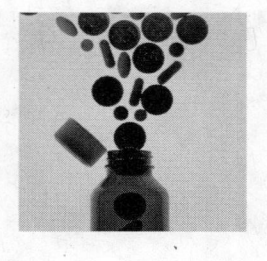
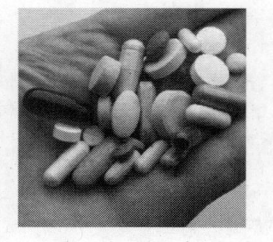
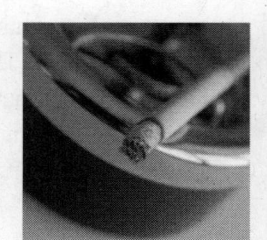

Q   **I thought I'd heard good things about something called leptin. Any truth in them?**

How did it go?

A   *This goes back a few years and relates to some research in rodents in which those with a lack of leptin had increased appetites. The idea was that obese people may be lacking leptin, so if you gave them more, their appetite should reduce. However, leptin is rarely deficient in humans. In fact, obese people can have high levels, though it's mooted that there could be a case for leptin-resistance. The jury is still out. And the researchers are still researching.*

Q   **OK, so if I can't take any pills, how else can I control my appetite?**

A   *Eat little and often to keep your blood sugar levels stable and ward off uncontrollable hunger pangs. Try drinking plenty of fluids to fill you up – anything from water to a bowl of tomato soup. Eat slowly when you have a meal to allow your brain to register more quickly that you are full, and try to sit down rather than eat standing up for the same reason. Avoid sugary snacks that will give you a quick hit, but soon leave you wanting more. Remember to distract yourself from thinking about food. Try doing anything that will take your mind off it!*

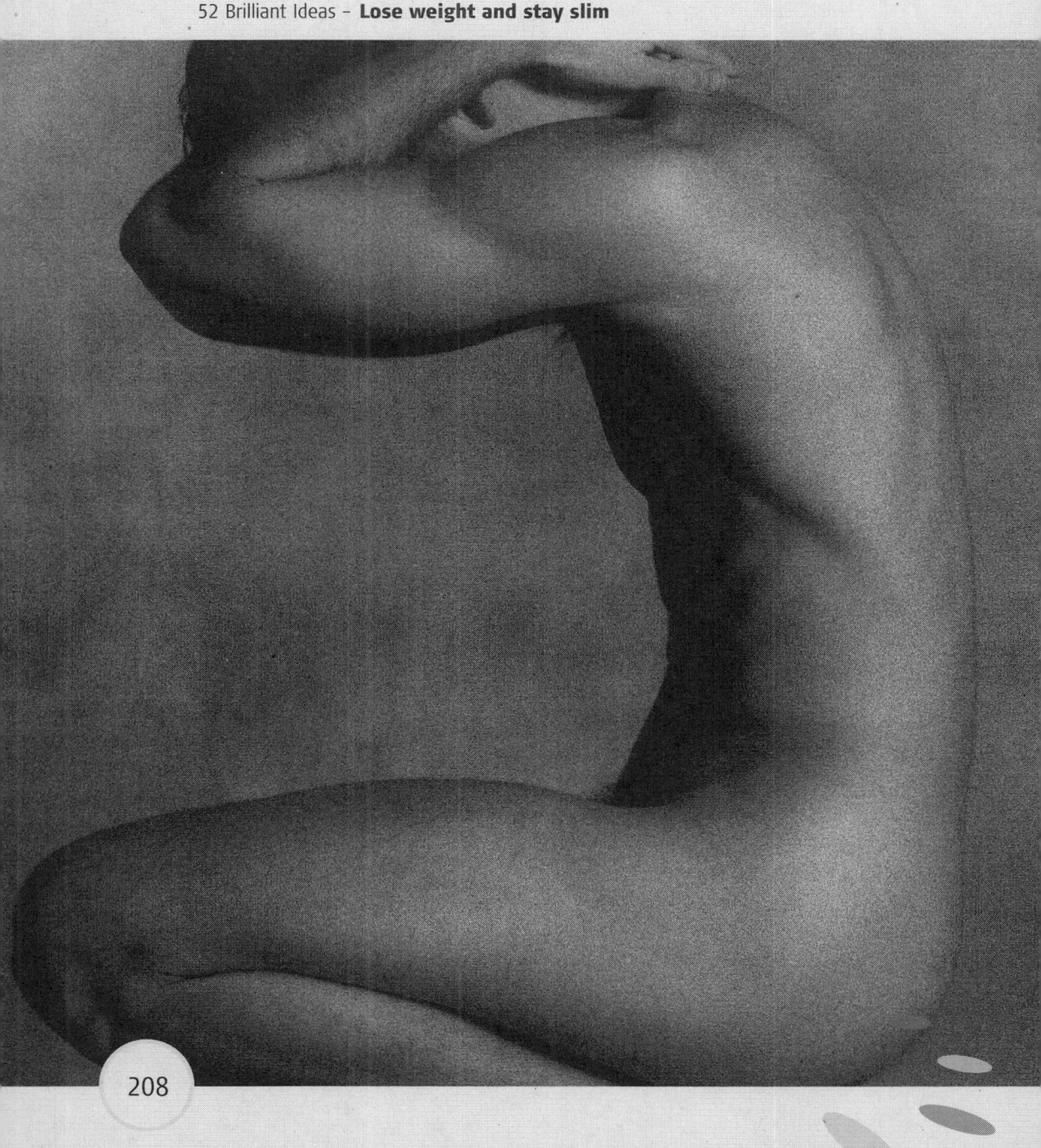

Spot reduction: the facts and the fiction

How much can you change your natural shape? Is it possible to lose weight from specific areas of your body? There are many myths surrounding those questions. Here's the truth.

What did you inherit? I don't mean a cottage by the sea or your Great Uncle Stan's stamp collection — I'm talking about things like Mum's thighs and Dad's height.

As well as your gender and your nutrition in childhood, the main influence on your body shape comes from your parents. You can take after one or other of them, or be a mix of both.

Broadly speaking, human shapes can be split into three main types, ectomorphs, mesomorphs and endomorphs. Ectomorphs are tall and thin and are often quite angular or even delicate-looking. They have a low body fat percentage and not

Here's an idea for you...

To get an idea of whether you really need to lose weight or indeed to track your progress, you can have your body fat measured electronically. A harmless electric current is passed through your body which estimates body water, showing the amount of muscle you have. The difference between your overall weight and lean tissue weight gives an idea of your body fat. Gyms and health centres usually offer this service (for a price) or you can also buy special scales to use at home.

much muscle, either. Although they usually have few weight problems when young, they are likely to put on weight around the stomach area as they age. Mesomorphs tend to have quite a bit of muscle and indeed a higher muscle to fat ratio than the other two types. They appear well-built with strong arms and legs. A mesomorph stays in good shape if active. However, a sedentary mesomorph will gain body fat. The endomorph is altogether rounder and softer looking, with more fat than muscle. They put weight on easily, but with regular physical activity can achieve good muscle tone.

As well as the basic shapes, you can have an android or gynoid influence. The android is an apple shape, with most weight carried on the top half of the body (and of course, sooner or later around the abdominal area). This shape is more closely associated with ectomorphs and mesomorphs as they age and especially men, while it affects endomorphs more generally. The gynoid influence, which is a pear shape, i.e. heavier on the bottom half, is a more female shape and can occur across the three groups. While we can be a combination of the groups, most of us do tend to fall into one identifiable type. The key is to identify the closest to your shape and work with it, rather than battling against it, to be in the best possible shape you can be.

MOVERS AND SHAPERS

You cannot spot reduce and lose weight from specific areas of the body. Research has shown that we all tend to lose weight from the top down, so, first it shows in your face, then your chest and stomach area, followed by hips, thighs and legs. Abdominal fat seems to be fairly easy to shift – good news for apple shapes, less good for pear shapes. But of course as abdominal fat is a risk factor in heart disease, pear shaped people can afford to be a little smug. But I'd rather be slim and in proportion, I hear the pear shapes say. A fat pear shaped person will slim into, well, a slimmer pear shaped person. And there's not a lot more you can do about your basic shape apart from surgery, which I don't recommend, but it's up to you. There is also exercise, which I do strongly recommend. One of the best tips for the pear-shaped person is to focus your strength training efforts on your top half to create more balance.

How much can exercise change your shape? Toning exercises certainly work to either increase your muscle bulk or streamline your muscles. However, if you've got lots of fat covering your muscles it will be harder to see muscle definition, plus you could just end up looking bigger. It's best to lose some body fat first. Contrary to popular myth it's not possible to turn fat into muscle or the other way around. Fat is fat and muscle is muscle.

What has sleep got to do with weight control? More than you might think! See IDEA 29, *Snooze and lose.*

Try another idea…

'I'm in shape. Round is a shape, isn't it?'
ANONYMOUS

Defining idea…

211

How did it go?

Q I'm losing weight...and my bust. Can you help?

A *This is a hard one to get around. Just as you can't lose weight from specifically targeted areas, you can't put weight back on selectively either! The best course of action is to do plenty of chest exercises (press ups and the pec dec machine in the gym for example) to work your pectoral muscles around the breast area. While this sort of exercise won't increase the size of your breasts, it will keep them uplifted and perky. Other than that, you can create cleavage using a good push-up bra, one that is filled with gel, or 'chicken fillets', those rubbery shapes to slip inside your bra.*

Q Is there anything I can do to help give a better shape to my waist?

A *Your waist should decease in size as you lose weight overall. Good posture helps too, as do specific Pilates and yoga moves. You can also work your waist with toning exercises that target your oblique muscles that run down the sides of your torso. Talk to a trainer at your local gym or health club and ask to be shown a selection of moves. I have also heard that exercising for ten minutes a day with a hula hoop can whittle inches from your waistline.*

The incredible bulk

It comes from plants and cannot be digested, nor does it provide any calories or energy. So what, you may well ask, is the point of fibre? Actually it's fascinating. How long have you got?

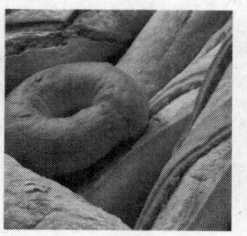

Fibre is about a lot more than chewing on bran flakes to keep you regular. As well as its myriad health benefits, fibre can also help you stay slim.

Generally people with high fibre diets weigh less than those who don't each much fibre. This could be due to the fact that fibre-rich foods are filling. And if you're full you don't feel the need to overeat or snack on treats. A recent paper on weight loss in the US confirmed that low fat diets with plenty of complex carbohydrates, fruit and vegetables are naturally high in fibre and low in calories and as such lead to weight loss. One study even reported that following this kind of eating model, the carbohydrates could be consumed freely and weight would still be lost.

Drink a litre of juice a day: it's around 400 calories. Drink a litre of water and eat a couple of oranges instead. It will save you calories and give you more fibre. Fruit juice is healthy and full of vitamins and counts as one of five a day fruit and vegetable portions. It's also high in sugars, albeit natural ones.

The benefits of fibre, or to give it its new, proper name, non-starch polysaccharides, have been known for thousands of years. Hippocrates (known as the father of medicine) advised his wealthy patients to follow the example of their servants and eat brown bread rather than white for example, "for its salutary effect on the bowel". Now we now more about fibre itself.

There are two kinds of fibre, soluble and insoluble. They are not nutrients in themselves as they are not digested for the most part, but both have important jobs to do. Soluble fibre lowers blood cholesterol levels and also slows the absorption of glucose into the blood stream ensuring there isn't a sudden rise in blood sugar levels. Although most plant foods combine soluble and insoluble fibre, the former is found particularly in oats and oat bran, barley, brown rice, beans and pulses, and fruit and vegetables. Insoluble fibre keeps things moving along in your digestive system. Look away now if bottom and bowel business makes you feel a little uncomfortable and fidgety. It acts a bit like a sponge and soaks up water to expand the bulk of your waste products (the faeces). Basically with dietary fibre your stools are softer and move along easily, which helps to avoid constipation and piles and also protects against rectal and colon cancers. The best sources of insoluble fibre are wheat, whole grain breads and cereals, corn, green beans and peas and the skins of fruits such as apples.

'A fruit is a vegetable with looks and money.'
P. J. O'ROURKE

CAN YOU HAVE TOO MUCH OF A GOOD THING?

It's recommended that we eat around 18 g of fibre a day, which most of us barely manage. We don't manage it because we eat more refined carbohydrates (white, processed foods and sugars) and don't eat enough fruit and vegetables. But the benefits are clear to see. When you increase your fibre consumption, make sure you drink plenty of water. You might also find that you retain some fluid at first, making you look and feel a little heavier. And there may be a bit of wind! This is temporary though as you get used to the new foods in your diet. Increasing your activity levels helps as it stimulates the muscles in the torso, helping speedier elimination – you don't want all that waste hanging around. There's some evidence that very high intakes of wheat bran can interfere with the absorption of iron and calcium, but it would need to be consistently high to really cause problems (though it can be a big issue for children and pregnant women). As new research suggests that high fibre consumption from a variety of sources affords a 40 per cent lesser risk of bowel cancer and that women who eat plenty of fruit and vegetables and wholegrain cereals have a lower incidence of breast cancer, it makes sense to increase your dietary fibre and start chewing for health. And of course to keep hunger pangs at bay!

Try another idea…

As well as plenty of fibre, you can discover what else a balanced diet should contain in **IDEA 4, *Pyramid selling*.**

Defining idea…

'**There are food scares in Belgium involving everything from poultry to chocolate. To the despair of many worldwide, however, another millennium ends without any bad news about Brussels sprouts.**'
FRANK McNALLY

How did
it go?

Q **I've got irritable bowel syndrome and I don't know whether to eat more bran and fibre or whether that will make it worse. Which is it?**

A *A high-fibre diet has always been recommended for IBS, but it doesn't work for everyone. Just as the actual symptoms of IBS can vary, so can the effects of fibre – it can make both diarrhoea and constipation worse for example. Mostly it seems that the problem is with wheat fibre, found in wholemeal bread and often in biscuits and cereal too. The only way to find out if it is this that's making things worse is to cut it out for at least a month, then slowly reintroduce some wholewheat into your diet and see what happens. You'll find you probably won't have problems with refined wheat products, such as white bread and pasta.*

Q **Could I take a fibre supplement?**

A *I wouldn't. Besides there are so many other nutrients in high fibre foods that you'd be missing out on – phytochemicals, minerals and antioxidants that all pack big health benefits.*

Q **Is there any way to avoid the windiness you get after eating pulses?**

A *If you're preparing them yourself, just make sure that they are thoroughly cooked (and, except for lentils and split peas, soaked overnight before cooking). I buy my pulses in cans because I can't be bothered with the lengthy preparation process. Just check they're canned in water only and don't have added sugar or salt. You could also try adding certain herbs to the pulse dishes you're making. Herbs that are claimed to help with wind include thyme, fennel, caraway, rosemary and lemon balm.*

Stuck on those last 7lb?

That stubborn half a stone is hard to shift whether you are near the end of your weight loss programme or when 7 lb is all you want to lose to begin with.

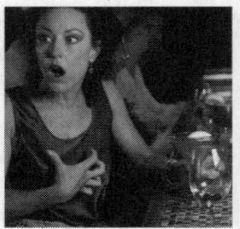

It's such a small amount, you'd think it would pack its bags and leave without a whimper. But no, that half a stone always seems to be trickiest to shift.

I don't know why, but what I do know is that to make it go away you have to re-double your efforts and have more tricks up your sleeve than a magician. Make a start with my ten-point checklist.

1. Be honest with yourself about what you're eating. Keep a food diary for a week and note down everything that you consume. You might think you're eating sensibly, but a diary could help you spot the source of those extra kilos.

2. Do you suffer from portion distortion? Even healthy diet-friendly foods such as fruits have calories. If you eat vast amounts of anything and it exceeds your calorie output, you'll put on weight. Match it and you'll maintain that extra half stone.

Here's an idea for you...

Limit your food options: too many choices can make you eat more. Research has shown that volunteers ate 44% more than a control group when offered a variety of dishes rather than the same amount of one dish.

Defining idea...

'Habit, if not resisted, soon becomes a necessity.'
ST AUGUSTINE

3. How consistent are you? There are some experts who say as long as you eat sensibly for 80% of the time, you can relax a little for the other 20%. This could translate as making the healthiest choices all week and then eating whatever you like at the weekend. However, there's a big difference between relaxing a little and having a total blow-out every weekend. If you opt for the blow-outs, your week's calorie intake will stack up and your healthful efforts will be for nothing. That dull word 'moderation' springs to mind, but it really is a good concept to live by.

4. Be more active, whatever your current levels of activity, to rev up your rate of weight loss. If you are sedentary start walking or swimming, ideally for at least half an hour five times a week. They are both safe effective exercises that, if done regularly, will pay dividends. If you are reasonably active, or even if you think you work out a lot, try to incorporate some new activities into your week to challenge your mind and body. Try working out for longer, more frequently or harder – or all of these together!

5. A simple way to cut a few calories is to cut out carbohydrates with your evening meal. You could try it every night for a couple of weeks, or every other night if that's more convenient. As long as your other meals and snacks are nutrionally balanced with some carbohydrate, you won't be missing out and you'll definitely see a difference of the scales.

6. Have healthy snacks. If you eat regular well-balanced meals and have a few in-between snacks that are also healthy – not a packet of crisps or bar of chocolate – your blood sugar levels will remain stable and you won't ever feel ravenously hungry, so you're less likely to binge or overeat.

Could alcohol be contributing excess calories? Check out IDEA 32, *High spirits*

Try another idea...

7. Spice up your life with a few hot peppers in your lunch or dinner. Pepper eaters have less of an appetite and feel full quicker according to Canadian research. The compound capsaicin that is found in peppers temporarily speeds your metabolism.

8. Include calcium in your diet, as, along with other substances in dairy foods, it seems to help your body burn excess fat faster. In a study, women who ate low fat yoghurt and cheese and drank low fat milk three or four times in a day lost 70% more body fat than women who didn't eat dairy at all.

9. Get your rest. Sleep deprivation and a stressed out lifestyle can boost levels of cortisol in your body, which is associated with higher levels of insulin and fat storage. We can interpret the body's cues for sleep as hunger and end up snacking or drinking gallons of coffee to stay awake…and then not be able to sleep.

10. Don't eat when you're not hungry. It seems obvious, but think about it next time you put your food in your mouth. Ask yourself "Am I really hungry?" before that second mouthful.

'It's OK to let yourself go, just as long as you let yourself back.'
MICK JAGGER

Defining idea...

219

How did it go?

Q **Are there some quick-fix beauty treatments that would help shed a few kilos?**

A *Yes, but they'll only help you lose inches by losing water, so won't have anything more than a temporary effect. Still, if you need a boost, I think they're great. Look out for the Universal Contour Wrap, Ionithermie and Shape Changers Detox Wrap Mini Home Kit. Looking after your body and nurturing it, even just by say massaging in body lotion, is a psychologically healthy thing to do. It indicates that you're not at war with your body, which is a positive attitude for diet success.*

Q **Should I cut out all fat to speed up my weight loss?**

A *No! A moderate consumption of fat gives you taste and variety and besides, we need fats for health. You do need to choose your fats wisely though. They are all calorific, but some bring health benefits to the party too. Trans fats should be avoided as far as possible and you should also try to cut down on saturated fats. Plant oils, oily fish, nuts and avocados are all packed with the beneficial fats that protect against heart disease and other diseases and conditions, so when you do eat fat, choose those.*

What's your excuse?

We all have them – perfectly good reasons why our diet has failed, where it went wrong, why we can't exercise and so on. Only they're not reasons, they're excuses. Let's expose them one by one.

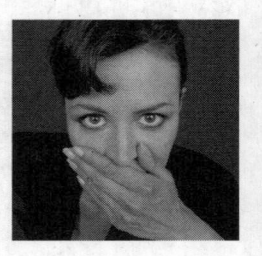

It's my glands! It's my knees! It's because I have to wait for a phone call from my granny to let me know if she needs a lift to the hairdresser's.

Whether they are plausible reasons or fictional tales worthy of Hollywood's finest, the trouble with excuses is that they are stopping you from achieving your goals. Usually there are some powerful emotions struggling underneath these excuses. If you can unravel what they are, it could help you to move on. For example, you may be fearful of failing or of loooking silly. Maybe there's anger inside you, manifesting itself as "I have too many commitments to others to make time for myself". If you can get to the root of negative emotions, you can develop strategies to deal with them. Here's a selection of the excuses we've all heard (and used?!) a million times before, with ideas on how to overcome them:

Here's an idea for you...

Eating carbohydrates before you exercise can reduce the amount of fat you burn for hours afterwards. Instead, researchers recommend having a high protein snack, such as a handful of nuts, before your workout.

'I don't have time to exercise.'

This is the commonest excuse that people give for avoiding physical activity. But ask yourself if your life is really that different to people who do exercise. How do they manage? It's so important to exercise both from a weight loss and fitness point of view that you really should try to give it priority. So, if it's childcare that's an issue, could your partner watch the kids, a neighbour or perhaps a fellow mum would be willing to barter babysitting hours with you? Many health clubs also offer crèches. Perhaps you could get up earlier or work out at lunchtime? You don't have to do all your exercise at once either – you could split it into smaller chunks throughout the day.

'Everyone puts on weight as they get older.'

It's not inevitable, unless you consistently overeat whilst being inactive.

'I never had a weight problem until I had children.'

Well give them back then! No, just kidding. Baby weight is lost through sensible eating and physical activity, but you also need to look at your habits. Do you eat up the kids' leftovers or snack constantly because you're so busy rushing around that you don't make time to prepare yourself a nourishing meal? Do you eat with the kids and then later with your partner too? Do you treat yourself at the end of day when kids are packed off to bed with a few glasses of wine or tub of ice-cream?

Defining idea...

'The only way to get rid of a temptation is to yield to it.'
OSCAR WILDE

'I don't feel like exercising.'

If you need motivation, make a commitment to working out with a friend or group. It's hard to let the side down, even if you feel OK about letting yourself down. If you don't feel like it because you don't like exercise, what have you tried? Just because you may not fancy the gym with all its machinery, doesn't mean you wouldn't enjoy classes, sports, swimming or walking. You might love dancing for example, so make a workout out of it by joining a salsa club or even just dancing to all your favourite music in your living room.

If you've ever considered cosmetic surgery as an answer to weight loss, read IDEA 34, *Suck it out*, first.

Try another idea…

'Exercise hurts!'

If it hurts so much you hate it, get dizzy or exhausted, stop. However, if you simply feel some muscle soreness afterwards, it is normal – assuming you warmed up, cooled down and didn't actually injure yourself. The key is not to overdo things, especially if you're new to exercise and have been very sedentary, both to not put yourself off for good and also to avoid injury. Little and often is a good beginning. As you get fitter – and you'll see results in a few weeks – you can push yourself harder.

'I just end up bingeing on all the foods I can't have.'

Well don't deny yourself anything. Have a small amount of your craved food stuff as soon as you want it. Just make sure it is a small amount and then go and do something else. Denial is a recipe for weight gain.

'People are always blaming circumstances for what they are. I do not believe in circumstances. The people who get on in this world are the people who get up and look for the circumstances they want, and if they cannot find them, make them.'
GEORGE BERNARD SHAW

Defining idea…

223

How did it go?

Q **I'm a morning person, but when is the best time to exercise?**

A *When you feel motivated, I'd say! Research on athletes has shown that the best time for training is actually in the evening, as this is when flexibility, heart rate and body temperature are at their peak. Of course, if you exercise too late, you'll probably be too full of energy to get to sleep for a while. Ultimately, to keep it up, exercise has to fit in to your lifestyle, so whether that means you do it in the morning, at lunchtime or in the evening, it is entirely up to you. The benefits of exercising every day, or most days, are much greater than the time of day at which you do it – so don't use the idea that you have missed the right time of day as an excuse not to exercise!*

Q **Couldn't there be something wrong with my glands?**

A *It's just possible that you have thyroid problems. The symptoms of hypothyroidism, when not enough of the hormone thyroxine is produced, include weight gain, feeling tired all the time and feeling cold. If that sounds familiar, do go to see your doctor and have yourself tested. Fluid retention can also make you gain weight and can be connected to the menstrual cycle or taking the Pill in women, or the use of corticosteroids. Again, a conversation with your doctor would probably be useful.*

51

Support act

Only you can lose your excess weight, but it's a whole lot easier if you have a support team to help. From formal support to the goodwill of family and friends, it's essential to feel you're not alone.

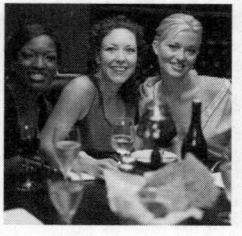

I don't like my partner to do the food shopping because he ignores my list. It is not his fault, it turns out — it is mine for not enlisting him as an ally. It's up to you to rally your supporters and keep them on side.

When my partner goes shopping, instead of bringing back lots of fruit and vegetables, low-fat dairy products, brown bread, rice and lean cuts of meat, he'll just bring a few of those, plus lots of 'extras' like full-fat cheeses, quiches, ice-cream and sausages. At first it was quite funny and endearing. Now it's getting expensive and annoying. I thought perhaps it was a deliberate ruse to get out of doing the supermarket run, but then I realised I'd never told him why I wanted the produce on the list and what wasn't good about all the fatty stuff he liked to bring back home.

'Ask your child what he wants for dinner only if he's buying.'
FRAN LEBOWITZ

Defining idea...

Here's an idea for you... **Improving your posture can make you look slimmer instantly. Relax your shoulders and draw them down and slightly back. Your chest should then naturally lift. Investigate Pilates or Alexander technique classes for more posture skills.**

You've got to communicate your weight loss ambitions and plans to your partner and family. You need to sit them down and explain why you want to lose weight and also how you're going to go about it. It's important to ask for their help at this stage too. It could be for example that you'll need help with childcare, running errands, cooking or shopping. Perhaps you'd like them to exercise with you. Could they be eating more healthily too? If they're slim, they could eat the healthier foods you'll be choosing, but in larger quantities. If they're carrying a little excess baggage themselves, your motivation could well inspire them. At the very least the praise and encouragement of your nearest and dearest will be vital during your battle with the bulge.

Of course it's not unknown for those closest to you to be unenthusiastic, even obstructive, about you wanting to slim down. They're used to the cuddly you and fear that you'll change personality as well as size. Partners can harbour worries that the new slim you will run off with someone else. All you can do is be reassuring, but if they continue to be unsupportive, you'll just have to get on with it quietly. Try making new friends too. Meeting people in the same position as you is terrific for moral support. It's the contact and understanding that counts, not to mention the sharing of tips and advice.

Defining idea... **'It is the friends you can call up at 4 a.m. that matter.'** MARLENE DIETRICH

As well as the support structure of family and friends, a more formal arrangement might suit you even better. Slimming clubs, such as WeightWatchers, Slimming World and Rosemary Conley have meetings nationwide, not to mention internet services and magazines. As well as the actual diets themselves, which are all basically healthy eating with slightly different approaches, the community spirit is great, high on support, motivation and inspiration. Research also confirms that your chances of losing weight and keeping it off are higher if you join a club.

Is it really a lack of support or just a handy excuse? Don't sabotage yourself! See IDEA 50, What's your excuse?

Try another idea...

Depending on your financial circumstances, you could also go for one-to-one help and support. A personal trainer could devise a tailor-made exercise plan for you and really help with your commitment to exercise – there's nothing like your personal trainer calling you through your letterbox to get you out of bed in the morning! You could also see a dietician for nutrition advice as well as ongoing support. There are diet coaches who are like life coaches but specialise in weight loss. They mostly work on the phone, though some do face-to-face as well. They are marvellous for helping you draw up an action plan and stick to it. Ultimately, it's your determination that will help you succeed, but you should also take all the help you can get.

'People change and forget to tell each other.'
LILLIAN HELLMAN

Defining idea...

227

How did it go?

Q **We have dinner with a couple we're friendly with quite often. She knows I'm trying to lose weight, but serves up really fatty foods. What should I do?**

A *Is she not thinking, or is she a bitch? If you enjoy their company, I'd attempt to grin and bear it and just eat small portions. Have a salad or bowl of soup before going over to their place. You have to be gracious and well-mannered, but that doesn't mean you can't pass up pudding: say the main course was so delicious and filling that you simply can't eat any more.*

Q **My partner and kids are overweight. How can I avoid giving the children a complex about weight issues?**

A *This is a tricky one, but to be blunt, obesity is a bigger problem for teenagers today than eating disorders. Seventy per cent of overweight teens grow into overweight adults. I think the way to deal with it is subtlety. Get more active as a family and make small changes in your eating habits. Cut down on junk and processed foods and swap to low fat dairy products and sugar free drinks and spreads. The fewer tempting snacks you have in the house, the less easy it is for them to grab one and slump in front of the TV. I'd also encourage them to learn more about food basics, either from websites such as the Food Standards Agency, the British Dietetic Association or food books. Kids enjoy learning; they may even end up teaching you a thing or two!*

Zen and the art of weight loss maintenance

We can all lose weight, at least in the short term, but the greatest challenge is keeping it off. What are the secrets of success?

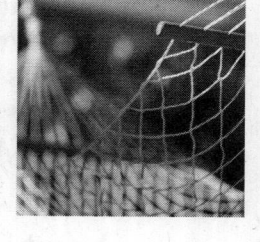

There's an often-quoted figure that 90% of people who lose weight put it all back on within a year. Estimates vary from 95 to 80%, but at any level above zero, it's too high.

However you look at it, there are a lot of people who don't keep up their weight loss. Rather than dwelling on the reasons for this 'failure', try to figure out how the 10, 5 or indeed 20% of people who have lost weight and kept it off have done it. Using studies, research and anecdotes, the reasons they succeed where others don't looks something like this:

Here's an idea for you...

Get a life! Successful dieters don't say 'When I lose weight, I'll take that holiday/get a new job/sort out my love life.' They just carry on with living alongside losing weight. So don't put your life on hold: do what you have to do and the rest will follow. It really will, honestly!

SUCCESS STRATEGY 1

People who keep weight off link their positive healthy behaviours with other areas of their lives. For instance, eating sensibly not only helps your health and weight, but it could set a good example to children. Exercise becomes not simply physical activity, but also a way of spending time with your partner, friends, kids and the dog! Many people also find that having started to take a real interest in nutrition and fitness for dieting reasons, they're inspired to build new careers as dieticians, fitness instructors and complementary medicine practitioners. Any change is great, but if it has a powerful effect on other areas of your life, it's more likely to stick.

SUCCESS STRATEGY 2

Small changes over a long period of time will become an integral part of your lifestyle, unlike short-termist tactics. Short-term plans only work in the short term, which is why for example crash dieting ultimately fails. Once you've lost your excess weight, the slimmer you will need fewer calories for maintenance. If you go back to your old eating habits, you'll put weight back on.

If your eating habits are changed gradually, you'll lose weight slowly and safely and the new habits will start to become second nature – the recipe for permanence.

SUCCESS STRATEGY 3

People who lose weight and keep it off know the value of exercise, combining both aerobic activity with resistance training. Not only does exercise help burn off calories – and fat if you do it for long enough – but it will also build muscle, which uses up more calories than fat does. It keeps you in shape from a health perspective too, protecting against osteoporosis, cardiovascular disease, high blood pressure and depression to name but a few. People who exercise also tend to have greater self-esteem than non-exercisers. As with healthy eating habits, exercise has to be consistent and regular to deliver benefits.

SUCCESS STRATEGY 4

Research has found that if your weight loss is motivated by health reasons, it's more likely to stay off long term than if it's motivated by looks alone.

SUCCESS STRATEGY 5

Long-term weight losers have also developed a well-balanced approach to food and themselves in relation to it. They know they can get themselves back on track if they gain weight and that is by forgiving themselves rather than dwelling on the potential consequences of eating another slice of chocolate cake. Ultimately the consistency (albeit with occasional lapses allowed) of eating low fat, low, but not too low, calorie, with a balance of protein, carbohydrates and plenty of fruit and vegetables is the eating pattern that generates long-term success.

Would a detox diet help you stay trim? See IDEA 20, *Detox diets – con or cure?*

Try another idea…

'Success is getting what you want. Happiness is wanting what you get.'
DALE CARNEGIE

Defining idea…

Q I've heard about a 'set point' theory that we all have a natural weight which you can't change. Is this true?

A It is a theory and it's still being debated. The idea is if you lose weight below your set point, your body will do everything it can to get you back to your former weight – it could explain why so many of us find weight loss hard to maintain. How annoying it is that the theory doesn't work in reverse – if you put too much weight on, your body doesn't fight to get it off! Even if it is found to be true, exercise is still the way to regain control as it can raise your metabolism and encourages fat to be used up.

Q Can I lose weight without dieting – say with exercise alone?

A Yes, you can lose weight just with a regular exercise routine, as long as you don't also eat more. To lose a significant amount you'd have to work out hard. I suggest you get a trainer in your local gym or health club to help you devise a programme, but you could also achieve a slower loss over time by burning up just a few hundred calories extra a day than you currently do. However, just because you burn off your calories doesn't mean you're well-nourished. It's important to eat healthily too!

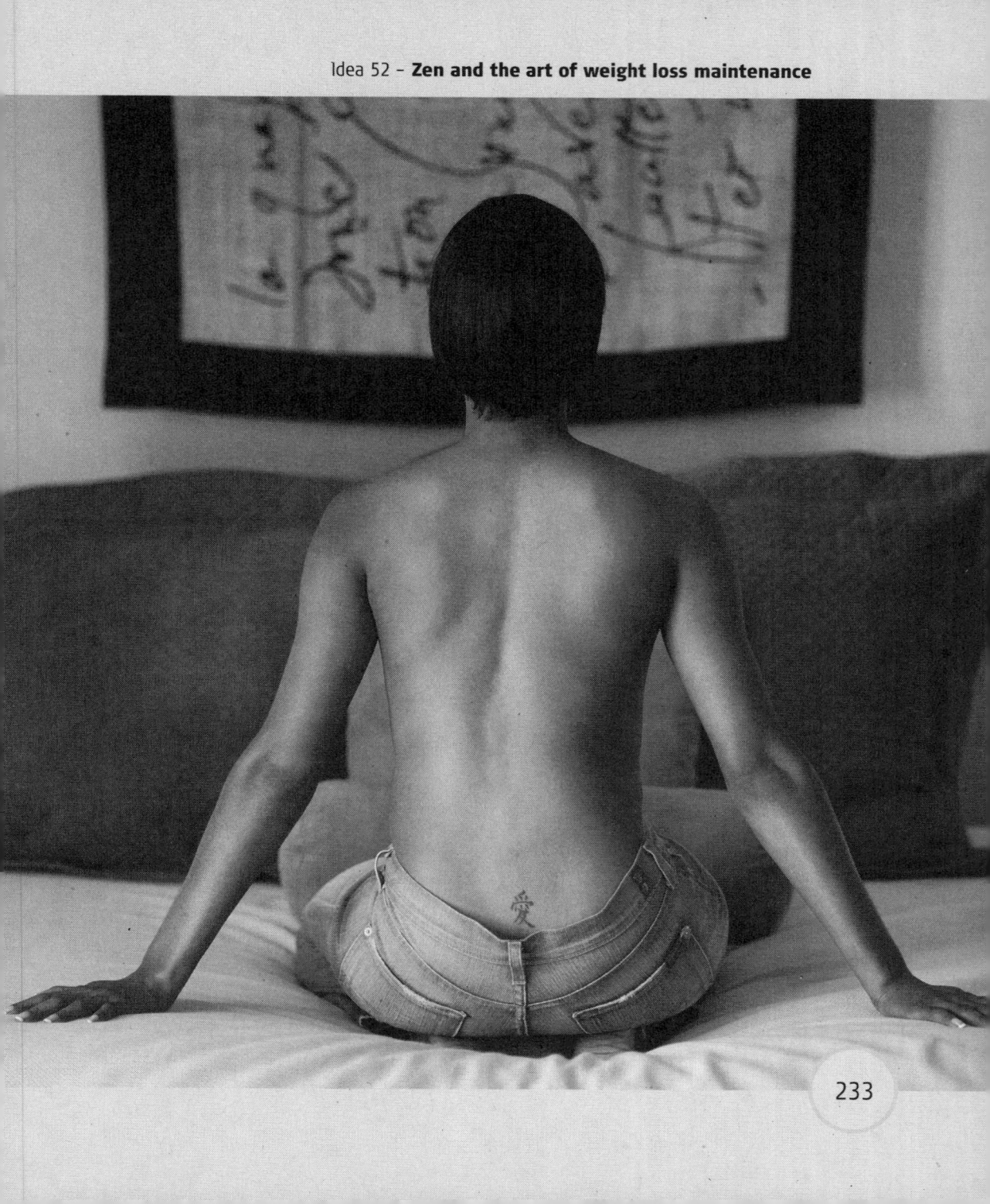

The end...

Or is it a new beginning?

We hope that the ideas in this book will have inspired you to try some new things. You should be well on your way to a slimmer you. And you can look also forward to a healthier, fitter, more fulfilled and balanced you, brimming with good intentions.

You're mean, you're motivated and you don't care who knows it.

So why not let *us* know all about it? Tell us how you got on. What did it for you – what helped you beat the cravings? What got you back on your bike after years of motoring? Maybe you've got some tips of your own you want to share (see next page if so). And if you liked this book you may find we have even more brilliant ideas that could change other areas of your life for the better.

You'll find the Infinite Ideas crew waiting for you online at www.infideas.com.

Or if you prefer to write, then send your letters to:
Lose weight and stay slim
The Infinite Ideas Company Ltd
Belsyre Court, 57 Woodstock Road, Oxford OX2 6HJ, United Kingdom

We want to know what you think, because we're all working on making our lives better too. Give us your feedback and you could win a copy of another *52 Brilliant Ideas* book of your choice. Or maybe get a crack at writing your own.

Good luck. Be brilliant.

Offer one

CASH IN YOUR IDEAS

We hope you enjoy this book. We hope it inspires, amuses, educates and entertains you. But we don't assume that you're a novice, or that this is the first book that you've bought on the subject. You've got ideas of your own. Maybe our author has missed an idea that you use successfully. If so, why not send it to info@infideas.com, and if we like it we'll post it on our bulletin board. Better still, if your idea makes it into print we'll send you £50 and you'll be fully credited so that everyone knows you've had another Brilliant Idea.

Offer two

HOW COULD YOU REFUSE?

Amazing discounts on bulk quantities of Infinite Ideas books are available to corporations, professional associations and other organizations.

For details call us on:
+44 (0)1865 292045
fax: +44 (0)1865 292001
or e-mail: info@infideas.com

Where it's at...